Emergency and Critical Care

Editors

MARGARET FORDHAM
BRIAN K. ROBERTS

VETERINARY CLINICS OF NORTH AMERICA: EXOTIC ANIMAL PRACTICE

www.vetexotic.theclinics.com

Consulting Editor
JOERG MAYER

May 2016 • Volume 19 • Number 2

ELSEVIER

1600 John F. Kennedy Boulevard • Suite 1800 • Philadelphia, Pennsylvania, 19103-2899
http://www.vetexotic.theclinics.com

VETERINARY CLINICS OF NORTH AMERICA: EXOTIC ANIMAL PRACTICE Volume 19, Number 2
May 2016 ISSN 1094-9194, ISBN-13: 978-0-323-44486-6

Editor: Patrick Manley
Developmental Editor: Meredith Clinton

Veterinary Clinics of North America: Exotic Animal Practice (ISSN 1094-9194) is published in January, May, and September by Elsevier, Inc., 360 Park Avenue South, New York, NY 10010-1710. Subscription prices are $260.00 per year for US individuals, $438.00 per year for US institutions, $100.00 per year for US students and residents, $305.00 per year for Canadian individuals, $528.00 per year for Canadian institutions, $340.00 per year for international individuals, $528.00 per year for international institutions and $165.00 per year for Canadian and foreign students/residents. To receive student/resident rate, orders must be accompanied by name of affiliated institution, date of term, and the *signature* of program/residency coordinator on institution letterhead. Orders will be billed at individual rate until proof of status is received. Foreign air speed delivery is included in all *Clinics* subscription prices. All prices are subject to change without notice. **POSTMASTER:** Send address changes to *Veterinary Clinics of North America: Exotic Animal Practice*, Elsevier Health Sciences Division, Subscription Customer Service, 3251 Riverport Lane, Maryland Heights, MO 63043. **Customer Service: Telephone: 1-800-654-2452** (U.S. and Canada); **1-314-447-8871** (outside U.S. and Canada). **Fax: 1-314-447-8029. E-mail: journalscustomerservice-usa@elsevier.com (for print support); journalsonlinesupport-usa@elsevier.com (for online support).**

Reprints. For copies of 100 or more of articles in this publication, please contact the Commercial Reprints Department, Elsevier Inc., 360 Park Avenue South, New York, New York 10010-1710. Tel.: 212-633-3874; Fax: 212-633-3820; E-mail: reprints@elsevier.com.

Veterinary Clinics of North America: Exotic Animal Practice is covered in *MEDLINE/PubMed (Index Medicus).*

Contributors

CONSULTING EDITOR

JOERG MAYER, Dr.med.vet, MSc
Diplomate American Board of Veterinary Practitioners (Exotic Companion Mammals); Diplomate European College of Zoological Medicine (Small Mammals); Diplomate American College of Zoological Medicine; Associate Professor of Zoological Medicine, Department of Small Animal Medicine and Surgery, College of Veterinary Medicine, University of Georgia, Athens, Georgia

EDITORS

MARGARET FORDHAM, DVM
Mount Laurel Animal Hospital-Exotics, Mount Laurel, New Jersey

BRIAN K. ROBERTS, DVM
DACVECC; Head, Department of Clinical Sciences; Professor, Small Animal Medicine, School of Veterinary Medicine, St. Matthew's University, West Bay, Cayman Islands

AUTHORS

SANDRA I. ALLWEILER, DVM
Diplomate of the American College of Veterinary Anesthesia and Analgesia; Department of Clinical Sciences, Colorado State University, Fort Collins, Colorado

HEATHER BARRON, DVM
Diplomate American Board of Veterinary Practitioners (Avian); Clinic for the Rehabilitation of Wildlife, Sanibel, Florida

ANAÏS BOYEAUX, DVM
Department of Emergency and Critical Care, Centre Hospitalier Vétérinaire Frégis, Arcueil, France

DANIEL CALVO CARRASCO, LV, CertAVP, MRCVS
Great Western Exotics, Vets-Now Referrals, Swindon, United Kingdom

JULIE DECUBELLIS, DVM, MS
Calgary Avian and Exotic Pet Clinic, Calgary, Alberta, Canada

NICOLA DI GIROLAMO, DMV, GPCert(ExAP), MSc(EBHC)
Clinica per Animali Esotici, Centro Veterinario Specialistico, Roma, Italy

CHRISTINA D. HILDRETH, BA, AAS, RVT
Avian and Exotic Pet Service, Carolina Veterinary Specialists, Huntersville, North Carolina

MINH HUYNH, DVM
Diplomate European College of Zoological Medicine (Avian); Exotic Department, Centre Hospitalier Vétérinaire Frégis, Arcueil, France

JEFFREY ROWE JENKINS, BS, DVM
Diplomate, American Board of Veterinary Practitioners (Avian Practice); Chief Officer/
Veterinarian, Avian and Exotic Animal Hospital, Inc, San Diego, California

SIMON Y. LONG, MS, VMD
PhD Candidate, Viral Oncology Under the Cellular and Molecular Medicine Graduate
Program, Pathology Postdoctoral Fellow, Department of Molecular and Comparative
Pathobiology, Johns Hopkins University School of Medicine, Baltimore, Maryland

CINTHIA MARNELL, BS, BVMS
Supervisory Public Health Veterinarian, Salisbury, Maryland

ALICIA McLAUGHLIN, DVM
Center for Bird and Exotic Animal Medicine, Bothell, Washington

MEERA KUMAR MUSIC, BVM&S, MRCVS
Center for Bird and Exotic Animal Medicine, Bothell, Washington

CHARLY PIGNON, DVM
Diplomate European College of Zoological Medicine (Small Mammals); Exotics Medicine
Service, Alfort National Veterinary School, Maisons Alfort, France

JENNIFER RILEY, DVM
Lion Country Safari, Loxahatchee, Florida

BRIAN K. ROBERTS, DVM
DACVECC; Head, Department of Clinical Sciences; Professor, Small Animal Medicine,
School of Veterinary Medicine, St. Matthew's University, West Bay, Cayman Islands

MIKEL SABATER GONZÁLEZ, LV, CertZooMed
Diplomate European College of Zoological Medicine (Avian); Exoticsvet, Valencia, Spain

PAOLO SELLERI, DMV, PhD
Diplomate of the European College of Zoological Medicine (Herpetology and Small
Mammals); Clinica per Animali Esotici, Centro Veterinario Specialistico, Roma, Italy

JANE D. STOUT, VMD
Associate Veterinarian, Avian and Exotic Animal Hospital, San Diego, California

ANNELIESE STRUNK, DVM
Diplomate, American Board of Veterinary Practitioners (Avian Practice); Medical Director,
Center for Bird and Exotic Animal Medicine, Bothell, Washington

Contents

> Small animal veterinary hospitals will have exotic animal emergencies. Preparing the hospital space, equipment, and staff will provide optimal exotic animal emergency medicine and care. A well-gathered history can be more valuable in exotic pet medicine than most diagnostics. A gentle, well-planned approach, combined with common sense and focused observational skills, is necessary for avian and exotic patients.

> Veterinarians who are practicing emergency medicine, and/or working with exotic animals must be well versed in the pathophysiology of shock because many exotic pets present with an acute crisis or an acute manifestation of a chronic process causing poor organ perfusion. This article discusses the pathophysiology of shock and the systemic inflammatory response syndrome, which may lead to organ dysfunction, organ failure, sepsis, and death. The physiology of perfusion, perfusion measurements, categories of shock, and altered function of the immune system, gastrointestinal barrier, and coagulation system are discussed. Veterinarians providing emergency care to patients with shock must also be aware of comorbidities.

> The routine use of cardiovascular and respiratory monitor devices is essential for a good outcome in small mammal anesthesia. Physiologic differences between species and variation between individual animals should be considered when choosing an anesthetic protocol. The development of new pain assessment tools (eg, mouse grimace scale) can help recognize and alleviate pain.

> Rabbits have the ability to hide their signs and often present in a state of decompensatory shock. Handling can increase susceptibility to stress-induced

cardiomyopathy and specific hemodynamic changes. Careful monitoring with a specific reference range is important to detect early decompensation, change the therapeutic plan in a timely manner, and assess prognostic indicators. Fluid requirements are higher in rabbits than in other small domestic mammals and can be corrected both enterally and parenterally. Critical care in rabbits can be extrapolated to many hindgut fermenters, but a specific reference range and dosage regimen need to be determined.

Rabbits, guinea pigs, and chinchillas are some of the more common exotic pets seen in emergency clinics. They frequently present with acute illnesses that are the result of several chronic conditions, most related to inadequate diet and husbandry. This article reviews the diagnosis and treatment of some of the more common acute illnesses. It also discusses the predisposing factors that culminate in acute presentations, so that emergency providers can recognize and be mindful of underlying causes of disease before treatment of acute illnesses.

 Video content accompanies this article at http://www.vetexotic. theclinics.com

In the last few years, significant improvement in diagnosis and treatment of ferret emergencies has occurred. Scientific advances demonstrated the need of specific practices when dealing with emergencies in ferrets. The risk of overdiagnosis of hypoglycemia with human portable blood glucose meters is a clear example. The purpose of this article is to describe the current approach to common medical and surgical emergencies in ferrets.

Small exotic mammal pets such as rats, mice, hamsters, gerbils, degus, hedgehogs, and sugar gliders are becoming more popular. Because these animals are prone to a variety of health problems, and require specialized husbandry care to remain healthy, they may present to emergency hospitals in critical condition. This article provides a basic overview of common emergency presentations of these species.

Successful care of the critical pet bird patient is dependent on preparation and planning and begins with the veterinarian and hospital staff. An understanding of avian physiology and pathophysiology is key. Physical preparation of the hospital or clinic includes proper equipment and understanding of the procedures necessary to provide therapeutic and supportive care to the avian patient. An overview of patient intake and assessment, intensive care environment, and fluid therapy is included.

Treating avian emergencies can be a challenging task. Pet birds often mask signs of illness until they are critically ill and require quick initiation of supportive care with minimal handling to stabilize them. This article introduces the clinician to common avian emergency presentations and details initial therapeutics and diagnostics that can be readily performed in the small-animal emergency room. Common disease presentations covered include respiratory and extrarespiratory causes of dyspnea, gastrointestinal signs, reproductive disease, neurologic disorders, trauma, and toxin exposure. The duration and severity of the avian patient's disease and the clinician's initiation of appropriate therapy often determines clinical outcome.

Fowl are birds belonging to one of the two biological orders, the game fowl, or land fowl (Galliformes), and the waterfowl (Anseriformes). Studies of anatomic and molecular similarities suggest these two groups are close evolutionary relatives. Multiple fowl species have a long history of domestication. Fowl are considered food-producing animals in most countries and clinicians should follow legislation regarding reportable diseases and antibiotic use, even if they are pets. This article reviews aspects of emergency care for most commonly kept fowl, including triage, patient assessment, diagnostic procedures, supportive care, short-term hospitalization, and common emergency presentations.

This article summarizes the physiology and anatomy of reptiles, highlighting points relevant for emergency room veterinarians. Other systems, such as the endocrine and immune systems, have not been covered. The many other aspects of reptile species variation are too numerous to be covered. This article provides an overview, but encourages clinicians to seek additional species-specific information to better medically diagnose and treat their reptile patients.

Reptile emergencies are an important part of exotic animal critical care; both true emergencies, and those perceived as emergencies by owners. The most common presentations for reptile emergencies are addressed here, with information on differential diagnoses, helpful diagnostics, and approach to treatment. In many cases, reptile emergencies are actually acute presentations originating from a chronic problem, and the treatment plan must include both clinical treatment and addressing husbandry and dietary deficiencies at home. Accurate owner expectations must be set in order to have owner compliance to long-term treatment plans.

VETERINARY CLINICS OF NORTH AMERICA: EXOTIC ANIMAL PRACTICE

RELATED INTEREST

Veterinary Clinics of North America: Small Animal Practice
September 2015 (Vol. 45, Issue 5)
Perioperative Care
Lori S. Waddell, *Editor*

THE CLINICS ARE NOW AVAILABLE ONLINE!
Access your subscription at:
www.theclinics.com

Foreword

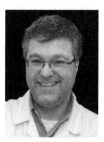

Joerg Mayer, Dr.med.vet, MSc
Consulting Editor

It is my distinct pleasure to be writing this foreword as the new Consulting Editor for *Veterinary Clinics of North America: Exotic Animal Practice*. Needless to say, I have large shoes to fill. Dr Agnes Rupley has done an amazing job in guiding this section of the *Veterinary Clinics of North America* series to the level of being a "must read" for any clinic that is involved with exotic patients. I seriously hope I can keep up the level of great contributions and help to guide the senior editors through the process of producing great new issues for years to come. One of the great advantages of the series is that the reader gets a flow of fresh and novel information, which is constantly updated over the years. This current issue is a great example, as we all know how fast treatments and management ideas change in exotic animal medicine, and emergency medicine is part of this evolution. With access to more and more scientific literature and great research being conducted on exotic animal species, the body of knowledge grows constantly. Updating the treatment approaches and introducing new ideas/thoughts are key features of the *Veterinary Clinics of North America: Exotic Animal Practice*, and this is why I always recommend everyone subscribe to this important part of the growing body of literature in exotic animal medicine. I hope that we can find a good balance between addressing important but older aspects of health care, and introducing new insight and novel approaches. As the body of knowledge continues to grow, we see new specialties and areas of interest form a development, which mirrors the evolution in human medicine. It is my sincere hope that I can help to contribute to this evolution in our exotic animal medicine specialty. I encourage readers to contact me directly in case they would like to see a special topic covered or have a topic reviewed that was covered in the distant

Vet Clin Exot Anim 19 (2016) xi–xii
http://dx.doi.org/10.1016/j.cvex.2016.03.001
1094-9194/16/$ – see front matter © 2016 Published by Elsevier Inc.

vetexotic.theclinics.com

past. I am looking forward to this exciting challenge, and I am sure that together with the publisher, the editors, the authors, and the readers we can create many exciting issues of this series in the future.

Yours sincerely,

Joerg Mayer, Dr.med.vet, MSc
Department of Small Animal Medicine & Surgery
College of Veterinary Medicine
University of Georgia
2200 College Station Road
Athens, GA 30605, USA

E-mail address:
mayerj@uga.edu

Preface

Exotic Pet and Wildlife Emergency Medicine for the Small Animal Practitioner

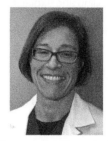 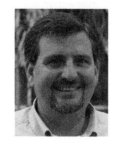

Margaret Fordham, DVM   Brian K. Roberts, DVM, DACVECC
Editors

The practice of emergency medicine has advanced greatly over the last several decades, corresponding to the increasing demand by pet owners for high-quality, 24-hour care of their pet. It is not surprising that exotic pet owners demand the same level of care for their pet that is available to humans, and dogs and cats. Given this expectation, it is likely that, at some point, a small animal emergency hospital or small animal practitioner will be presented with a rabbit, parrot, or snake for emergent care.

Exotic animal medicine is a unique challenge for the small animal emergency veterinarian for many reasons. The different groups of exotic animals vary greatly in their anatomy and physiology as well as in disease processes and treatment. Husbandry plays a vital role in the health of most exotic pet species, and inadequacies in care commonly lead to a chronic disease that can present with an acute manifestation. Exotic pets are often prey species that have subtle signs of illness that are easily missed by owners so that the pet presents to the emergency room in an advanced stage of illness. The high metabolic rate of many species can lead to a rapid decline in their condition, making effective intervention by the veterinarian even more difficult. Providing emergency care for wildlife presents other unique concerns, including knowledge by the veterinarian of basic federal and state regulations.

In addition to the challenges inherent in providing medical care for these species, veterinarians often get minimal training during their veterinary education in exotic animal medicine and surgery. There are hundreds of exotic species that can be kept as pets, with major anatomic and physiologic differences, and different disease processes and treatments. In addition, emergency room facilities may not be set up to receive or care for exotic pets or wildlife.

Vet Clin Exot Anim 19 (2016) xiii–xiv
http://dx.doi.org/10.1016/j.cvex.2016.02.001
1094-9194/16/$ – see front matter © 2016 Published by Elsevier Inc.

Our purpose in this issue of *Veterinary Clinics of North America: Exotic Animal Practice* was to provide a concise and thorough resource for emergency room veterinarians and practitioners seeking to add exotic pet care to their emergency service. While the presentation of the information is geared to the small animal emergency veterinarian who may not have extensive training or familiarity with each species, we think it is valuable to any veterinarian seeking to advance their knowledge in exotic pet care, or learn of recent advances in exotic animal emergency and critical care.

We cannot thank our authors enough for the excellent job they have done in so succinctly and effectively presenting their expert experience, compiling and explaining previously published information, providing quick and easy guides for disease recognition and treatment, all in the goal of advancing our understanding of exotic pet and wildlife emergency and critical care.

Margaret Fordham, DVM
Mount Laurel Animal Hospital- Exotics
220 Mount Laurel Road, Mount Laurel, NJ 08054, USA

Brian K. Roberts, DVM, DACVECC
School of Veterinary Medicine
St. Matthew's University
West Bay, Cayman Islands

E-mail addresses:
mpmf410@gmail.com (M. Fordham)
broberts@stmatthews.edu (B.K. Roberts)

Preparing the Small Animal Hospital for Avian and Exotic Animal Emergencies

Christina D. Hildreth, BA, AAS, RVT

KEYWORDS

- Emergency medicine • Equipment • Exotic pets • Husbandry • Psittacine birds
- Staff training • Technicians • Wildlife

KEY POINTS

- There are many aspects of small animal emergency medicine that can be applied to the exotic animal patient.
- It is important for the entire hospital staff to work as a team for providing optimal care for avian and exotic patients.
- Because of the variety of species that may be seen, organization of supplies, designated areas, policies regarding wildlife or more dangerous species, should be addressed before the intake of exotic emergencies.
- In a fast-paced emergency setting, a gentle, well-planned approach, combined with common sense and focused observational skills, is necessary for avian and exotic patients.
- Although there are a variety of diagnostic and treatment options available for exotic pets, it is important to approach these patients with intentional handling that avoids overstressing or injuring the patient.

INTRODUCTION

Emergency and critical care for exotic animals is a complex topic because of the variety of species that may be seen. Any veterinary practice should expect to receive at least the occasional exotic emergency. Most hospitals that provide emergency and critical care for small animals comprise highly trained and educated technical staff that has access to critical care monitoring and diagnostics. Most of the technical skills familiar to clinicians and technicians can be transferred to exotic patients. Transferring those skills is often accomplished by not getting overwhelmed by the unknown and always pursuing knowledge and combining it with experience. It is beyond the scope of this article to cover all the intricacies of working with exotic animals. However, some of the logistics

The author has nothing to disclose.
Avian and Exotic Pet Service, Carolina Veterinary Specialists, 12117 Statesville Road, Huntersville, NC 28078, USA
E-mail address: Childreth@carolinavet.com

and strategic approaches for exotics in the small animal emergency hospital will help prepare the hospital staff to be effective and prepared for exotic animal emergencies.

MAKING THE DECISION TO SEE EXOTICS IN THE SMALL ANIMAL PRACTICE

Exotic pets are frequently obtained without thought to the when and where of veterinary care needed for these unique animals. When an emergency arises, owners will often seek veterinary care with their local small animal hospital. Unfortunately, a visit to the veterinary hospital for an emergency may be the first and only time an exotic pet may ever receive veterinary care. Small animal hospitals may decide to take on these challenging emergencies for a variety of reasons:

- The community has a need for an emergency veterinary hospital that will also see exotic pets.
- The community frequently contacts the veterinary hospital for valuable information about the care and health of exotic pets.
- The hospital provides triage to sick or injured wildlife and provides the community with recommendations and support for native wildlife concerns and rehabilitation options within the bounds of state and federal laws and regulations.
- Veterinary clinicians and technicians enjoy working with a variety of species, and providing emergency veterinary care for these patients is a bonus to the joy and fulfillment of their career.
- Exotic pets will be brought to veterinary hospitals in an emergency whether advertised for or not.

If the hospital decides to accept exotic patients, it is usually because a clinician has a strong interest in practicing exotic animal medicine. For some staff, the variety of species and fear of the unknown may make them hesitant to join the team in this endeavor. Veterinary technicians with a strong interest in exotic animal medicine can play a leading role in helping set up the animal hospital to accept a variety of patients. In order for the hospital staff to work together, training plans should be set in place so that all of the staff, from the receptionists to assistants to technicians to clinicians, can be prepared. Veterinary technicians can provide client education, create entrance history forms, create training plans for coworkers, and set up hands-on training for clinicians and technicians. Compiling a collection of information resources for the hospital, such as bookmarked online educational and informational Web sites, journal articles, and textbooks, is recommended.[1–12]

POLICIES AND PROCEDURES

Once a hospital has decided to accept exotic patients, policies should be designed that address several aspects of this endeavor. The practice will need to decide what species it will and will not accept. Some species are a greater risk physically to humans, such as primates and venomous species. Large exotic cats may present safety concerns, and the hospital facility may not have the necessary equipment and space required for these species. If the hospital does decide to see some of these more inherently dangerous species, policies regarding handling and when they will be seen should be communicated with all hospital staff. For certain exotic species such as falconry birds, state and federal permits to possess these animals should be presented at the time of admission.

PROFESSIONAL STAFF INTEREST AND TRAINING

Working with exotic patients may be a completely new experience or a limited past experience for many and may be something that encourages an individual to learn as much as possible, or something that causes fear and retreat. It is important to encourage coworkers to move past possible fears or uncertainties and to challenge everyone within the practice to have a basic knowledge of avian and exotic species. Using local wildlife rehabilitators or wildlife centers may help with some of the more technical training. Many rehabilitators are willing to provide cadavers that can be used for teaching purposes; this is an excellent way to become familiar with the anatomy and to try out some techniques for nursing and emergency care. Cadavers from wildlife rehabilitators or centers can be used to practice examination skills, restraint, tube feeding, injections, intraosseous (IO) catheters, intravenous (IV) catheters, and bandaging techniques. These cadavers can also be used to create a chart of appropriate kilovolt (peak) and milliampere second settings for radiographs of smaller species. Of course, no one can learn and retain everything about every species, but an effort to have the most basic understanding should be the goal. The basic understanding will vary with each staff worker's position. When all of the staff has some knowledge of exotic animals, it will encourage the client to entrust the hospital with care of their pet (**Table 1**).

BENEFITS OF ACHIEVING BASIC GOALS FOR HOSPITAL STAFF

- Clients feel reassured by recognition or knowledge of the species.
- Recognizing common psittacine species communicates experience with avian patients.
- The human-animal bond between exotic pet owners and their pets is often as strong as the bond between owners and traditional domestic pets.
- Recognizing that most exotic patients are prey species that require quiet, separation from predators, and gentle and calm interaction reassures clients their pet will receive appropriate care.

INITIAL WELCOME FOR THE EXOTIC ANIMAL

Receptionists are usually the first staff members to interact with clients, so they should be involved in the training also. Providing resources, booklets, and Web sites to help

Table 1
Basic goals for emergency exotic animal hospital staff

Receptionists	Technicians	Clinicians
Recognize common species	Identify common species and possess working knowledge of basic husbandry needs	Be able to perform physical examination and clinical assessment on a variety of species
Have familiarity with state and federal laws and regulations regarding native wildlife	Be able to properly restrain avian, reptile, and small exotic mammal species	Possess working knowledge of most common emergency presentations and diseases & disorders of exotic pets
Know hospital policies and procedures for primates, venomous species, and other inherently dangerous species	Understand anatomy and basic physiology of commonly presented exotic animal species	Able to create appropriate diagnostic and treatment plans
	Be familiar with basic techniques (eg, venipuncture, IV and IO catheter placement, intramuscular & subcutaneous injection)	Able to evaluate historical findings and interpret diagnostic results

receptionists learn some of the most common exotic species kept as pets, especially some of the psittacine species, could be beneficial. (For psittacine birds, the World Parrot Trust provides an online encyclopedia of a wide variety of species and is a useful resource.[3]) Creating a notebook that contains information such as contact information for local wildlife centers and rehabilitators, hospital wildlife policies and procedures, quick answers for questions about wildlife, and certain applicable state and federal laws and regulations regarding native wildlife for receptionists and technicians will help with continuity in the practice. Veterinary technicians can create detailed history forms that can be provided online or for receptionists to hand out when new patients are admitted.

THE IMPORTANCE OF A THOROUGH HISTORY

Exotic patients often take more time for client interaction than dogs and cats in part because of the uniqueness of the variety of species seen. Husbandry and nutrition are vital to the well-being and survival of these patients. Husbandry concerns are related to most problems seen in exotic animals, especially in reptiles. Therefore, gathering a detailed and thorough history is critical for all cases; this can pose a challenge because some patients come in to the emergency hospital barely hanging on to life. At this time, several things need to happen almost simultaneously: the patient needs to be stabilized; a detailed history needs to be gathered; and a plan of action needs to be formed based on the client's budget and emotional attachment in combination with the patient's prognosis. Creating an avian, reptile, and small mammal history questionnaire for clients to fill out may help in this process (**Table 2**).

The veterinary technician can then focus on specifics when speaking with the owner:

- In the owner's words, why have they brought the pet to the hospital?
- Timeline for this concern: When did the problem start? Was it gradual or immediate?
- Did the client see the accident, trauma, self-mutilation, etc?

Table 2 General history questions	
Background	• Source of pet • Length of ownership • Exposure to other animals of same and different species • Previous preventative care, vaccines • Prior illness, treatment, response to treatment
Diet/environment	• Food offered, supplements offered, diet actually eaten • Source of drinking water and method of delivery • Cage material, dimensions, bedding, cage furniture • Supervision level, toxin exposure • Travel and boarding history
Presenting complaint	• Onset and duration • Progression • Treatment and response
Systems review	• Appetite, thirst • Regurgitation or vomiting • Polyuria, diarrhea, melena, other • Coughing, sneezing, nasal or ocular discharge • Attitude and level of mentation, strength, responsiveness • Reproductive history

- What is the animal actually eating currently? (This is a challenging question to get an accurate response. Many clients say the animal is not eating ANYTHING, but in reality the animal may still be eating some things.)
- Any changes around the home: construction, new pet, visitors, etc? (This is important because with most exotics being prey species, stress or change can greatly factor into their health.)
- Describe the droppings: frequency, consistency, size and shape, colors. (This also can be difficult for the client to describe. For example, many bird owners may say the bird has diarrhea, but when questioned further and specifically, the technician may be able to determine the owner is actually seeing polyuria rather than diarrhea.)

PREPARING THE HOSPITAL SPACE FOR EXOTIC ANIMAL PATIENTS

Most small animal and emergency hospitals will have most of the supplies needed to begin accepting exotic patients. However, the hospital may need to gather additional supplies and designate a working space specifically for exotic patients. Ideally, a separate room away from loud noises, without windows, and having the cabinets closed should be designated for exotic patients. This area will allow exotic patients to be examined and housed away from predatory species and loud noises that may increase stress and reduce further injury. By having items stored in closed cabinets, disinfecting regularly will be more practical and effective. Native wildlife species should not be allowed in the room designated for exotic pets due to the possibility of transmission of infectious diseases (**Fig. 1**).

Working with such a variety of species may require creativity and ingenuity to make size-appropriate supplies. Perches can be made with polyvinyl chloride (PVC) pipes and various plumbing supplies. Induction or weighing boxes can be basic small plastic boxes with a drilled hole and insulation stripping along the edges. Small head masks can be made with a drilled hole in plastic containers and veterinarian wrap, or an examination glove can create the seal. There are a wide variety of brands of 18-gauge thermoplastic polymer IV catheters that can be used as endotracheal tubes for very small birds by adding an adaptor. Also, cutting Kendall Argyle pediatric PVC nasogastric feeding tube without a radiopaque line, 5 FR and 8 FR, and adding an adaptor creates endotracheal tubes for small birds (Medtronic, Minneapolis, MN, USA). Toolboxes or craft boxes with dividers can be repurposed to store endotracheal tubes or to create a small exotic crash kit. Labeled airtight containers can be used to store a

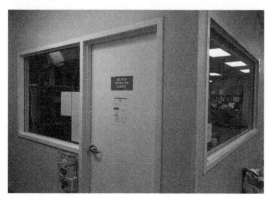

Fig. 1. Isolation room.

variety of diets to offer hospitalized patients. Emptied and thoroughly cleaned plastic cat litter containers with lids make great storage containers for hay. Foam pipe wrap insulation can be cut to appropriate sizes to create extensions for E-collars on birds (**Figs. 2–5**).

Table 3 provides some items that may already be in a small animal hospital. However, some items may not already be in the hospital and should be considered for providing effective and optimal care for avian and exotic pet emergencies. Current hospital supplies should be evaluated, and certain items should be designated for use in critical exotic patients (**Figs. 6–15**).

DIETS

Nutrition for exotic pets that may be hospitalized must be addressed. Ideally, the owner can provide some favorite foods or the normal diet, but often that is not possible in an emergency situation. Again, the history gathered will be important to properly set up the animal in the hospital. It is better to keep the animal eating during this critical time even if the pet is on a poor diet or inappropriate diet (**Figs. 16** and **17**). Transitioning to a healthy diet should not be attempted when an animal is weak or debilitated. Offering foods that are more appealing may be necessary to keep some of these patients eating in the stressful hospital environment. It is also important to note from the owner if the animal normally drinks water from a bowl or bottle. Both can be provided if it is not known. Most exotic patients need free choice of food because of faster metabolisms and physiology. Even if a patient is presented for anorexia, food should be made available after evaluation by the clinician. It is not practical to keep every type of food available for the variety of exotic pets, but keeping a general supply is necessary (**Table 4**).

THE EMERGENCY EXOTIC ANIMAL PATIENT ARRIVES

Exotic animal pets may be brought in for emergency care because of a true emergency, or sometimes for a behavior or characteristic that the client did not realize is normal for that species. Because most exotic pets are prey species, they hide signs of illness as long as possible or owners are not familiar with signs of sickness in exotics. Often the animal is in critical condition and may not be stable enough for an immediate examination with restraint. Owners may not realize that a fluffed, lethargic,

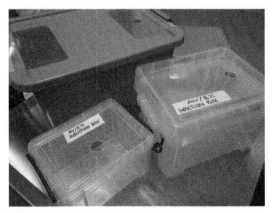

Fig. 2. Example of induction boxes.

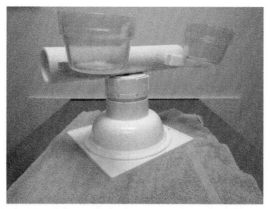

Fig. 3. Example of perches 1.

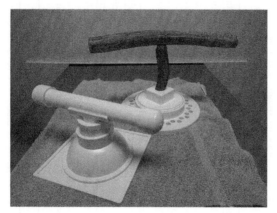

Fig. 4. Example of perches 2.

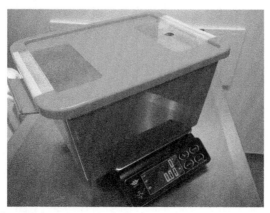

Fig. 5. Example of weigh box on gram scale.

Table 3
Designated equipment for exotics

Examination Supplies	Examples
Pediatric or infant stethoscope	3M Littmann Classic II Infant Stethoscope (3M Littmann, St. Paul, MN, USA)
Gram scales	Variety of types available; ideally have a scale that weighs in 0.1-g increments for patients that weigh <100 g
Plastic boxes with lids	Variety of sizes; can be used for weighing or anesthesia induction of mammals
Small hand towels/washcloths/fleece pieces	Used for collecting the animal out of the cage or carrier
Leather gloves/welding gloves	Used for raptors, large lizards, or some exotic mammals; smaller leatherwork gloves may be used for hedgehogs
Nail clippers: dog, cat, and human varieties are used	Variety available; extralong nails can get caught in bedding and other cage belongings
Styptic powder	Always have it available; the quick in birds' nails tend to be longer and almost always bleed if the nail is cut to appropriate length
Small clippers/beard trimmer	Variety available; ideal for shaving small areas (The Wahl Lithium Ion Trimmer; Wahl Clipper Corporation, Sterling, IL, USA)
Disinfectant	F10 SC Veterinary Disinfectant (Health and Hygiene [Pty] Ltd, Florida Hills, South Africa)
Wing wraps/AviStraint	Used rather than towels to keep birds' wings from flapping while examining; sizes L, XL, XXL, used most commonly (AviStraint; Diamond Avian Distributors, Hurdle Mills, NC, USA)
Dental speculum for oral examination on rabbits and rodents	3.5-V bivalve nasal speculum (Welch Allyn Inc, Skaneateles Falls, NY, USA)
Identification reference books	Especially useful for wildlife; many choices available: native birds, reptiles, mammals, sometimes include natural history

Diagnostics	Examples
Insulin syringes	These are used frequently for blood draws in small patients; insulin syringes can be used for more accurate measurement of medication injections: 3/10-mL U-100 insulin syringe with 29-G × ½-inch needle (BD, Franklin Lakes, NJ, USA)
Microtainer blood tubes	Terumo Capiject Micro Collection Tubes (Capiject Terumo Medical Corporation, Somerset, NJ, USA)
Bench top biochemistry analyzer that requires small volumes of blood	Abaxis VetScan VS2 provides results in 12 min from 100 μL of blood, serum, or plasma (Abaxis Inc, Union City, CA, USA)

Dental radiography	This could be used for patients <100 g
Radiation attenuating surgical gloves	Very helpful protection from scatter radiation when restraining exotic patients for radiographs; provides greater flexibility, dexterity, and sensitivity; can be disinfected and reused; various types available (International Biomedical, Austin, TX, USA)

Treatment	Examples
24-gauge and 26-gauge IV catheters	Various available
22-gauge 1.5-inch (0.72 mm to 3.81 cm) spinal needles	Various available to use for IO catheters
Insulin syringes or 0.5-mL oral dosing syringes	3/10-mL U-100 insulin syringe with 29-g × ½-inch needle (BD); this particular insulin syringe can have the needle twisted off with cat nail clippers (even though it states the needle is not removable) and can be used to administer oral medicine (Baxa Exactamed 0.5-mL syringes; Baxter Healthcare Corporation, Round Lake, IL, USA)
Compounding supplies or trusted local compounding pharmacy	Exotics frequently need medications compounded into liquid for administration and more appropriate dosing; some common medications can be compounded in the hospital; Mortar & Pestle, Ora-Plus Oral Suspending Vehicle, and Ora-Sweet Flavored Syrup Vehicle (Orion Laboratories Pty Ltd, trading as Perrigo, Balcatta, WA, Australia).
IV fluid pumps & syringe pumps	Various available
Perches of various sizes and diameters	Make or purchase
Cages with narrow space between bars	—
Incubator(s)	Variety of sizes and models; oxygen support ideal; Lyon ProCare CCU for critical care patients (Lyon Technologies, Inc, Chula Vista, CA, USA)
Aquariums with lids	—
Thermostats/rheostat	ReptiTemp500R (Zoo Med Laboratories, Inc, San Luis Obispo, CA, USA)
Heat lamp/ceramic heat emitter	Zoo Med Repticare Ceramic Infared Heat Emitter 60w (Zoo Med Laboratories, Inc)
Temperature/humidity gauges for indoor/outdoor	Variety available; does not have to be designed just for reptiles (AcuRite Digital Thermometer with Indoor/Outdoor Temperature and Humidity [various models]; Chaney Instrument Co, Lake Geneva, WI, USA)
Small bowls/shallow dishes/heavy ceramic bowls/attachable bowls	—

(continued on next page)

Table 3
(continued)

Treatment	Examples
Attachable water bottles	—
Avian E-collars	VSP restraint collars and extensions in multiple sizes (Veterinary Specialty Products, Shawnee, KS, USA); Saf-T Shield Bird E-collar in various sizes (KVP International Inc, Chino, CA, USA); foam pipe wrap insulation can be used as extensions needed for birds
Feeding tubes	Gavage/crop tubes variety of sizes available (Non-Flexible Stainless Steel Needles [Reusable]; Cadence, Staunton, VA, USA) can be used with psittacines; red rubber catheters can be cut to appropriate length and used in raptors, waterfowl/poultry, snakes, lizards, and turtles

Anesthesia	Examples
Non-rebreathing systems with 0.5-L bag	—
Variety of sizes of masks	Bird's entire head needs to fit in the mask; small masks can be made from containers with a hole drilled for the hose connection; rabbits, guinea pigs, and chinchillas are obligate nasal breathers and only need masks that cover the nose
Small boxes for anesthesia induction	Make by drilling a hole for the hose in the lid and weather-stripping can be along the lid to help decrease gas leaks
Tracheal tubes for intubation	Variety available; choose noncuffed or pediatric Cole tubes; V-gel for rabbits may be useful for emergency airway access (Docsinnovent Ltd, London, England)
Semiflexible 1.9-mm-diameter endoscope for intubation	Used for intubation of rabbits (FM-1.9×6 Semi-Flexible, 1.9-mm-diameter endoscope; MDS, Incorporated, Brandon, FL, USA)
Crash kit for exotic emergencies	Include insulin syringes, 1-mL syringes, emergency room drugs, spinal needles, IV catheters, and small endotracheal tubes; a quick reference chart for exotic emergencies can be laminated and attached to the kit[13]
Heating pad/hot water blanket/3M Bair Hugger	Patients <1000 g are generally light enough to use with heating pads on low; the Sunbeam King Size Xpress Heat Heating Pad has an option to select hour auto-off or leave on continuously (Sunbeam Products, Inc, Jarden Consumer Solutions, Boca Raton, FL, USA). Nails or a bite can easily puncture hot water blankets; small patients often get "lost" in a 3M Bair Hugger but could still be modified and used (3M Bair Hugger, St. Paul, MN, USA)

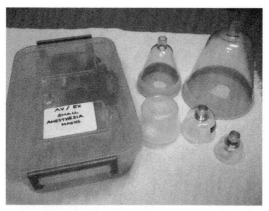

Fig. 6. Example of induction masks.

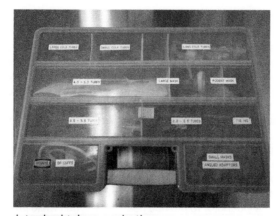

Fig. 7. Example endotracheal tube organization.

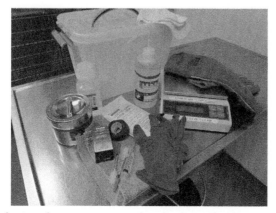

Fig. 8. Example of set up for emergency exotic animal examination.

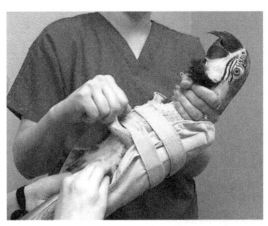

Fig. 9. Example of macaw being examined in an AviStraint. Invented and developed by Greg Burkett, DVM, DABVP(Avian) (drb@thebirdvet.com, www.avistraint.com).

quiet bird staying on the bottom of the cage is very sick, and it may not be a quick fix. Rabbits that present lying on their side, or those who have not eaten or defecated, are also very sick. Severe trauma is often a more recognizable emergency to the owner and usually they are more aware of the risk of losing their pet. However, during this time, it should be gently explained to the owner that when an exotic pet is very sick or injured, it might not be able to survive handling.

Exotic pets should be observed first in the carrier or enclosure. Based on the history and observation, supplies should be gathered in anticipation of possible work to be done while restraining the animal. It should be determined if the animal seems stable enough to handle restraint and an examination. Always be prepared for diagnostics, but ready to abort if the patient is not handling the restraint and examination well. For patients that seem extremely weak or in respiratory distress, place the entire carrier (if possible) in the incubator to provide heat and oxygen while preparing for the examination and/or diagnostics. Always be thinking about minimal handling with any exotic or wild species brought to the hospital. Once the animal is being restrained, it is critical to work thoroughly, gently, and quickly. It is not an ideal time for a clinician

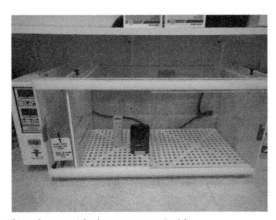

Fig. 10. Example of incubator with thermometers inside.

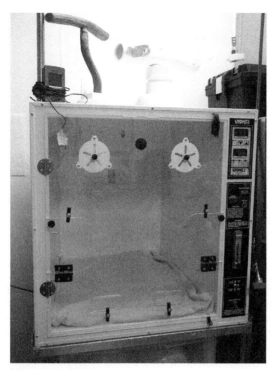

Fig. 11. Example of larger incubator.

to be interrupted, deal with other cases, or take phone calls. Keep voices low and movements slow and gentle and avoid staring directly at prey species (**Table 5**).

THE AVIAN EMERGENCY PATIENT

There are a wide variety of avian patients that may be seen in the emergency setting. Personal effort to learn the various species and unique characteristics will benefit the hospital. A working knowledge of a variety of species will allow the individual to observe and assess each patient relative to what is normal for particular species (**Figs. 18–20**).

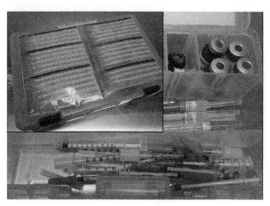

Fig. 12. Example of exotic patient emergency crash kit.

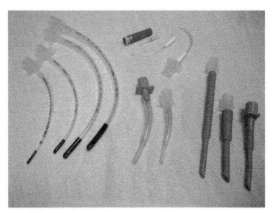

Fig. 13. Example of endotracheal tubes.

THE HERBIVORE EMERGENCY PATIENT (RABBITS, GUINEA PIGS, AND CHINCHILLAS)

Rabbits exhibit illness and pain in body posture very different that cats and dogs. It is important to handle high-stress rabbits on the floor in a quiet, safe room to avoid further injury. Less is more in terms of restraint. Covering their eyes gently with hands often helps keep them calmer. Always remind owners that extremely critical patients may not survive handling.

The following list is applicable to rabbits, guinea pigs, and chinchillas in terms of triaging the critical status of a patient:

- Has the patient eaten in the past 24 hours? Food should be moving through the gastrointestinal (GI) tract at all times.
- Position of the ears? Ears down or back indicates illness, pain, or annoyance/agitation.
- Eye position? Closed, semiclosed, dull, or wide open in fear or pain?
- Teeth grinding? May indicate pain.
- Sitting up or lying down? Laying down on side in emergency situation means immediate intervention is necessary.

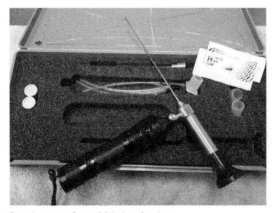

Fig. 14. Example of endoscope for rabbit intubation.

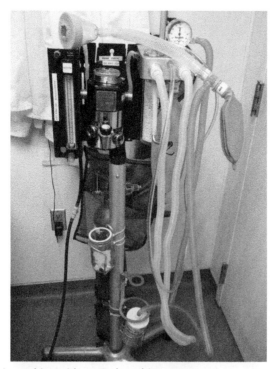

Fig. 15. Anesthesia machine with non-rebreathing system.

- Is the stomach hard? Possible gas bloat, which is life-threatening.
- Respiratory effort and appearance? If the head is raised, neck extended, nostrils flaring widely, or mouth opening with breaths, the patient is in respiratory distress and should be place in oxygen immediately.
- Body temperature? If low, most likely will require IV catheter and fluids as soon as possible.

THE FERRET EMERGENCY PATIENT

Ferrets are energetic carnivores with fast metabolisms. They are not legal in every state, but are relatively easy to work with for the small animal clinician or technician. A ferret should not be allowed to sniff one spot on an individual because it is often followed by a bite. Check state laws regarding rabies vaccination and always ask the owner the vaccine status. Ferrets should be housed away from rabbits, guinea pigs, chinchillas, and birds because they are considered a predator to these smaller species. Housing for the hospitalized ferret requires narrow cage bars and sleep sacks to crawl inside or under. An abnormal or sick ferret may be referred to as a "flat" ferret. They may exhibit the following:

- Lethargy
- Anorexia
- Teeth grinding (indicates pain)
- Vomiting
- Diarrhea

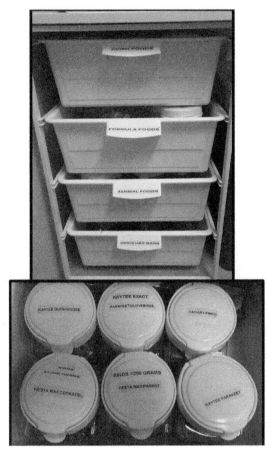

Fig. 16. Example of organizing diets.

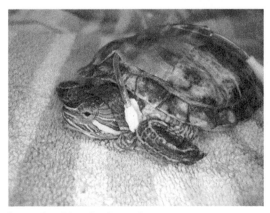

Fig. 17. Example of a turtle with a feeding tube.

Table 4
Ideas for diets to keep in hospital

Avian Diets	Examples
Parrot seed (for birds >200 g)	High-quality seed mix (Kaytee Fiesta Max Parrot Food; Kaytee Products, Inc, Chilton, WI, USA; Lafeber's Classic Nutri-berries Parrot Food; Lafeber Company, Cornell, IL, USA)
Cockatiel seed (for birds 200–65 g)	Kaytee Fiesta Max Cockatiel Food can be offered to a wide variety of birds in the 200–65-g weight range (Kaytee Products; Lafeber's Classic Nutri-berries Cockatiel Food; Lafeber Company)
Parakeet seed (for birds <65 g)	Kaytee Fiesta Max Parakeet Food (Kaytee Products, Inc)
Pellets for parrots (small and large)	Variety available; choose natural colored pellets (Harrison's Bird Foods, Brentwood, TN, USA; Lafeber Company; Roudybush, Woodland, CA, USA)
Millet spray for birds <100 g	Cockatiels and Budgerigars can benefit from this high-energy treat when sick or energized (Kaytee Natural Spray Millet (Kaytee Products, Inc)
Formula food for tube feeding psittacines	Kaytee exact Hand Feeding Formula
Chicken and/or duck feed if possibility of patients in hospital location	Variety available (Purina Scratch Grains; Purina Animal Nutrition LLC, Gray Summit, MO, USA; Mazuri Exotic Animal Nutrition Waterfowl Maintenance; Land O'Lakes Purina Feed LLC, PMI Nutrition International, Richmond, IN, USA)

Mammals	Examples
Ferrets	Variety of diets; most ferrets do not accept new foods; sometimes ferret shelters will make mixes of a variety of dry kibble diets and donate to the hospital (Marshall Pet Products, Wolcott, NY, USA)
Rabbits	Always need hay; high-quality timothy hay is a most common type; alfalfa hay ideal for young (<1-y-old pets) or thin animals; provide hay-based pellets (Oxbow Essentials Adult Rabbit Food & Oxbow Essentials Young Rabbit Food; Oxbow Animal Health, Murdock, NE, USA)

(continued on next page)

Table 4
(continued)

Mammals	Examples
Guinea pigs	Always need hay; High-quality timothy hay is a most common type; pellets available (Oxbow Essentials Guinea Pig Food & Oxbow Cavy Performance Food)
Chinchillas	Always need hay; High-quality timothy hay is a most common type; pellets available (Oxbow Essentials Chinchilla Food; Oxbow Animal Health)
Formula food for syringe feeding for various species	Oxbow Critical Care Anise or Apple-Banana flavors or Oxbow Critical Care Fine Grind for herbivores and Oxbow Carnivore Care for ferrets (Oxbow Animal Health); Lefeber's Emeraid Carnivore and Herbivore are also choices (Emeraid, LLC, Cornell, IL, USA); some ferret owners will bring in homemade ferret gravy/soup; meat baby foods could be tried for short-term nutrition

Reptiles	Examples
Variety of species; many do not need to eat every day; research appropriate diets	Owners may need to bring prey items or fresh food (salads), if hospitalized pet is likely too sick to eat and may need to be tube fed (Lefeber's Emeraid Omnivore (Emeraid, LLC); mixtures of Oxbow Critical Care Fine Grind for herbivores and Oxbow Carnivore Care can be also be used for omnivores

Table 5
Common emergencies

Emergency	Examples
Trauma	Birds may fly into windows, ceiling fans, etc; feather destruction and self-mutilation common in psittacines; broken blood feathers; wild birds may be hit by car; attacks by other animals; thermal burns (reptiles); outdoor animals: wounds of unknown origin, maggots
Anorexia	Life threatening in many exotic species; can be a nonspecific sign of a variety of problems
Not moving/lethargy	Nonspecific sign of variety of illnesses and injuries
Respiratory issues	Bacterial infections, fungal infections, chronic infections, may also be associated with other systemic diseases
GI issues	Very common in many herbivore exotic mammals: GI stasis, bloat, anorexia, decreased or no defecation; vomiting, diarrhea; obstructions/foreign bodies in ferrets
Reproductive issues	Egg-binding: life-threatening; cloacal prolapses in birds

THE REPTILE EMERGENCY PATIENT

Just like with avian species, there are a wide variety of reptile species that may be seen. It is important to be familiar with basic anatomy of snakes, lizards, and chelonians. Reptiles are ectothermic, and patients should be placed in incubators or enclosures that have ambient temperature control. Posting a chart of preferred optimum temperature zones for common pet reptiles in the designated exotic ward is a helpful quick reference.[12] Knowledge of a reliable resource for basic husbandry and requirements will allow the hospital to work with a variety of species.[2–4] A thorough history is critical because most emergencies are from ongoing deficiencies in diet, housing, and overall care.

WILDLIFE EMERGENCIES

Along with seeing captive commonly owned exotic species, the small animal hospital may have to provide care for injured or sick native wildlife brought in by concerned citizens. Vehicles, predators, or habitat disturbances may be the cause of injuries to native wildlife. Orphaned native wildlife is common during certain seasons, and it should be determined if the animal is truly "orphaned" before the finder leaves it at the hospital. It is important that these animals be kept away from other patients, and excessive handling and viewing should be avoided. The following should be followed concerning wildlife presentations:

- Attempt to identify the species and life stage.

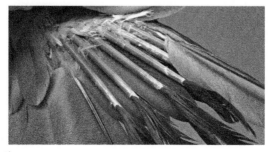

Fig. 18. Blood feathers.

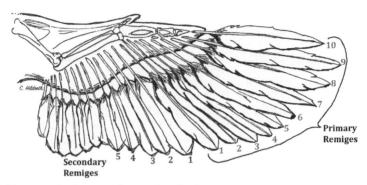

Fig. 19. Diagram of primary and secondary feathers.

- Set up an area/box/enclosure before handling the animal.
- Limit handling. Be prepared with equipment for examination, bandaging, and stabilization before restraint.
- Use appropriate safety protection—welder's gloves or small leather gloves for animals that may talon or bite; safety glasses for many shore birds or birds with sharp beaks; towels for restraint.
- Familiarize yourself with applicable local/state laws regarding native wildlife.
- Familiarize yourself with applicable federal laws—that is, protected species, Migratory Bird Treaty Act, the Bald and Golden Eagle Protection Act, rabies vector species.
- Create a list of local rehabilitators and the species they are permitted to rehabilitate.

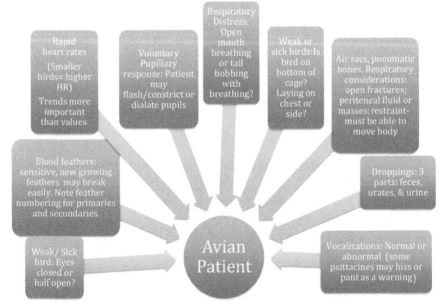

Fig. 20. Assessment of the avian patient. HR, heart rate.

- Triage the patient. Coordinate transferring the animal to a local rehabilitator if prognosis is good or determine if humane euthanasia is in the best interest of the animal.

SUMMARY

There are many techniques and basic knowledge of small animal emergency medicine that can be transferred to the exotic patient. Although the exotic patient needs a gentle, well-planned approach, common sense and observation can lead the small animal hospital to provide excellent care for a variety of species. Knowledge of where to obtain accurate information on different species quickly will help the technician and staff answer emergency questions and communicate with clients effectively. Continuing education, the support of the hospital team, and determination can help the small animal technician and clinician transition to provide emergency care for the exotic patient. Learning to be very observant of behaviors in a variety of species will allow the technician to identify critical situations and to avoid overstressing or injuring the patient during examinations, diagnostics, and treatments. Although the emergency environment is fast paced and often full of distractions, work with the exotic patient always requires full attention, intentional handling, gentleness, and a slower approach. Remembering to combine technical skills with gentleness and patience, along with strong observational skills, will create an effective exotic emergency medicine team.

REFERENCES

1. World Parrot Trust encyclopedia of species profiles. Available at: http://www.parrots.org/encyclopedia. Accessed November 29, 2015.
2. Melissa Kaplan's herp care collection. 2014. Available at: http://www.anapsid.org. Accessed November 29, 2015.
3. Reptile care series and small mammal health series, 1991-2015. Veterinary Information Network, Inc. Available at: http://www.veterinarypartner.com. Accessed November 29, 2015.
4. LafeberVet. Available at: http://lafeber.com/vet/. Accessed November 29, 2015.
5. Orosz SE. Clinical avian nutrition. Vet Clin North Am Exot Anim Pract 2014;17: 397–413.
6. Ballard B, Cheek R. Exotic animal medicine for the veterinary technician. 2nd edition. Ames (IA): Wiley-Blackwell; 2010.
7. Muir WW, Hubbell JAE. Handbook of veterinary anesthesia. 5th edition. St Louis (MO): Elsevier Mosby; 2013.
8. Longley LA. Anaesthesia of exotic pets. London: Saunders; 2008.
9. Quesenberry K, Carpenter J. Ferrets, rabbits, and rodents clinical medicine and surgery. 3rd edition. St Louis (MO): Elsevier Saunders; 2012.
10. Mayer J, Donnelly T. Clinical veterinary advisor birds and exotic pets. St Louis (MO): Elsevier Saunders; 2013.
11. Carpenter J. Exotic animal formulary. 4th edition. St Louis (MO): Elsevier Saunders; 2013.
12. Mader D. Reptile medicine and surgery. 2nd edition. St Louis (MO): Elsevier Saunders; 2006. p. 26.
13. Kottwitz J, Kelleher S. Emergency drugs: quick reference chart for exotic animals. Exotic DVM Magazine 5.5 2003;23–5.

Basic Shock Physiology and Critical Care

Brian K. Roberts, DVM, DACVECC[a,b,*]

KEYWORDS

- Shock • Physiology • Critical care • Exotic animals

KEY POINTS

- Most of the literature discussing shock, systemic inflammation, and sepsis relates to experimental studies using small mammals such as rodents and rabbits; there is a paucity of research of these syndromes in other species, such as ferrets, birds, and reptiles.
- Although small mammals, experimentally, have a similar autonomic response to dogs during induced hemorrhage and shock states, this response is not noted in the clinical setting, in which decompensated shock is more commonly reported.
- Poor perfusion affects every major organ system, but particular attention should be given to the immune system, coagulation system, cardiovascular system, gastrointestinal tract, and kidneys.
- Knowing how these systems are affected helps explain to clinicians why patients with shock can later become septic or coagulopathic.
- To ensure the best outcomes in patients who have shock or systemic inflammatory response syndrome, early recognition and intervention by provision of supplemental oxygen and fluid resuscitation is essential.

DEFINITIONS

1. Shock is the clinical expression of dysoxia. Dysoxia is lack of oxygen supply to, or use by, the cells, limiting energy production.[1] Poor perfusion and diminished oxygen delivery to the tissues with resulting signs of pallor, tachycardia, tachypnea, and altered pulse quality is another way to describe shock.
2. Oxygen delivery (Do_2) is the amount of oxygen delivered to tissues as determined by cardiac output and oxygen carrying capacity.[2] It is described best by the equation $CO \times Cao_2$, in which CO is cardiac output (the heart rate multiplied by stroke

Disclosure: The author has nothing to disclose.
[a] Department of Clinical Sciences, School of Veterinary Medicine, St Matthew's University, PO Box 32330, Grand Cayman KY1-1209, Cayman Islands; [b] Small Animal Medicine, School of Veterinary Medicine, St Matthew's University, PO Box 32330, Grand Cayman KY1-1209, Cayman Islands
* Department of Clinical Sciences, School of Veterinary Medicine, St Matthew's University, PO Box 32330, Grand Cayman KY1-1209, Cayman Islands.
E-mail address: broberts@stmatthews.edu

Vet Clin Exot Anim 19 (2016) 347–360
http://dx.doi.org/10.1016/j.cvex.2016.01.010
vetexotic.theclinics.com
1094-9194/16/$ – see front matter © 2016 Elsevier Inc. All rights reserved.

volume) and Ca_{O_2} is the oxygen carrying capacity of arterial blood, which is determined by the saturation of oxygen bound to hemoglobin, the amount of hemoglobin, and the small amount of dissolved oxygen in the serum (**Fig. 1**).

3. Oxygen consumption (V_{O_2}) is the amount of oxygen used by the tissues after being delivered and off-loaded from hemoglobin.[3] It can be determined by using the equation $CO \times (C_aO_2 - C_vO_2)$ which is cardiac output multiplied by the difference between arterial oxygen content (C_aO_2) and venous oxygen content (C_vO_2).

4. Systemic inflammatory response syndrome (SIRS) is a condition characterized by changes in heart rate, body temperature, and respiration rate with either leukocytosis or leukopenia.[4] SIRS can be caused by trauma; organ inflammation, such as pancreatitis; infection; and environmental stressors, like heat stroke.[5] Criteria for SIRS have been described for humans and extrapolated for small animal veterinary medicine.[6] SIRS has been described experimentally using similar criteria in rabbits[7] and in rodents.[8] SIRS in reptiles, amphibians, and other exotic species has not been characterized to the author's knowledge.

5. Sepsis is defined as SIRS secondary to infection. An infection is a pathologic process caused by the invasion of microorganisms that cause disease of normally sterile tissue or fluid.[9] The term has been used since Hippocrates' time to describe putrefaction and decomposition.[10] Many clinicians use terminology such as sepsis syndrome, bacteremia, and SIRS interchangeably with sepsis. Note that SIRS can occur without infection.

6. Multiple organ dysfunction syndrome is a condition whereby disease, injury, lack of perfusion, and so forth cause at least 1 vital organ (heart, lung, kidney, nervous system) to no longer function normally. Failure of multiple organs (>1) is multiple organ failure (MOF).[11]

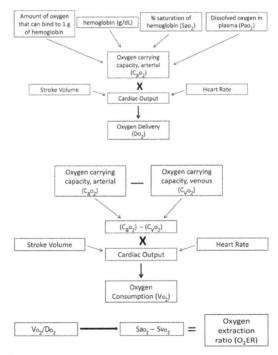

Fig. 1. Perfusion dynamics.

PHYSIOLOGY OF PERFUSION

To provide oxygen to tissues and their cells, there are 3 basic requirements: functional cardiovascular system comprising a pump (heart) and responsive vasculature, the ability of the fluid pumped to carry oxygen (red blood cells, normally working hemoglobin, and saturation of the hemoglobin), and a way for the oxygen to become bound to hemoglobin through a normally working respiratory system.

Oxygen delivery (Do_2) is the amount of oxygen carried to the tissues in blood by hemoglobin. It is determined by cardiac output and oxygen carrying capacity (see **Fig. 1**). In rats, normal Do_2 is approximately 1.8 ± 0.2 mL O_2/min/kg.[12] In rabbits, the normal Do_2 reference range is 27.1 ± 2.7 mL/kg/min.[13]

Determination of oxygen delivery is more difficult in reptiles because of the various species and slow heart rates. Instead of Do_2, researchers sometimes measure oxygen pulse (OP), which was used in several tissue oxygenation studies summarized by Gleeson and Bennett.[14] OP is the amount of oxygen delivered per heartbeat, which differs among turtles, snakes, and lizards according to their body temperature, with values ranging between 1 and 4 mL $O_2 \times 10^{-5}$/g/beat. In turtles, as body temperature increased, so did OP,[15] whereas in lizards[16] and snakes[17] OP decreased with increasing body temperature. Therefore, species differences and habitat affect emergency treatment such as warming or not warming a reptile in shock.

Oxygen use by the tissues, termed Vo_2, has a direct association with the amount of oxygen being delivered and extracted by cells. The ratio of arterial oxygen delivery to oxygen consumption is the oxygen extraction ratio (o_2ER) (see **Fig. 1**). Approximately 20% to 30% of the oxygen delivered to tissues is extracted in mammals under normal conditions.[18] During periods of increased oxygen need caused by changes in metabolism, such as fever, the tissues can extract more oxygen. This ability also occurs during times when there is diminished oxygen delivery caused by hypovolemia, bradycardia, dyshemoglobinemia, pulmonary disease, and so forth. Therefore, the cells, and specifically the mitochondria of cells, can still produce enough ATP despite diminished hemoglobin saturation and lowered cardiac output by extracting more oxygen.

During exercise, acute hypoxia, and acute anemia, Do_2 is maintained by increasing cardiac output.[19] However, once a critical point is reached, the tissues can no longer extract enough oxygen unless more is delivered. For example, you are stocking up on water because of an impending hurricane. You fill up a whole shopping cart with bottles of water. Because you have a big family, you need more than 1 cart-full, so you fill another cart. Soon, the bottled water shelves become sparse. The only way you can extract more water (ie, put more in the cart) is if more is delivered and stocked on the shelves.

During states in which the tissues and cells cannot extract enough oxygen and more must be delivered, anaerobic metabolism ensues. This critical point is termed oxygen supply dependency.[20] It is at this point that symptoms of shock are seen; a response that tries to increase oxygen delivery. Physiologic changes that occur include tachycardia, tachypnea, and vasoconstriction of peripheral and splanchnic vessels. This condition is shown in **Fig. 2**; once the Do_2 cannot be maintained at greater than or equal to twice the level of Vo_2, biochemical changes associated with shock, such as hyperlactatemia and acidemia, ensue. Not only does inadequate Do_2 result from hypovolemia, pulmonary disease, and dyshemoglobinemia but it can also be caused by altered cellular function, as seen with sepsis and mitochondrial dysfunction in the critically ill. During such insults, the cell's machinery, cell membrane, protein receptors, and genes become dysfunctional, leading to apoptosis and loss of integrity.[21]

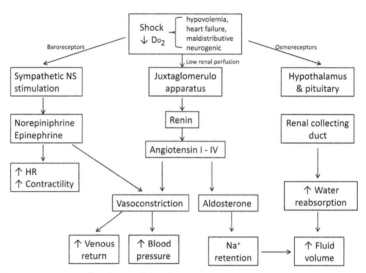

Fig. 2. Compensatory mechanisms of shock.

Nonmammalian species such as reptiles and birds have different values for Do_2, Vo_2, and o_2ER because of slower or faster heart rates, hemoglobin concentration, and saturation of hemoglobin. Reptiles, depending on the species, balance oxygen delivery during exercise differently. Iguanas maintain Do_2 primarily by increasing heart rate because stroke volume decreases by 20% from a resting state during exercise. However, *Varanus* spp such as monitor lizards increase stroke volume and heart rate to normalize oxygen delivery during exercise.[22] Reptiles also tend to have lower oxygen saturation of arterial blood. Most reptiles have Sao_2 of 70% to 90%, with turtles at the higher end of the range and lizards at the lower end.[23] Reptiles differ from birds and mammals in their higher reliance on anaerobic metabolism, which can make evaluation of the importance of oxygenation and perfusion more challenging. Another feature that affects reptile oxygen dynamics is blood shunting. Reptilian hearts (other than those of the Crocodylia) have an incomplete interventricular septum. In these animals, both left-to-right shunting and right-to-left shunting can occur. With intracardiac left-to-right shunting, areas of the myocardium that are normally oxygen poor receive more oxygen.[24] Reduction of right-to-left shunting of deoxygenated blood leads to an increase in oxygen carrying capacity. It is thought that alteration of the shunt fraction is controlled by changes in physiologic conditions. This change, along with a right-shift to the oxygen dissociation curve, maintains oxygen delivery in reptiles that have been studied.[25] Studies in turtles have shown right-to-left shunting facilitates warming while left-to-right shunting improves systemic oxygen transport. Left-to-right shunting is partly responsible for increasing myocardial oxygenation, which is needed for the tachycardic response to hemorrhage.[26]

PATHOPHYSIOLOGY OF SHOCK

During episodes of decreased tissue oxygenation, or shock, cells try to maintain homeostasis by altering their metabolism to create ATP anaerobically via glycolysis. It is thought that, in mammals, the stimulus for anaerobic glycogenolysis is not oxygen deficiency but stimulation of sarcolemmal $Na^+/K^+/ATPase$ secondary to stress hormone release (ie, epinephrine).[27] Stimulation of the sympathetic nervous system

(SNS) occurs through baroreceptor-mediated response to poor cardiac output and decreased tissue oxygen delivery.[28] The increase of sympathetic activity results in tachycardia, increased contractility, and vasoconstriction. Fluid shifts from the interstitial and extravascular space to the intravascular space occur following the Starling law, especially during episodes of diminished hydrostatic pressure.[28] Activation of the rennin-angiotensin-aldosterone system (RAAS) also occurs because of reduced renal perfusion and also sympathetic system–induced vasoconstriction of the splanchnic vasculature. RAAS activation results in sodium and water retention, vasoconstriction, more upregulation of the sympathetic response, and release of antidiuretic hormone (ADH).[29] The purpose of RAAS activation is to increase effective circulating volume, increase cardiac output, and shunt blood to the heart and brain. A summary of compensatory mechanisms is outlined in **Fig. 2**.

SHOCK STAGES
Compensatory Shock

The stimulation of the SNS and release of RAAS and ADH result in classic clinical signs of dull mentation, pallor, and tachycardia. During this stage, capillary refill time may be normal and blood pressure is preserved.[30]

Decompensatory Shock

If perfusion, effective circulating volume, cardiac output, and/or oxygen delivery do not improve from compensatory mechanisms, additional symptoms of prolonged capillary refill, poor pulse quality, and hypotension occur. As poor perfusion persists, the eventual result of this phase is unresponsive hypotension.[31] This final phase of decompensatory shock results from hemodynamic collapse of the autoregulatory escape mechanism. As organs are starved of oxygen, fluid, and nutrients, arterioles dilate to increase flow. This process is a global phenomenon that leads to systemic hemodynamic collapse and death.[32] Intervention (fluid therapy, oxygen supplementation, pressor drugs, transfusion, and so forth) does not reverse this reflexive mechanism.

SYSTEMIC INFLAMMATORY RESPONSE SYNDROME

As previously defined, SIRS is a state in which there is clinical and clinicopathologic evidence of systemic inflammation, characterized by tachycardia, tachypnea, hypothermia or hyperthermia, and leukocytosis or leukopenia. Insults causing SIRS, such as trauma, neoplasia, immune-mediated disease, can progress to cause shock, multiple organ dysfunction, and MOF.[33] The underlying cause of SIRS is the immune system's lack of balance between the activators of inflammation and inhibitors of inflammation. If the balance is tipped in either direction, organ damage occurs. Injury to organs occurs from activated leukocytes' release of damaging cytoplasmic granules, microcirculatory ischemia from leukocyte obstruction, altered apoptosis, and production of reactive oxygen species.[34] Infection causing sepsis is the classic example of SIRS and results in the production of inflammatory mediators, called cytokines, such as tumor necrosis factor-alpha, interleukin-1, and interleukin-6. Cytokines are produced by immunocytes, especially B lymphocytes, T lymphocytes, and macrophages.[35] There are more than 20 different cytokines and many more non–immunocyte-produced inflammatory proteins, such as platelet activating factor, interferons, and products of the arachidonic acid cascade.[36] These inflammatory mediators bind to receptors of endothelial cells, other immunocytes such as neutrophils, and mast cells. Effects of cytokine binding include alteration of vascular permeability, increased chemotaxis of immunocytes, and activation of the coagulation cascade.

To limit this robust inflammatory response, many of the same cells that produce inflammatory cytokines also produce antiinflammatory molecules known as the compensatory antiinflammatory response syndrome (CARS). Antiinflammatory mediators include interleukin 10, Transforming growth factor-beta, and interleukin-13.[37] SIRS and CARS are balanced to produce enough inflammation to respond to an insult, such as an infection or a neoplasm, whereby the inflammatory mediators attack the infectious agent/neoplastic cell and activate the complement cascade while sparing noninfected/nonneoplastic tissue. If the inflammatory response overwhelms the counteractive antiinflammatory response, SIRS progresses, causing organ damage, cellular apoptosis, and a hypermetabolic state. In contrast, if the antiinflammatory response is too forceful, a syndrome of immunoparalysis develops, increasing the likelihood of dying of something like a simple infection.[38]

Pathogen recognition through receptor activation is a key factor in how the immune system responds to infection and targets the organism. Receptors against pathogens are expressed by immunocytes and other cells, such as the endothelium. Targets of pathogen recognition are called pathogen-associated molecular patterns (PAMPs). These signaling molecules are produced by microbial pathogens and are structures that give the pathogen the ability to survive and cause disease. The classic example of a PAMP is lipopolysaccharide from gram-negative bacteria. PAMPs bind to many different receptors, the largest class being Toll-like receptors, of which there are more than 10 described in the literature.[39] Once bound to a pattern recognition receptor, internal signaling pathways result in a change of cellular metabolism, protein production, or other cell activation, such as chemotaxis. PAMP production is influenced by genetic factors and aging. In dogs, one study noted that the cytokine response to PAMPs alters with age and is likely a contributing factor to morbidity in geriatric dogs with gram-negative sepsis.[40]

Danger-associated molecular patterns (DAMPs) are similar to PAMPs. These molecules also can initiate and perpetuate the inflammatory response by binding to many of the same receptors of PAMPs found on leukocytes. The main difference is that DAMPs are proteins and molecules from host cells, not the pathogen. DAMPs constitute molecules from the plasma membrane, endoplasmic reticulum, nucleus, and cytosol from apoptotic cells and damaged cells.[41] For this reason, noninfectious sources of injury, such as trauma, pancreatitis, and heat stroke, can lead to SIRS.

Another organ system heavily involved in the pathophysiology of SIRS is the endothelial system. Activation of endothelial cells from trauma, infection, or inflammation results in expression of receptors (P and L selectins, endothelial cell immunoglobulin adhesion molecules).[42] Leukocytes, namely neutrophils, bind to expressed endothelial receptors, adhering to the wall of the vessel lumen. As this process continues with more neutrophils binding and rolling, microvascular flow can be disrupted, causing changes in capillary integrity and vascular tone.[43] In addition, cytokines cause changes in vascular tone, resulting in contraction of arteries but not venules. This process, mediated by tumor necrosis factor-alpha, interleukin-6, and other cytokines, modifies the blood supply to ischemic and inflamed tissues.[44] Interstitial edema, especially that of the pulmonary parenchyma, occurs as the result of cytokines and inducible nitric oxide which is a potent vasodilator. Several studies have found that acute lung inflammation, known as acute respiratory distress syndrome, is in part caused by activation of immunocytes, their production of cytokines, and the response by the pulmonary microvascular system.[45,46] This type of edema, termed capillary leak syndrome, not only affects the lungs but also other organ systems, causing interstitial edema, which makes it more difficult to deliver oxygen from the capillaries to their target cells. As this process progresses, multiple organ system failure ensues.[47]

The coagulation system is also altered during the SIRS cascade. Tissue factor expression by monocytes, and its expression from activated platelets and endothelial cell microparticles, results in thrombin formation. Thrombin formation leads to additional thrombin activation and the final formation of cross-linked fibrin.[48] Fibrin and activated platelets form thrombi in the microvasculature, disrupting blood flow and oxygen delivery. Protection against thrombin formation is overwhelmed during states of SIRS, exhausting stores of endogenous anticoagulants such as activated protein C, antithrombin, and protein S. As this process becomes more systemic, no longer isolated to the site of inflammation or infection, disseminated intravascular coagulopathy (DIC) occurs. DIC is an independent predictor of mortality and its diagnosis is often a poor prognostic sign.[49]

An overview of some of the pathways of SIRS, with resulting effects on target organs, is provided in **Fig. 3**.

Clinically, 2 common effects of poor perfusion and the subsequent sympathetic response are alteration of the gastrointestinal tract and the renal system. When there is significant hypovolemia, trauma, or sepsis with resultant sympathetic-induced vasoconstriction, the splanchnic vasculature is affected,[50] leading to ischemic injury and loss of the protective gastrointestinal barrier, which is primarily sustained because of normal capillary mucosal blood flow. Once the barrier is compromised, commensal pathogenic bacteria have the ability to increase in number and translocate. Primarily, translocation occurs via lymphatic vessels but can also occur through the blood supply via the portal system.[51] This process is one reason whereby patients who present for trauma or hypovolemic shock from an inflammatory, noninfectious process can become septic without being inoculated with bacteria.

The main effect of poor perfusion on the renal system is a decrease in glomerular filtration rate (GFR). This phenomenon is now termed acute kidney injury, in contrast with the older terminology of acute renal failure.[52] However, traditional biochemical methods of estimating GFR using blood urea nitrogen and creatinine concentrations do not alert clinicians to the injury until 75% of functioning nephrons are no longer working. In humans, sepsis accounts for 50% of acute kidney injury and some degree of acute kidney injury is documented in up to 20% of persons hospitalized in intensive care units.[53] Acute kidney injury has been described in birds with both viral and bacterial infections.[54] Small mammals, mainly rodents, have served as models of acute kidney injury secondary to sepsis for some time. It is well recognized that sepsis and septic shock induced through cecal ligation result in renal injury.[55] Although chronic renal failure is more commonly reported in reptiles, acute renal injury has been reported and is more likely to occur because of injected medications to the hind limbs. The reptile renal-portal system allows circulation from the hind limbs and tail to traverse directly to the kidneys.

SPECIES DIFFERENCES OF SHOCK AND SYSTEMIC INFLAMMATORY RESPONSE SYNDROME
Mammals

Overall, there is a paucity of clinical data regarding shock and SIRS in the clinical setting. Much of the shock research on pocket pets, rabbits, and rodents are controlled experiments. Rodents and rabbits have served as research animals in this field of study for many decades, and there are numerous reports inducing shock, sepsis, and SIRS in rats, mice, and rabbits.[56–58] In rats, typical increases in heart rate

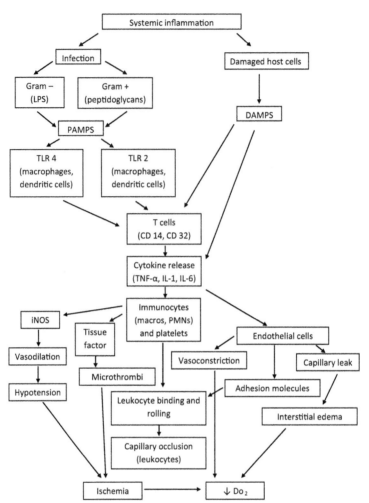

Fig. 3. SIRS cascade. IL, interleukin; iNOS, inducible nitric oxide; Macro, macrophage; PAMPS, pathogen-associated molecular pattern; PMNs, polymorphonuclear leukocytes; TNF-α, tumor necrosis factor-alpha.

and sympathetic response occur during sepsis and shock, characterized by tachycardia and decreased mean arterial pressure.[59] Rats also develop hypothermia associated with shock, similar to dogs, cats, and humans.[60] Hamsters have been used to study sepsis and, similar to rats in shock, develop hypotension and leukocyte activation with vessel margination.[61] Similarly, in a ferret model of SARS –coronavirus, hyperthermia associated with viremic sepsis progressing to hypothermia associated with decompensatory shock was described. That same study also showed leukopenia in moribund ferrets on day 2 after infection.[62] One study of rabbits that underwent experimental hemorrhagic shock by removing 26% of blood volume noted tachycardia, hypotension, and significantly decreased cardiac output versus controls.[63] That same study, by Chalmers and colleagues,[63] which compared normal rabbits with adrenalectomized rabbits, noted that the sympathetic response in normal animals minimized reductions in CO and blood pressure. Contrasting this research, clinical reports note the difficulty in resuscitating hypotensive rabbits and small mammals because of vagal stimulation, which becomes active simultaneously with sympathetic activity.[64] Rabbits in an uncontrolled hemorrhage shock study required 123 to 133 mL/kg of crystalloid fluid in attempts to control hypotension.[65] The aforementioned dose is significantly higher than crystalloid shock dose recommendations for lagomorphs in the literature, which are 15 mL/kg or initial boluses of 3 to 5 mL/kg.[66]

Reptiles

There is limited experimental research on hypovolemia and its effects on cardiovascular measurements in reptiles. Reptiles have vascular adaptations allowing blood shunting, known as the renal-portal system. During periods of dehydration and prolonged hypovolemia, blood from their hind limbs and tail traverses to the afferent renal portal veins, preserving renal perfusion.[67] One study noted that, during acute hemorrhage, snakes were able to maintain their blood volume by restoring up to 90% of deficit within 2 hours of hemorrhage by shifting extravascular fluid to the intravascular space.[68] Although snakes are able to restore their circulating volume after hemorrhage, their autonomic response is minor and does not allow compensation of hypotension.[69] Because of their body configuration, environmental temperature effects on metabolism, and cardiovascular anatomy (3-chambered heart), snakes have highly variable blood pressure. Depending on their habitat (arboreal vs terrestrial vs aquatic), systemic blood pressures in snakes correspond with gravitational stress. Arboreal snakes have higher arterial pressures than aquatic snakes. Blood pressure in these species also depends on body mass, with larger snakes having higher blood pressure.[70]

Turtles also have temperature and habitat influences on their cardiovascular system. Turtles that underwent controlled hemorrhage had significantly increased heart rates and hypotension. In that same study, turtles were able to restore prehemorrhage blood volume 2 hours after hemorrhage, which is similar to snakes.[71] The ability of turtles to recover from hemorrhage is not highly dependent on vasoconstriction but depends on increased heart rate. Baroreceptor response occurs in these species, resulting in tachycardia and increased contractility. Catecholamine effects on their vasculature causes accelerated resorption of interstitial fluid versus increased pressure.[72]

Lizards, specifically the green iguana, have undergone similar controlled hemorrhage studies to determine cardiovascular responses. Progressive hemorrhage resulted in tachycardia, decreased femoral blood flow, and hypotension. Changes in body position affect arterial pressure, and passive, head-up tilting induce reflexive cardiovascular changes to regulate blood pressure.[73] Hemorrhage and subsequent clot formation takes significantly longer in iguanas than in mammals. Higher temperatures have been shown to improve blood clotting in iguanas.[74]

Birds

Much of the scientific literature discussing hypotension and shock in avian species uses poultry as models. One article compared fluid types for resuscitation in leghorn chickens. That study only used colloidal-type fluids (hetastarch) and a hemoglobin-based oxygen carrier (HBOC) (Hemospan) to resuscitate chickens that had undergone experimentally induced hemorrhage of 50% of their blood volume. Surprisingly, there were no significant differences found between those two fluids and autotransfusion with respect to heart rate, respiratory rate, and systolic blood pressure.[75] In a similar study by Lichtenberger and colleagues,[76] mallard ducks underwent controlled hemorrhage and fluid resuscitation with either crystalloid (Plasmalyte A), colloid (Hetastarch), or an HBOC (Oxyglobin). Tachycardia was not noted until 25% to 45% of blood volume was lost. There was no statistical difference in mortality among the different types of fluid. However, Oxyglobin is no longer commercially available.

Birds tolerate hypovolemia secondary to hemorrhage very well. Clinical signs of anemia and shock are not seen until 50% to 60% of blood volume is lost. In pigeons, loss of 60% of blood volume resulted in no clinical signs and their hematocrits returned to normal within 7 days. The ability of birds to tolerate such large volumes of blood loss is thought to be caused by 3 adaptations. There is rapid extravascular fluid resorption from muscles that have a large capillary surface area, which then replenishes the intravascular deficit. In addition, birds have blunted autonomic response, resulting in fewer clinical signs of tachycardia, tachypnea, and hypothermia. The ability to mobilize large numbers of immature red blood cells is a third adaptation to hemorrhagic shock that birds possess.[77] This unique response to hemorrhage was also noted in a study that compared the hemodynamics of hemorrhage in chicks with that of rats. Controlled hemorrhage caused significant reduction of mean arterial pressure and cardiac output in rats, by 23% and 43% respectively. In the chicks, mean arterial pressure was only reduced by 15% and cardiac output reduced by 4% because of their ability to maintain stroke volume. The investigators concluded that chicks were able to maintain mean arterial pressure independently of changes in peripheral vascular tone.[78]

SUMMARY

In conclusion, most of the literature discussing shock, systemic inflammation, and sepsis relates to experimental studies using small mammals such as rodents and rabbits. There is a paucity of research of these syndromes in other species such as ferrets, birds, and reptiles. Although small mammals, experimentally, have a similar autonomic response to dogs during induced hemorrhage and shock states, that response is not noted in the clinical setting, in which decompensated shock is more commonly reported. Poor perfusion affects every major organ system, but particular attention should be given to the immune system, coagulation system, cardiovascular system, gastrointestinal tract, and kidneys. Knowing how these systems are affected helps to explain to clinicians why patients with shock can later become septic or coagulopathic. To ensure the best outcomes in patients who have shock or SIRS, early recognition and intervention by provision of supplemental oxygen and fluid resuscitation is essential. Treatment to combat shock in exotic species is discussed elsewhere in this issue.

REFERENCES

1. Marino P. Tissue oxygenation. In: The ICU book. Philadelphia: Lippincott Williams & Wilkins; 2007. p. 193–207.
2. Mazzaferro E. Oxygen therapy. In: Silverstein DC, Hopper K, editors. Small animal critical care medicine. 2nd edition. St Louis (MO): Elsevier; 2014. p. 77–80.
3. Klabunde RE. Cardiovascular physiology concepts. Available at: http://www.cvphysiology.com/CAD/CAD003.htm. Accessed November 9, 2015.
4. Marino P. Inflammation and infection in the ICU. In: The ICU book. Philadelphia: Lippincott Williams & Wilkins; 2007. p. 737–47.
5. Rangel-Frausto MS, Pittet D, Costigan M, et al. The natural history of the systemic inflammatory response syndrome: a prospective study. JAMA 1995; 273(2):117.

6. Byers CG. Principles of fluid therapy in sepsis & SIRS in dogs & cats. In: American College of Veterinary Internal Medicine (ACVIM) Proceedings 2014. Nashville (TN): 2014.

7. Jackubrovsky J, Brozman M, Chorváth D, et al. A comparative study of the morphology of the systemic anaphylactic reaction (SAR) and the shock reaction induced by antigen-antibody complexes in rabbits. Virchows Arch A Pathol Anat Histol 1981;394(1–2):97–108.

8. Jackubrovsky J, Brozman M. Morphology of haemorrhagic shock, systemic immunocomplex reaction and systemic anaphylactic reaction. A comparative study. Czech Med 1984;7(4):215–37.

9. American College of Chest Physicians/Society of Critical Care Medicine Consensus Conference: definitions for sepsis and organ failure and guidelines for the use of innovative therapies in sepsis. Crit Care Med 1992;20:864–74.

10. Geroulanos S, Douka ET. Historical perspective of the word "sepsis". Intensive Care Med 2006;32:2077.

11. Osterbur K, Mann FA, Kuroki K, et al. Multiple organ dysfunction syndrome in humans and animals. J Vet Intern Med 2014;28:1141–51.

12. Edmunds NJ, Marshall JM. Vasodilatation, oxygen delivery and oxygen consumption in rat hindlimb during systemic hypoxia: roles of nitric oxide. J Physiol 2001;532(1):251–9.

13. Matsuyama S, Hayakawa K, et al. Vasodilating prostaglandin E1 does not reproduce interleukin-1B-induced oxygen metabolism abnormalities in rabbits. Acute Med Surg 2015;2:40–7.

14. Gleeson TT, Bennett AF. Respiratory and cardiovascular adjustments to exercise in reptiles. In: Raymond G, editor. Circulation, respiration, and metabolism: current comparative approaches. Berlin: Springer-Verlag; 1985. p. 34–5.

15. Gatten RE Jr. Effects of temperature and activity on aerobic and anaerobic metabolism and heart rate in the turtles *Pseudemys scripta* and *Terrapene ornate*. Comp Biochem Physiol 1974;8A:619–48.

16. Bennet AF. Blood physiology and oxygen transport during activity in two lizards, *Varanus gouldii* and *Sauromalus hispidus*. Comp Biochem Physiol 1973;46A: 673–90.

17. Dmi'el R, Borut A. Thermal behavior, heat exchange and metabolism in the desert snake *Spalerosophis cliffordi*. Physiol Zool 1972;223(3):510–6.

18. McLellan SA, Walsh TS. Oxygen delivery and haemoglobin. Crit Care Pain 2004; 4(4):123–6.

19. Bartlett RH. Oxygen kinetics. In: Critical care physiology. Little, Brown and Co; 1996. p. 1–23.

20. Bakker J, Vincent J-L. The oxygen supply dependency phenomenon is associated with increased blood lactate levels. J Crit Care 1991;6(3):152–9.

21. Rocha LL, Pessoa CM, Corrêa TD, et al. Current concepts on hemodynamic support and therapy in septic shock. Rev Bras Anestesiol 2015;65(5):395–402.

22. Gleeson TT. Metabolic recovery from exhaustive activity by a large lizard. J Appl Physiol Respir Environ Exerc Physiol 1980;48(4):689–94.

23. Plough FH. Summary of oxygen transport characteristics of reptilian blood. Smithson Herp Inf Serv 1979;45:1–18.

24. Farmer CG, Hicks JW. The intracardiac shunt as a source of myocardial oxygen in the turtle, *Trachemys scripta*. Integr Comp Biol 2002;42:208–15.

25. Wood SC. Effect of O2 affinity on arterial PO2 in animals with central vascular shunts. J Appl Physiol Respir Environ Exerc Physiol 1982;53:1360–4.

26. Farmer CG, Hicks JW. The intracardiac shunt as a source of myocardial oxygen in a turtle, Trachemys scripta. Integr Comp Biol 2002;42:208–15.

27. Levy B. Lactate and shock state: the metabolic view. Curr Opin Crit Care 2006; 12(4):315–21.

28. Hopper K, Silverstein D, Bateman S. Shock syndromes. In: Dibartola, editor. Fluid, electrolyte and acid-base disorders in small animal practice. 4th edition. St Louis (MO): Elsevier; 2012. p. 557–61.

29. De Laforcade A, Silverstein D. Shock. In: Silverstein D, Hopper K, editors. Small animal critical care medicine. 2nd edition. St Louis (MO): Elsevier; 2015. p. 26–7.

30. Garreston S, Malberti S. Understanding hypovolaemic, cardiogenic and septic shock. Nurs Stand 2007;50(21):46–55.

31. Bonanno FG. Clinical pathology of the shock syndromes. J Emerg Trauma Shock 2011;4(2):233–43.

32. Raffe MR, Wingfield W. Hemorrhage and hypovolemia. In: Raffe MR, Wingfield W, editors. The veterinary ICU book. Jackson (WY): Teton NewMedia; 2002. p. 455.

33. De Laforcade A. Systemic inflammatory response syndrome. In: Silverstein D, Hopper K, editors. Small animal critical care medicine. 2nd edition. St Louis (MO): Elsevier; 2015. p. 30–1.

34. Binkowska AM, Michalak G, Słotwiński R. Current views on the mechanisms of immune responses to trauma and infection. Cent Eur J Immunol 2015;40(2): 206–16.

35. Lund FE. Cytokine-producing B lymphocytes – key regulators of immunity. Curr Opin Immunol 2008;20(3):332–8.

36. Zhang J-M, An J. Cytokines, inflammation and pain. Int Anesthesiol Clin 2007; 45(2):27–37.

37. Adib-Conquy M, Cavaillon JM. Compensatory anti-inflammatory response syndrome. Thromb Haemost 2009;101:36–47.

38. Ward NS, Casserly B, Ayala A. The compensatory anti-inflammatory response syndrome (CARS) in critically ill patients. Clin Chest Med 2008;29(4):617–25, viii.

39. Lewis DH, Chan DL, Pinheiro D, et al. The immunopathology of sepsis: pathogen recognition, systemic inflammation, the compensatory anti-inflammatory response, and regulatory T cells. J Vet Intern Med 2012;26:457–82.

40. Deischel SJ, Kerl ME, Chang CH, et al. Age-associated changes to pathogen-associated molecular pattern-induced inflammatory mediator production in dogs. J Vet Emerg Crit Care (San Antonio) 2010;20(5):494–502.

41. Krysko DV, Agostinis P, Krysko O, et al. Emerging role of damage-associated molecular patterns derived from mitochondria in inflammation. Trends Immunol 2011;32(4):157–64.

42. Granger ND, Senchenkova E. Leukocyte-endothelial cell adhesion. In: Inflammation and the microcirculation. San Rafael (CA): Morgan and Claypool Life Sciences; 2010. Chapter 7.

43. Hatakeyama N, Matsuda N. Alert cell strategy: mechanisms of inflammatory response and organ protection. Curr Pharm Des 2014;20(4):5766–78.

44. Iversen PO, Nicolaysen A, Kvernebo K, et al. Human cytokines modulate arterial vascular tone via endothelial receptors. Pflugers Arch 1999;439:93–100.

45. Abraham E, Araroli J, Carmody A, et al. Cutting edge: HMG-1 as a mediator of acute lung inflammation. J Immunol 2000;165(6):2950–4.

46. Abraham E, Bursten S, Shenkar R, et al. Phosphatidic acid signaling mediates lung cytokine expression and lung inflammatory injury after hemorrhage in mice. J Exp Med 1995;181(2):569–75.

47. Su J, Zhan Y, Hu W. The current opinions of capillary leak syndrome. J Clin Diag 2015;5:14–9.

48. Choi G, Schultz MJ, Levi M, et al. The relationship between inflammation and the coagulation system. Swiss Med Wkly 2006;136:139–44.

49. Gando S, Kameue T, Nanzaki S, et al. Disseminated intravascular coagulation is a frequent complication of systemic inflammatory response syndrome. Thromb Haemost 1996;75(2):224–8.

50. Fink MP. Gastrointestinal mucosal injury in experimental models shock, trauma, and sepsis. Crit Care Med 1991;19(5):627–41.

51. Magnotti LJ, Upperman JS, Xu DZ, et al. Gut-derived mesenteric lymph but not portal blood increases endothelial cell permeability and promotes lung injury after hemorrhagic shock. Ann Surg 1998;228(4):518–24.

52. IRIS Guidelines. Available at: www.iris-kidney.com.

53. Wan L, Bagshaw SM, Langenberg C, et al. Pathophysiology of septic acute kidney injury: what do we really know. Crit Care Med 2008;36(4):S198–203.

54. Eisbruch A, Zevin D, Djaldetti M. Acute renal failure due to combined infection with psittacosis and salmonellosis. Harefuah 1981;100(10):460–1.

55. Zhou F, Zhi-yon P, Bishop JV, et al. Effects of fluid resuscitation with 0.9% saline versus a balanced electrolyte solution on acute kidney injury in a rat model of sepsis. Crit Care Med 2014;42(4):e270–8.

56. Dowie HG, Stevenson JA. A standardized method for the production of hemorrhagic shock in the rat. Can J Biochem Physiol 1955;33(3):436–7.

57. Millican RC, Tabor H, Rosenthal SM. Traumatic shock in mice: comparison of survival rates following therapy. Am J Physiol 1952;170(1):187–95.

58. Fine J, Rutenbug S, Schweinburg FB. The role of the reticulo-endothelial system in hemorrhagic shock. J Exp Med 1959;110:547–69.

59. Palsson J, Ricksten SE, Delle M, et al. Changes in renal sympathetic nerve activity during experimental septic and endotoxin shock in conscious rats. Circ Shock 1988;24(2):133–41.

60. Stoner HB, Little RA. Studies on the mechanism of shock. The effect of catecholamines on the temperature response to injury in the rat. Br J Exp Pathol 1969;50:107–24.

61. Villela NR, Maia Teixeira dos Santos AO, de Miranda ML, et al. Fluid resuscitation therapy in endotoxemic hamsters improves survival and attenuates capillary perfusion deficits and inflammatory responses by a mechanism related to nitric oxide. J Transl Med 2014;12:232.

62. Chu Y-K, Ali GD, Jia F, et al. The SARS-COV ferret model in an infection-challenge study. Virology 2008;374(1):151–63.

63. Chalmers JP, Korner PI, White SW. The effects of haemorrhage in the unanaesthetized rabbit. J Physiol 1967;189:367–91.

64. Lichtenberger M. Monitoring and treatment of hypovolemic shock in small mammals. In: Proceedings of the SCIVAC. Rimini (Italy): 2007. p. 323–4.

65. Rezende-Neto JB, Rizoli SB, Andrade MV, et al. Rabbit model of uncontrolled hemorrhagic shock and hypotensive resuscitation. Braz J Med Biol Res 2010;43(12):1153–9.

66. Lennox AM. Emergency and critical care in exotic companion mammals. SCIVAC International Congress. 2012. Rimini (Italy).

67. Holz PH. The reptilian renal portal system – a review. Bull Assoc Reptil Amphib Vet 1999;9(1):4–9.

68. Smits AW, Lillywhite HB. Maintenance of blood volume in snakes: transcapillary shifts of extravascular fluids during acute hemorrhage. J Comp Physiol B 1985; 155(3):305–10.
69. Lillywhite HB, Pough FH. Control of arterial pressure in aquatic sea snakes. Am J Physiol 1983;244(1):R66–73.
70. Mosley CA. Anatomic and physiologic considerations for reptile anesthesia. In: Proceedings of the North American Veterinary Conference. Orlando (FL): 2006. p. 1643–5.
71. Smits A, Kozumbowski MM. Partitioning of body fluids and cardiovascular responses to circulatory hypovolaemia in the turtle, Pseudemys scripta elegans. J Exp Biol 1985;116:237–50.
72. Millard RW, Moalli R. Baroreflex sensitivity in an amphibian, Rana catesbeiana, and a reptilian, Pseudemys scripta elegans. J Exp Zool 1980;213:283–8.
73. Hohnke LA. Regulation of arterial blood pressure in the common green iguana. Am J Physiol 1975;228(2):386–91.
74. Kubalek S, Mischke R, Fehr M. Investigations on blood coagulation in the green iguana (Iguana iguana). J Vet Med A Physiol Pathol Clin Med 2002;49:210–6.
75. Wernick MB, Steinmetz HW, Martin-Jurado O, et al. Comparison of fluid types for resuscitation in acute hemorrhagic shock and evaluation of gastric luminal and transcutaneous PCO2 in Leghorn chickens. J Avian Med Surg 2013;27(2): 109–19.
76. Lichtenberger M, Orectt C, Cray C, et al. Comparison of fluid types for resuscitation after acute blood loss in mallard ducks (Anas platyrhynchos). J Vet Emerg Crit Care (San Antonio) 2009;19(5):467–72.
77. Morrisey JK. Practical hematology and transfusion medicine in birds. Western Veterinary Conference. 2013, Indianapolis (IN).
78. Ploucha JM, Fink GD. Hemodynamics of hemorrhage in the conscious rat and chicken. Am J Physiol 1986;251(5):R846–50.

How to Improve Anesthesia and Analgesia in Small Mammals

Sandra I. Allweiler, DVM, DACVAA

KEYWORDS

- Small mammals • Anesthesia • Analgesia • Pain assessment

KEY POINTS

- The routine use of cardiovascular and respiratory monitor devices is essential for a good outcome in small mammal anesthesia.
- Physiologic differences between species and variation between individual animals should be considered when choosing an anesthetic protocol.
- The development of new pain assessment tools (eg, mouse grimace scale) can help recognize and alleviate pain.

In 2008, Broadbelt and colleagues[1] stated the overall risk of anesthetic and sedation-related death in rabbits to be 1.39% in the United Kingdom. That is more than 8 times the anesthetic risk in dogs. In this study, the risk in healthy rabbits was estimated to be 0.73% and in sick rabbits it was 7.37%. Postoperative death accounted for 64% in rabbits. Most other small animal species also had higher mortality risks. Due to the increased risks, careful selection of an appropriate anesthetic protocol is needed and continuous monitoring of the patient under anesthesia until fully recovered is mandatory. The advancement in patient monitoring and supportive care has substantially improved the safety of anesthesia in small mammals and is discussed in this article.

The overall goal is to focus on a practical clinical approach to anesthesia and pain management in small mammals. It should be understood that because of the limited number of published studies related to anesthesia and analgesia in small mammals, the author is drawing from her own clinical experience and extrapolating from what is known in other species. Whenever possible, reference is made to published information.

PREANESTHETIC EVALUATION

A thorough physical examination, including accurate body weight, and baseline values for heart rate, respiration rate, and body temperature (if possible without causing too

The author has nothing to disclose.
Department of Clinical Sciences, Colorado State University, 300 West Drake Road, Fort Collins, CO 80523, USA
E-mail address: sandraallweiler@gmail.com

much stress for the patient) are obtained for reference during anesthesia. Reviewing the medical history and a minimum diagnostic panel including packed cell volume, total protein, glucose and urea nitrogen should be included to determine the patients "fitness" for anesthesia (**Box 1**).

FASTING

Fasting times depend on species, clinical status, and the potential for regurgitation. Rabbits do not regurgitate or vomit so fasting is not recommended. It does not significantly reduce gastrointestinal volume and may cause ileus in guinea pigs and other herbivores.[2] High metabolic rates and small glycogen reserves predispose to hypoglycemia.[3] In ferrets, vomiting and aspiration can occur, so fasting is warranted but should not exceed 4 hours unless the presence of an insulinoma has been ruled out.[4] Small rodents should not be fasted because vomiting does not occur and hypoglycemia is a consequence.

STABILIZATION

Ideally, all patients should be physically stable before anesthesia induction. If sufficient time is available, abnormalities, such as dehydration, anemia, hypoglycemia, electrolyte imbalance, and acid-base disturbances, should be corrected. Vascular access (intravenous [IV] or intraosseous) should be attained in unstable patients and in those undergoing prolonged procedures or invasive procedures that may lead to significant blood loss. Unfortunately, small animal size and difficulties in catheter placement often require continuing the procedure without vascular access.

MONITORING

Patient monitoring helps detect early homeostatic imbalance before damage to organ systems become irreversible. The cardiovascular, respiratory, and central nervous systems are the essential body systems, and failure of one usually leads to failure of the others and consequently patient death. The small patient size, physiologic features, and unfamiliarity and limited information accessible for each species make monitoring more difficult. Higher metabolic rates and increased tissue oxygen consumption in smaller patients reduce the tolerance to even brief hypoxemia. Irreversible central nervous system damage occurs within less than 30 seconds of respiratory arrest.[4] Despite these challenges, similar principal and technique used in dogs and cats can be extrapolated to the small mammal.

Box 1
ASA physical status classification system

  I Normal healthy patient

  II Patient with mild systemic disease

  III Patient with moderate to severe systemic disease, or multisystem disease

  IV Patient with severe systemic disease that is a threat to life

  V Patient is moribund and not expected to live 24 hours with or without intervention

Abbreviation: ASA, American Society of Anesthesiologists.
Adapted from ASA. New classification of physical status. Anesthesiology 1963;24:111.

Most commonly used perfusion parameters in clinical practice are mucous membrane color, capillary refill time, auscultation of heart rate, pulse rate, rhythm and strength, mentation, and temperament.

Mucous Membrane

The mucous membrane color is an indirect measurement of peripheral tissue perfusion. Pink and moist mucous membranes indicate good perfusion and hydration status. Anatomic locations are gums, rectal mucosa, and sclera.

Capillary Refill Time

Capillary refill time should be less than 2 seconds. Prolonged capillary refill time indicates poor tissue perfusion.

Heart Rate

The resting heart rate for small mammals is calculated using the allometric evaluation: Heart rate = $241 \times M_b^{-0.25}$ (M_b is body weight in kg). A heart rate greater than or less than 20% of the calculated value is considered tachycardia or bradycardia.[5]

Electrocardiogram

Electrocardiogram (ECG) is useful to detect and diagnose cardiac arrhythmias. It is important to remember that electrical activity does not ensure mechanical (pumping) activity of the heart. Lead II is used most commonly to determine rate, rhythm, and conduction abnormalities. Atraumatic alligator clips, ECG patches, or alligator clips attached to 25-gauge needles penetrating through skin can be used. ECG clips are placed on right and left forelimb and left hind limb.[6,7] Because of the fast heart rate, record speed should be set at 100 mm/second and the machine standardized at 1 cm equals to 1 mV. The number of complexes that occur in 3 seconds (markings on ECG paper) are counted and multiplied by 30 to estimate the heart rate in beats per minute.

Most commonly seen abnormalities during anesthesia before cardiac arrest is severe bradycardia, which becomes progressively slower before asystole occurs and should prompt the anesthetist to reduce or terminate anesthesia and administer atropine or glycopyrrolate.

Mentation

Mentation evaluation of the level of consciousness and arousability is important to evaluate brain function.

Body Temperature

Monitoring body temperature is very important in small animals because there is rapid heat loss in the first 10 minutes of anesthesia, which is contributed to by vasodilation from anesthetic drugs, which increases conduction heat loss and reduced muscle activity, which decreases heat production. Minimizing anesthesia time and providing supplemental heat (water blankets or forced-air warming blanket) and core body temperature warming using warm IV fluids is recommended. Aluminum foil or plastic bubble wrap is used to cover the head, extremities, and hairless tail in rats. Minimizing the amount of hair clipped and rinsing the surgery site with warm prep solutions and surgical flush instead of alcohol will prevent further heat loss. Warming of the small mammal patient should start at time of premedication if possible. Otherwise, immediately after induction of anesthesia and lasting until the patient has fully recovered and the body temperature has returned to normal. Prolonged recoveries can be associated with low body temperature, which reduces metabolism of anesthetic drugs. Hyperthermia has been described in ferrets during recovery if kept wrapped in a warming blanket for prolonged periods of time. Skin burns have been described with the use of electric heat blankets or heated fluid bags if used in direct contact with the skin. Heat lamps should remain at least 1 m from the patient to prevent burning.

Blood Pressure

Blood pressure provides a close correlation to cardiovascular function. Measuring pressure can be done either directly or indirectly.

Direct invasive measurements are done with an arterial catheter connected to either a manometer or electronic pressure transducer. Due to small patient size, catheterization of an artery can be technically difficult, time-consuming, and expensive. There are several risks associated with the placement of an arterial catheter, like excessive bleeding, infection, air embolism, and accidental injection of drugs into the arterial catheter. Benefits are beat-to-beat monitoring, ability to sample arterial blood for blood gas analysis, and continuous observation of arterial waveform.

In rabbits, catheters should not be placed in the central auricular artery except for direct blood pressure monitoring because of the risk for thrombosis and ischemic necrosis of the ear.

Indirect blood pressure is monitored with an appropriate-sized cuff placed on an appendage or tail, a sphygmomanometer with a Doppler ultrasound probe, or an oscillometric device.

As a general rule, the MAP (mean arterial pressure) should be greater than 60 mm Hg and systolic arterial pressure should be kept higher than 90 mm Hg to ensure adequate organ perfusion. The Doppler method is more versatile and the author's first choice for small mammals. Advantages are low cost, portability, and better reliability in small and hypotensive patients compared with oscillometric devices. Disadvantage is that it is intermittent and diastolic arterial pressure and MAP cannot be detected. To place the Doppler probe, the fur has to be shaved on the ventral carpus, tarsus, or tail in ferrets and on the medial midshaft of the radius-ulnar area in other small mammals.

Rabbits have coarse fur covering their toes and metatarsal area. Do not clip the bottom of their feet for a Doppler probe because it can cause skin irritation and often leads to pododermatitis.

The cuff size should be approximately 40% of circumference of the tarsus, carpus, humerus, or base of the tail. Unfortunately, the smallest available cuff size is a number 1 or infant-sized cuff, which is too large for many small mammals. A study in ferrets confirmed that a larger cuff gives a false low reading when compared with direct systolic blood pressure.[8] Another study in rabbits concluded that the forelimb cuff oscillometric method is accurate for evaluating arterial blood pressure at low and normal pressure ranges.[9] In rats and mice, a volume-pressure recording tail cuff has been shown to provide accurate blood pressure readings over the physiologic range.[10]

Pulse Oximetry

Pulse oximetry is a noninvasive method of estimating arterial hemoglobin saturation for oxygen. A clip contains an infrared light transmitter-detector system and by sensing the difference in the amount of light absorbed during arterial pulsation versus background absorption it reports the percent oxygen saturation of arterial hemoglobin and often reports a pulse rate. Most pulse oximeters provide a signal strength of pulsatile flow to help the clinician assess whether or not the number on display is correct. Limitations are poorly perfused, pigmented, or vasoconstricted areas. Pulse oximetry has been evaluated in rabbits and rats. It appears to be accurate at hemoglobin saturation levels greater than 85%.[11]

Position of the probe can be ear, tongue, buccal mucosa, vulva, prepuce, and proximal tail. A reflectance pulse oximeter sensor is used in either the esophagus or rectum or applied directly on the ventral aspect of the neck, overlying the carotid artery.

Respiratory Monitor

Respiratory monitors detect exhaled warm air and give an audible signal for each exhalation. Some machines have an audible alarm (apnea alert) if no exhalation is detected within 30 to 60 seconds. They can be useful tools in small patients where chest excursion or breathing bag movement cannot be easily seen. Limitations are no indication of adequacy of ventilation and carbon dioxide (CO_2) removal.

Capnography

Capnography is the graphic display of amount of exhaled CO_2.

End-tidal CO_2 ($ETCO_2$) refers to the amount of CO_2 measured at the end of exhalation when the gas being sampled originated from the alveoli. It is an estimate of arterial $Paco_2$ (partial pressure of arterial CO_2) and is normally approximately 2 to 5 mm Hg less than the normal $Paco_2$, which is 35 to 45 mm Hg in awake mammals.

A capnometer, by definition is either diverting (eg, sidestream) or nondiverting (eg, mainstream). A diverting capnometer transports a portion of the patient's respired gases from the sampling site, through a sampling tube, and into the sensor, whereas a nondiverting capnometer does not transport gas away from the sampling site.

In the sidestream method, the sampling rate should not exceed 25 to 50 mL/min, otherwise it may lead to artificially low $ETCO_2$ readings. Dead space associated with endotracheal tube (ETT) connection must be minimized. An 18-gauge needle can be inserted into the lumen of the ETT as long as it does not cause obstruction of air flow.

The mainstream method is not practical in small mammals because it adds more dead space, as it is connected directly to the ETT and is "top heavy" so accidental extubation can become a problem.

EQUIPMENT
Mask

Mask induction techniques are used in small mammals without IV access or if IV catheterization is difficult in the conscious patient. Masks can range from commercially available to homemade plastic bottles and syringe cases. The size and shape depends on the animal size and shape of the head and should be as small as possible. Disposable latex gloves can be placed over the opening and a central whole cut out large enough for the insertion of the nose to avoid waste gas contamination. Care should be taken to avoid direct contact of the mask or rubber diaphragm with the eyes. When maintaining anesthesia by mask, the head and neck have to be extended to facilitate air movement.

Induction Chamber

The induction chamber should be clear to allow visualization of the patient. It reduces risks of injury to handler and patient and reduces stress of handling to the animal. Disadvantages are the potential for environmental contamination, limited access, and difficulty in monitoring the patient.

Breath Holding

Apneic episodes can occur in rabbits with all of the commonly used inhalation agents, and this, coupled with possible catecholamine release, could increase the anesthetic risk. When inducing anesthesia in rabbits with a face mask, briefly removing the mask if an episode of apnea occurs and replacing the mask when respiration resumes will avoid the risk associated with prolonged breath holding.[12] Some degree of aversion to volatile agents has been demonstrated in rats and mice with isoflurane more pungent then sevoflurane.[13] Isoflurane appears particularly irritating to guinea pigs, triggering pronounced ocular and nasal discharge.

In all species, stress associated with induction can be minimized by use of preanesthetic medication.

Minimum Alveolar Concentration

Minimum alveolar concentration (MAC) for isoflurane is approximately 1.28% to 1.63%. The MAC for sevoflurane is between 2.3% to 2.7% in small mammals.

Breathing Circuits and Gas Flow

Breathing circuits and gas flow–non-rebreathing circuits, such as the modified Jackson Rees and Bain circuits, are typically used during small mammal anesthesia. These circuits rely on relatively high fresh gas flow to remove exhaled carbon dioxide. The oxygen flow rate should be 2 to 3 times the minute ventilation or 200 to 300 mL/kg per minute. For some vaporizers, the lower limit oxygen flow rate required to maintain vaporizer accuracy is approximately 500 mL/min and should be the lowest setting. An advantage of the non-rebreathing system is the instant change according to adjustment of the vaporizer setting and lower resistance to breathing. The disadvantage is that the relatively high fresh gas flow is uneconomical and the cold dry air will cool down body temperature.

Endotracheal Tube

A variety of commercially available ETTs are available; the smallest cuffed and uncuffed tubes have internal diameters (ID) of 3 and 1 mm, respectively, and will not fit in the smallest patients. ETTs can be constructed from over-the-needle catheters or urinary catheters and attached to commercial ETT adapters. Ideally, the ETT should be clear to allow visualization of condensation or occlusion with mucus or blood, and not too rigid or flexible to avoid trauma but allow guidance. Ideally a "Murphy eye" should be cut on the side of the ETT to prevent complete obstruction of the patient's airway, should the primary distal opening of the ETT become occluded.

V-Gel

V-gel is species-specific supraglottic airway device for general anesthesia and emergency resuscitation. Anatomic matching features combined with a soft gellike material to give a high-quality pressure seal that avoids laryngeal and tracheal trauma without the need for endotracheal intubation. V-gels are available for rabbits in 6 different sizes depending on patient body weight. The author feels the supraglottic airway device is useful if the veterinarian is unexperienced with endotracheal intubation in rabbits but recommends endotracheal intubation for procedures exceeding 1 to 2 hours. This recommendation is based on the author's observation of a rabbit developing ulceration and necrosis of the tongue after 5 hours of anesthesia with a supraglottic airway device.

INTUBATION
Ferrets

Intubation in ferrets is relatively simple and very similar to cats. Jaw tone is often still high at moderate levels of anesthesia and gauze placed around the upper and lower jaws is usually necessary to facilitate opening. Topical application of lidocaine reduces laryngeal spasm and the tongue should be pulled gently forward to visualize the glottis.

Rabbits

In rabbits, primarily 2 types of techniques are used: blind and direct visualization.

The blind technique requires spontaneous respiration for accurate ETT placement. The induced rabbit is placed in sternal recumbency and the animal's head and neck are hyperextended to align the larynx and the trachea with the oropharynx. The tip of the tongue must be gently pulled out of the mouth. Lidocaine topically applied to the glottis or tip of the ETT can reduce a vagal response during intubation. The rabbit's head is held with one hand, while the other hand guides the ETT through the diastema (opening behind the incisors) and toward the larynx. The tube clouds when in front of the larynx. No respiratory noise or gurgling sounds indicate the tube is in the esophagus. A stethoscope earpiece can be attached to an elbow connector on the ETT to facilitate listening for breathing sounds. Commonly the rabbit will cough when the ETT enters the trachea. Alternatively, a capnograph can be used to confirm the correct placement of the ETT. Excessive force should be avoided in any small mammal because the risk of laryngeal swelling and postoperative death increases dramatically. Intubation should not be attempted for more than a few minutes or when there is evidence of blood.

Direct technique requires an assistant to open the mouth. Because rabbits are obligate nasal breathers, the epiglottis must be displaced ventral to the soft palate to visualize the glottis through the oropharynx. A laryngoscope with a number 1 Miller blade can be used to depress the tongue and free the epiglottis. When the ETT is inserted into the oropharynx, visualization of the glottis is often lost. A urinary catheter can be used as a stylet and advanced between the arytenoid cartilages and into the trachea. The laryngoscope is removed after the guide is in place and the ETT is advanced over the guide into the trachea.

Endoscopic intubation can be achieved by placing the anesthetized rabbit in a dorsoventral position. A rigid endoscope can be inserted into the lumen of a 4.5-mm ET tube to advance under direct visualization. A semiflexible fiberoptic endoscope may be inserted into the ETT of 2.0 to 2.5 ID.

Guinea Pigs

In guinea pigs, the cheek pouches frequently contain stored food. Wet Q-tips can help remove the food before intubation. Guinea pigs often regurgitate if the oropharynx is stimulated and they salivate profusely, which can be controlled by adding glycopyrrolate to the anesthesia protocol. The soft palate is fused to the base of the tongue and the entry to the glottis is through a small opening of the palatal ostium.[14] The soft tissue at the base of the tongue is readily traumatized by a laryngoscope blade, resulting in profound bleeding. The author prefers to use a face mask in guinea pigs, but successful intubation in dorsal recumbency under direct visualization has been described.[15]

Palatal ostium is also present in Chinchillas.

Rodents

Prairie dogs, squirrels, Chinchillas, and medium to large rodents can be intubated using a blind technique. The anesthetized rodent is placed in lateral recumbency with the head and neck moderately extended. The tube is inserted into the space between the incisors and the first premolar and passed caudally over the base of the tongue.

Rats

Intubation in rats usually involves direct visualization of the glottis. This is made easier if a purpose-designed apparatus is used, like a modified otoscope speculum (Hallowell EMC [Pittsfield, MA]) or fiberoptic guide (Kent Scientific [Torrington, CT]).

Assessment of correct ETT placement is determined by (1) visualization of condensation on the inside of the ETT, (2) detecting air movement with a hair placed in front of the ETT, (3) a small mirror placed in front of the ETT to show condensation, (4) watching the non-rebreathing bag, (5) the cough responds to intubation, or (6) detecting exhaled CO_2 on a capnograph. Always premeasure the ETT before use to avoid single bronchus intubation and auscultate both lung fields for respiratory sounds (**Table 1**).

Eye Protection

Rodents have large protruding eyes and are subject to corneal dryness and abrasion. Protective eye drops should be applied after deep sedation and anesthesia induction. Nonadhesive tape can be used to keep the eye closed to prevent corneal injury during positioning. Ketamine causes the eye to remain open. Rats may get an ocular opacity that resolves after anesthesia.

Positioning

Rabbits and small mammals have very small chest cavities relative to body size and have a high prevalence of respiratory disease. Ventilation can be affected by body positioning and compression of lung tissue by distended viscera, obesity, or the surgeon's resting hands.

Checklist

Ensure that all equipment and medications deemed necessary for the procedure to be performed are readily accessible and in working order before induction of anesthesia. Regularly ensure proper maintenance and function of all anesthetic equipment (**Box 2**).

Table 1	
Guidelines for endotracheal tube size selection for small mammals	
Species	**Endotracheal Tube Internal Diameter, mm**
Ferret	2.0–3.5
Rabbit	2.0–3.5
Rat	16–18 gauge over-the- needle catheter
Guinea pig	14–16 gauge over-the- needle catheter, $\leq$2.0
Chinchilla	14–16 gauge over-the-needle catheter, $\leq$2.0
Hamster	16 gauge over-the-needle catheter
Squirrel	$\leq$2.0
Prairie dog	2.0–2.5
Hedgehog	14–16-gauge over-the-needle catheter, $\leq$2.0

From Heard DJ. Anesthesia, analgesia, and sedation of small mammals. In: Quesenberry KE, Carpenter JW, editors. Ferrets, rabbits and rodents clinical medicine and surgery. 3rd edition. Philadelphia: WB Saunders; 2012. p. 362; with permission.

Box 2
Anesthesia checklist for small mammals

Date: _____

Oxygen supply (high-pressure system)
☐ Open O_2 cylinder and log pressure _____
☐ Hoses connected and piped gas pressure less than 50 psi

Anesthesia delivery system (low-pressure system)
☐ Turn on machine's master switch (if applicable) and verify A/C power is present
☐ Test of flow meters

Induction chamber
☐ Tubing connected, positioned on stable, well-ventilated surface

Non-rebreathing circuit
☐ Outer tube occlusion test (>20 cm H_2O, acceptable drop 5 cm H_2O in 30 s)
☐ Inner tube occlusion test (drop of the float)

Ventilation System
☐ Leak test for bellows and transfer tubing
☐ Functional test of ventilator-setting appropriate for patient
☐ Verify gas flows properly through breathing circuit

Scavenging system and pressure relief valve
☐ Pressure relief valve open
☐ Scavenging transfer tube connected to scavenging system and scavenge system functioning

Monitors
☐ Inspect and turn on (electrical equipment requiring warm-up) and verify A/C power

All probes and cables necessary for patient present and functioning
☐ Electrocardiogram (pads/atraumatic alligator clips) ☐ Pulse Oximetry ☐ Capnograph
☐ Noninvasive Blood Pressure (oscillometric method) ☐ Temperature probe ☐ Arterial line (transducer)

Airway equipment available
☐ Endotracheal tubes/stylet/catheter
☐ Laryngoscope/Endoscope functioning
☐ Accessory intubation equipment (gauze to secure endotracheal tube, and so forth)
☐ Face mask

Other equipment
☐ Blood pressure cuff ☐ Doppler and crystal
☐ Sphygmomanometer ☐ Eye lubricant
☐ Intravenous fluids ☐ Infusion pump(s)
☐ Warming device (heating lamp/circulating water blanket/forced-air warmer)
☐ Incubator/Recovery box set up

Drugs

The high metabolic rate in small mammals results in a relatively high dose requirement of many of the agents commonly used in anesthesia and pain management.

Atropinase

Many but not all rabbits have circulating levels of atropine esterases so atropine only briefly induces a moderate tachycardia, and glycopyrrolate should be used if longer effects are desired.[16]

Intranasal Drug Administration

Intranasal drug administration can be an effective and rapid route described in rabbits. Nasal delivery is considered a promising technique because the nose has a large surface area available for drug absorption; the venous blood from the nose passes directly into the systemic circulation and therefore avoids loss of first-pass metabolism in the liver.[17,18]

Table 2 gives a short summary of the cardiovascular effects of common anesthetics.

Propofol

Propofol has a fast onset and short duration of action. Apnea after induction is seen with rapid IV administration of the drug. If administered slowly over 1 to 2 minutes, the incidence of apnea is greatly reduced. Propofol can be used in patients with liver disease because it is extrahepatically metabolized as well. The author uses propofol as an induction agent in stable ferrets at a dose of 4 to 6 mg/kg IV. In compromised patients, the dose of propofol can be greatly reduced by adding midazolam/diazepam 0.2 to 0.3 mg/kg IV. Propofol can be used in healthy rabbits if endotracheal intubation is achieved to avoid respiratory depression.[19,20]

Ketamine

The combination of ketamine with diazepam or midazolam is commonly used in ferrets, rabbits, and Guinea pigs. Ketamine will increase sympathetic response and increase myocardial oxygen demand. A normal stable animal can handle this sympathetic response, but in patients with preexisting cardiac disease, this drug may prove detrimental. Ferrets and rabbits can have underlying cardiac disease without outward clinical signs.

Etomidate

Etomidate induces minimal cardiovascular depression and undergoes rapid redistribution and hepatic metabolism after a single bolus. Its respiratory depressant effect is dose dependent and oxygen by mask or endotracheal intubation are recommended. Combinations with diazepam or midazolam reduce myoclonic twitching on induction and lower the dose of etomidate. Etomidate has to be given intravenously and it may cause lysis of red blood cells.[21]

Table 2
Cardiovascular effects of common anesthetics

Drug	Heart Rate	Blood Pressure	Vascular Resistance	HMV	Heart Contractility	Application
Benzodiazepine	=	=	=	=	=	IV, IM, SQ
α2-agonist	↓↓	↑a ↓b	↑a ↓b	↓	↓	IV, IM, SQ
Barbiturate	↑a =b	↓a =b	↓a =b	↓a =b	↓a =b	IV
Propofol	↑a =b	↓	↓	↓a =b	↓a =b	IV
Alfaxalone	↑a =b	=a ↓b	=	=	=	IV, IM
Etomidate	↑a =b	=	=	=	=	IV
Opioid	↓	↓a =b	=a ↓b	↓a =b	=	IV, IM, SQ
Ketamine	↑	↑	↑	↑	=	IM, IV
Isoflurane	↑	↓	↓	↓	↓	Inhalation
Sevoflurane	↑	↓	↓	↓	↓	Inhalation

Abbreviations: =, no change; ↑, increase; ↓, decrease; IM, intramuscular; IV, intravenous; SQ, subcutaneous.
[a] Initial effect.
[b] Prolonged effect.

Alfaxalone

Alfaxalone produces smooth, rapid induction of anesthesia. Its cardiovascular and respiratory effects seem to be similar to propofol with slightly less respiratory depression. Because of rapid metabolism, alfaxalone has minimal cumulative effects and can be used for maintenance of anesthesia without prolonging recovery. It has been used for intramuscular (IM) and IV anesthesia in rabbits with promising results.

Example for an anesthetic protocol in ferrets:
  Premedication: Atropine 0.02 mg/kg subcutaneously (SQ), hydromorphone 0.05 mg/kg SQ, ± midazolam 0.2 mg/kg SQ.
  Induction if IV access: Propofol 2 to 4 mg/kg IV, midazolam 0.2 mg/kg IV or ketamine 5 mg/kg IV, midazolam 0.3 mg/kg IV.
  No IV access: mask or chamber induction with sevoflurane or isoflurane.

Example for an anesthetic protocol in rabbits:
  Premedication: Glycopyrrolate 0.02 mg/kg SQ, butorphanol 0.2 mg/kg SQ or hydromorphone 0.05 mg/kg SQ, midazolam 0.3 mg/kg SQ.
  Induction with IV access: Ketamine 5 mg/kg IV, midazolam 0.3 mg/kg IV.
  No IV access: mask or chamber induction with sevoflurane or isoflurane.

Example for an anesthetic protocol in Chinchillas:
  Mask or chamber induction with sevoflurane or isoflurane or ketamine 40 mg/kg IM, midazolam 2 mg/kg IM.
  Only in healthy Chinchilla: Ketamine 20 to 40 mg/kg IM, dexmedetomidine 0.5 mg/kg IM.

Example for an anesthetic protocol in guinea pig:
  Premedication: Atropine 0.1 mg/kg IM, midazolam 1 to 2 mg/kg IM.
  Induction with IV access: Ketamine 5 to 10 mg/kg IV, midazolam 0.5 mg/kg IV.
  No IV access: Ketamine 20 to 40 mg/kg IM, midazolam 1 mg/kg IM.

Table 3 provides common drug dosages for injectable anesthesia in small mammals.

PAIN MEDICATION
Opioids

Opioids act centrally to limit the input of nociceptive information to the central nervous system, which reduces central hypersensitivity.[22] When used appropriately, opioids can be administered safely to small mammals to effectively alleviate pain. They have a wide margin of safety and excellent analgesic properties. Some examples of opioids used in small mammals are butorphanol, buprenorphine, morphine, hydromorphone, oxymorphone, and fentanyl.

The ileus-inducing effect of opioids are a major concern for practitioners working on rabbits; however, pain-induced ileus is much more difficult to treat than that brought on by administration of opioids. Forced feeding and adequate fluid therapy are usually enough to counteract the motility-slowing effects of opioids.

Ferrets seem especially sensitive to sedation and respiratory suppression. Preliminary work in our laboratory in a limited number of ferrets has demonstrated cardiorespiratory depression associated with morphine, hydromorphone, and butorphanol. It is advised to use the lower dose range and careful monitoring in this species.[23]

Buprenorphine is 35 times as potent as morphine and has a long duration of action (3–5 hours in mice, 6–8 hours in rats). Its poor oral bioavailability (5%–10%) coupled with a significant hepatic first-pass metabolism, makes oral administration of

Table 3
Drug dosage (mg/kg) for injectable anesthesia in small mammals

Drug + Combo	Ferret	Rabbit	Rat	Mouse	Gerbil/Chinchilla/Hamster	Guinea Pig
Ketamine (K)-acepromazine (A)	20 (K) + 0.2 (A) SQ, IM	25 (K) + 0.25-1 (A) IM, IV	75 (K) + 2.5 (A) SQ, IP	50 (K) + 2.5 (A) IM	40 (K) + 0.5 (A) IM	20-30 (K)+
Ketamine (K)-dexmedetomidine (D)	5 (K) + 0.03 (D) IM	15 (K) + 0.15-0.25 (D) IM	50-75 (K) + 0.25 (M) IM, IP	50-75 (K) + 0.5 (D) IP	50 (K) + 0.25 (M) SQ, IP	40 (K) + 0.25 (M) SQ, IP
Ketamine (K)-diazepam or midazolam (D/M)	5-10 (K) + 0.5 (D/M) IV 10-20 (K) + 1-2 (D/M) SQ, IM	10 (K) + 0.5 (D/M) IV 15 (K) + 0.3 (D/M) IM	50 (K) + 2 (D/M) SQ, IP	—	20-40 (K) + 1-2 (D/M) SQ/IM	20-30 (K) + 1-2 (D/M) IM
Propofol	5-8 IV	3-6 IV	7.5-10 IV	12-26 IV	3-5 IV	3-5 IV
Propofol (P)-diazepam or midazolam (D/M)	4-6 (P) + 0.3 (D/M)	2-4 (P) + 0.5 (D/M)	—	—	—	2-4 (P) + 0.5 (D/M)
Etomidate (E) - diazepam or midazolam (D/M)	1-2 (E) + 0.3 (D/M) IV	1-2 (E) + 0.3 (D/M) IV	—	—	—	—
Alfaxalone	—	4-6 IM	—	—	—	—

Abbreviations: IM, intramuscular; IP, intraperitoneal; IV, intravenous; SQ, subcutaneous.

Data from Carpenter JW. Exotic animal formulary. Philadelphia: Elsevier; 2012; and Mason DE. Anesthesia, analgesia and sedation for small mammals. In: Hillyer EV, Quesenberry KE, editors. Ferrets, rabbits, and rodents: clinical medicine and surgery. Philadelphia: WB Saunders; 1997. p. 378–91.

buprenorphine in rodents of limited value.[24] An unusual effect of opioids in rodents is the production of pica behavior. This is thought to be analogous to vomiting in other species and has been reported following use of buprenorphine in rats.[25] The incidence of pica appears very low, but if noted, analgesia should be provided using a nonopioid analgesic. Methadone has been shown to attenuate signs of neuropathic pain for 2 hours in mice.[26] This effect may be attributed to its μ-opioid receptor agonist action but also in part due to the N-methyl-D-aspartate (NMDA) receptor antagonism effect. Compared with other μ-opioid receptor agonists, methadone seems to produce less sedation and inappetence.

Nonsteroidal Anti-Inflammatory Drugs

Nonsteroidal anti-inflammatory drugs (NSAIDs) as a class share common therapeutic actions, including anti-inflammatory, analgesic, and antipyretic effects. They are the most commonly used analgesic drugs in veterinary medicine, because they are effective for acute and chronic pain. They exert their analgesic effect via inhibition of the cyclooxygenase enzyme. As in other species, there are concerns about preoperative use of NSAIDs and the author recommends reserving their use for postoperative administration. Meloxicam is a cyclooxygenase-2-selective NSAID, which means its side effects are minimal, although usually gastrointestinal when seen. Its ease of administration (owing to its commercially available liquid suspension), relative safety, and apparent effectiveness make meloxicam the most used NSAID in small mammals.

Local Anesthetic Agents

Local anesthetic agents can be administered topically (eg, as a cream to facilitate venipuncture), locally by infiltration at the surgery site, or around nerves and in epidural or spinal anesthesia. Most common local anesthetics in veterinary medicine are lidocaine and bupivacaine. Bupivacaine has a higher potency and longer duration of effect but greater cardiovascular toxicity, and should never be given intravascularly. Aspiration before injection of bupivacaine is strongly advised. Great care must be taken to calculate and prepare appropriate volumes of local anesthetic in small mammals. Dosages described in the literature are 2 to 4 mg/kg for lidocaine and 1 to 2 mg/kg for bupivacaine. Detailed description on dental nerve blocks, epidural anesthesia, and intratesticular block are described by Lichtenberger and Ko.[27]

α_2-Adrenergic Agonists

The α_2-adrenergic agonists, such as dexmedetomidine, possess analgesia, sedation, and muscle-relaxant properties. Microdose dexmedetomidine (1–3 μg/kg) minimally affects blood pressure in animals with normal cardiac output and provides good analgesia when used in combination with a tranquilizer and opioid but should be reserved for healthy patients. In conscious dogs, IV medetomidine (an analog to dexmedetomidine) at a rate of 1.25 μg/kg increased blood pressure by 15%, decreased heart rate by 26%, and decreased cardiac output by 35%.[28]

Ketamine

The NMDA receptor plays an important role in central sensitization (wind up). Ketamine is an NMDA receptor antagonist and it may be effective in preventing or lessening central sensitization at subanesthetic doses. Ketamine has been shown to be opioid sparing and inhalant-anesthetic sparing. Microdose ketamine does not appear to cause an increase in sympathetic tone and is frequently used for analgesia with a continuous rate infusion (CRI).

Gabapentin and Pregabalin

An MAC-sparing effect was demonstrated in rats with both sevoflurane and isoflurane.[29,30]

NONPHARMACOLOGIC INTERVENTION

Acupuncture as well as physical modalities have shown to gain an important place in the management of painful conditions in small mammals. Physical medicine is an all-encompassing term that refers to the use of mechanical touch and physical modalities including cryotherapy, heat therapy, laser therapy, massage, and rehabilitation. Acupuncture involves the use of solid, fine needles to diagnose, treat, and prevent disease by stimulating the body's own ability to heal.

PAIN ASSESSMENT

To effectively alleviate pain in animals we must first be able to recognize it.

Objective methods of assessing pain include monitoring food and water intake along with any changes in body weight.[31] Heart rate and respiration rate have been used as an indirect measure of pain, but many other factors can influence these parameters. Stress or excitement, even handling the animal will increase heart rate and respiration rate. Often the resting heart rate in small mammals is too high to assess by auscultation (eg, 300–400 beats per minute).[32]

As the response to pain varies considerably both between species and between individual animals, it is important that pain assessment is performed by clinicians with a comprehensive knowledge of the normal behavior and appearance of the species and animal concerned. Monitoring at regular intervals by the same observer is likely to provide the best insight into the improvement of an animal over time.

Pain Assessment Tools

A number of pain assessment tools have been developed, including body weight, food and water consumption, complex behavioral measures, such as nest building, specific pain-related behaviors, and changes in facial expression. Some of these assessment tools have been validated in mice, rats, and rabbits. A new potentially useful method of pain assessment is through analysis of facial expressions. Recently, the use of facial expressions has been assessed in mice, rabbits, rats, and horses during periods when pain has been induced. Orbital tightening, nose bulges, cheek bulges, and changes in ear and whisker position have been linked to the presence of pain in rodents.[33–35]

Table 4 provides common dosage for analgesics in small mammals.

Postoperative Care

A recovery area should be provided that is visible, quiet, and warm. The animal should be kept away from potential predators. Wet hair should be dried. Minimizing handling will reduce stress to the animal. Rats, mice, and hamsters are active during the dark phase of their photoperiod, whereas rabbits are most active at dawn and dusk. This should be considered when assessing normal behavior during their inactive phase of their diurnal rhythm. Almost all feeding and drinking by rats and mice occurs during the dark phase, and postsurgical pain and stress can suppress these activities. Consequently, voluntary oral intake may not resume for 24 hours or longer. This can have a detrimental effect in these animals because relatively short periods of fasting result in hypoglycemia and moderate dehydration. All of these species exhibit a degree of neophobia, so postsurgically their normal diet should be offered with palliative

Anesthesia and Analgesia in Small Mammals 375

Table 4
Analgesic drug dosages for small mammals

Drug, mg/kg	Ferret	Rabbit	Rat	Mouse	Gerbil/Chinchilla/Hamster	Guinea Pig
Butorphanol	0.1–0.5 q2–4h	0.5 q2–4h CRI 0.1–0.3 mg/kg/h	1.0–2.0 q4	1.0–2.0 q4	0.2–2.0 q2–4	1.0–2.0 q4
Buprenorphine	0.01–0.03 q6–10h	0.01–0.05 q6–10	0.01–0.05 q8–12	0.05–0.1 q12	0.01–0.05 q6–12	0.05 q8–12
Hydromorphone	0.1–0.2 q6–8h CRI 0.005–0.015 mg/kg/h	0.05–0.2 q6–8h	—	—	—	—
Oxymorphone	0.05–0.2 q6–8h	0.05–0.2 q6–8h	0.2–0.5	0.2–0.5	—	0.2–0.5
Morphine	0.2–2 sid 0.1 epidural	0.5–5 sid 0.1 epidural	2.0–5.0 q1h	2.0–5.0 q1h	—	2.0–5.0 q4
Fentanyl	CRI 0.02–0.03 mg/kg/h[a] 0.001–0.004 mg/kg/h[b]	0.005–0.01 loading dose CRI 0.01–0.04 mg/kg/h[a] 0.001–0.005 mg/kg/h[b]	—	—	—	—
Meloxicam	0.1–0.2 q24	0.1–1q12–24	1.0–2.0 q12–24	5.0 q24	0.1–0.3 q24	0.1–0.3 q24
Carprofen	—	1.0–2.0 q24	5.0	5.0	4.0 q24	4.0 q12–24
Tramadol	—	5.0 q12–24	5.0	5.0	5.0	—
Methadone	—	—	1–4	1–2	1–2	3.6 q4

Continuous rate infusion (CRI); Intravenous. Lower dosage for intravenous.
Abbreviations: q, every; SID, single dose.
[a] Intraoperative.
[b] Postoperative.

Data from Flecknell PA. Postoperative analgesia in rabbits and rodents. Lab Anim 1991;20:34; and Heard DJ. The Veterinary Clinics of North America - Exotic Animal Practice: Analgesia and Anesthesia, Volume 4, Issue 1. Philadelphia: Elsevier, 2001; or are based upon clinical experience and extrapolation from other species.

high-energy and high water content supplements. Coprophagia is a normal behavior and important for adequate nutrition. The use of Elizabethan collars to prevent interference with wounds could negatively affect their ability to perform coprophagia.

SUMMARY

The routine use of cardiovascular and respiratory monitor devices is essential for a good outcome in small mammal anesthesia. Physiologic differences between species and variation between individual animals should be considered when choosing an anesthetic protocol. The development of new pain assessment tools (eg, mouse grimace scale) can help recognize and alleviate pain.

REFERENCES

1. Broadbelt D, Blissett K, Hammond R. The risk of death: the confidential enquiry into perioperative small animal fatalities. Vet Anaesth Analg 2008;35:365–73.
2. Flecknell PA. Laboratory animal anaesthesia. San Diego: Academic press; 1996.
3. Heard DJ. Anesthesia, analgesia, and sedation of small mammals. In: Quesenberry KE, Carpenter JW, editors. Ferrets, rabbits and rodents clinical medicine and surgery. 3rd edition. Philadelphia: WB Saunders; 2012. p. 356–69.
4. Cantwell SL. Ferret, rabbit, and rodent anesthesia. Veterinary Clin North Am Exot Anim Pract 2001;4:169–91.
5. Schmidt-Nielsen K. Scaling. Why is animal size so important? New York: Cambridge University Press; 1984.
6. Sedgwick CJ. Allometrically scaling the database for vital sign assessment used in general anesthesia of zoological species. Proc Am Assoc Zoo Vets 1991;360:360–9.
7. Schoemaker NJ, Zandvliet MM. Electrocardiograms in selected species. Journal of Exotic Pet Medicine 2005;14:26–33.
8. Olin JM, Smith TJ, Talcott MR. Evaluation of noninvasive monitoring techniques in domestic ferrets (*Mustela putorius furo*). Am J Vet Res 1997;58(10):1065–9.
9. Ypsilantis P, Didilid VN, Politou M, et al. A comparative study of invasive and oscillometric methods of arterial blood pressure measurement in the anesthetized rabbit. Res Vet Sci 2005;78(3):269–75.
10. Feng M, Whitesall S, Zhang Y, et al. Validation of volume–pressure recording tail-cuff blood pressure measurements. Am J Hypertens 2008;21(12):1288–91.
11. Vegfors M, Sjoberg F, Lindberg LG, et al. Basic studies of pulse oximetry in a rabbit model. Acta Anaesthesiol Scand 1991;35:596–9.
12. Flecknell PA, Thomas AA. Comparative anesthesia and analgesia of laboratory animals, Veterinary Anesthesia and Analgesia, Fifth edition of Lumb and Jones. 2015. p. 754–63.
13. Leach M, Bowell V, Allan T, et al. Measurement of aversion to determine human methods of anesthesia and euthanasia. Anim Welfare 2004;13:S77–86.
14. Timm KI, Jahn SI, Sedgwick CJ. The palatal ostium of the Guinea pig. Lab Anim Sci 1987;37:801–2.
15. Kujime K, Natelson BH. A method for endotracheal intubation of Guinea pigs (*Cavia porcellus*). Lab Anim Sci 1981;31:715–6.
16. Olson ME, Vizzutti D, Morck DW, et al. The parasympatholytic effects of atropine sulfate and glycopyrrolate in rats and rabbits. Can J Vet Res 1994;58:254–8.
17. Robertson SA, Eberhart S. Efficacy of the intranasal route for administration of anesthetic agents to adult rabbits. Lab Anim Sci 1994;44:159–65.

18. Lindhardt K, Bagger M, Andreasen KH, et al. Intranasal bioavailability of buprenorphine in rabbit correlated to sheep and man. Int J Pharm 2001;217:121–6.
19. Aeschenbacher G, Webb AI. Propofol in rabbits. 1. Determination of an induction dose. Lab Anim Sci 1993;43(4):324–7.
20. Allweiler S, Leach MC, Flecknell PA. The use of propofol and sevoflurane for surgical anaesthesia in New Zealand White rabbits. Lab Anim 2010;44(2):113–7.
21. Janssen PA, Niemegger CJ, Marsboom RP. Etomidate, a potent non-barbiturate hypnotic. Intravenous etomidate in mice, rats, guinea pigs, rabbits and dogs. Arch Int Pharmacodyn Ther 1975;214(1):92–132.
22. Dobromylskyj P, Flecknell P, Waterman-Pearson A, editors. Pain management in animals. Philadelphia: WB Saunders; 2000. p. 81–145.
23. Johnston MS, Allweiler S, Smeak D. Cardiorespiratory effects of morphine, butorphanol and hydromorphone in conscious ferrets. In: Proceedings of the Association of Exotic Mammal Veterinarians Annual Conference. 2011. p. 137.
24. Leach MC, Forrester AR, Flecknell PA. Influence of preferred foodstuffs on the antinociceptive effects of orally administered buprenorphine in laboratory rats. Lab Anim 2010;44(1):54–8.
25. Clark JA Jr, Myers PH, Goelz MF. Pica behavior associated with buprenorphine administration in the rat. Lab Anim Sci 1997;47(3):300–3.
26. Erichsen HK, Hao J-X, Xu X-J, et al. Comparative actions of the opioid analgesics morphine, methadone and codeine in rat models of peripheral and central neuropathic pain. Pain 2005;116(3):347–58.
27. Lichtenberger M, Ko J. Anesthesia and analgesia for small mammals and birds. Veterinary Clin North Am Exot Anim Pract 2007;10(2):293–315.
28. Lamont LA, Tranquilli WJ. Alpha 2 agonists. In: Gaynor JS, Muir WW, editors. Handbook of veterinary pain management. St Louis (MO): Mosby; 2002. p. 199–220.
29. Boruta DT, Sotglu G, Golder FJ. Effects of intraperitoneal administration of gabapentin on the minimum alveolar concentration of isoflurane in adult male rats. Lab Anim 2012;46(2):108–13.
30. Aguado D, Abreu M, Benito J, et al. The effects of gabapentin on acute opioid tolerance to remifentanil under sevoflurane anesthesia in rats. Anesth Analg 2012;115(1):44–5.
31. Livingston A, Chambers P. The physiology of pain. In: Flecknell P, Waterman-Pearson A, editors. Pain management in animals. London: WB Saunders; 2000. p. 9–20.
32. Leach MC, Allweiler S, Richardson C, et al. Behavioral effects of ovariohysterectomy and oral administration of meloxicam in laboratory house rabbits. Res Vet Sci 2009;87(2):336–47.
33. Keating SC, Thomas AA, Flecknell PA, et al. Evaluation of EMLA cream for preventing pain during tattooing of rabbits: changes in physiological, behavioral and facial expression responses. PLoS One 2012;7(9):e44437.
34. Dalla C, Minero M, Lebelt D, et al. Development of the Horse Grimace Scale (HGS) as a pain assessment tool in horses undergoing routine castration. PLoS One 2014;9(3):e92281.
35. Langford DJ, Bailey AL, Chanda ML, et al. Coding of facial expressions of pain in the laboratory mouse. Nat Methods 2010;7:447–52.

Assessment and Care of the Critically Ill Rabbit

Minh Huynh, DVM, DECZM (Avian)[a],*, Anaïs Boyeaux, DVM[b],
Charly Pignon, DVM, DECZM (Small Mammals)[c]

KEYWORDS

- Rabbit • Critical care • Shock • Hypovolemia • Stress • Fluid therapy • Emergency

KEY POINTS

- Rabbits have the ability to hide their signs and often present in a state of decompensatory shock.
- Handling can increase susceptibility to stress-induced cardiomyopathy and specific hemodynamic changes.
- Careful monitoring with a specific reference range is important to detect early decompensation, change therapeutic plan in a timely manner, and assess prognostic indicators.
- Fluid requirements are higher in rabbits compared with other small domestic mammals and can be corrected both enterally and parenterally.
- Critical care in rabbits can be extrapolated to many hindgut fermenters, such as chinchillas and guinea pigs, but a specific reference range and dosage regimen need to be determined.

INTRODUCTION

Domestic rabbits are prey species and their medical management is particularly challenging because most clinical signs are hidden. Those subtle clinical signs make early recognition of illness and/or injury difficult for owners, resulting in them delaying while the health status deteriorates. For this reason, rabbit patients sometimes present in a critical stage. One other difficulty to consider is that rabbits are highly stress-sensitive animals, which must be kept in mind in an intensive care context whereby those patients may decompensate quickly during diagnostic procedures and examination. The physiology of shock in rabbits shares many common features with the other mammals, with a noticeable increased influence of stress and fear. Shock is defined by tissue hypoperfusion, decreased oxygen delivery, and insufficient cellular energy

[a] Exotic Department, Centre Hospitalier Vétérinaire Frégis, 43 Avenue Aristide Briand, Arcueil 94110, France; [b] Department of Emergency and Critical Care, Centre Hospitalier Vétérinaire Frégis, 43 Avenue Aristide Briand, Arcueil 94110, France; [c] Exotics Medicine Service, Alfort National Veterinary School, 7 avenue du Général de Gaulle, Maisons-Alfort 94700, France
* Corresponding author.
E-mail address: nacologie@gmail.com

Vet Clin Exot Anim 19 (2016) 379–409
http://dx.doi.org/10.1016/j.cvex.2016.01.011
1094-9194/16/$ – see front matter © 2016 Elsevier Inc. All rights reserved.
vetexotic.theclinics.com

production (See Brian K. Roberts: Basic Shock Physiology and Critical Care in this issue). There are several classifications of shock. A functional classification of shock usually includes cardiogenic, hypovolemic, distributive, and anaphylaxis.

The most common clinical types of shock in pet rabbits are hypovolemic and distributive shock. Maldistribution of fluid occurs in rabbits because of their digestive tract, which requires a lot of water and an adequate bacterial environment for normal function. The daily water intake of a rabbit ranges from 10% to 12% of the body weight, which is twice that of a small carnivore.[1] Rabbit digestion relies on hindgut fermentation and a well-established population of commensal microflora. When the normal balance of micro-organisms is disrupted, dysbiosis can occur, resulting in endotoxemia and bacterial translocation. This article mainly focuses on hypovolemic shock.

Cardiogenic shock is rarely seen because spontaneous primary heart disease is uncommon in pet rabbits, although reports of it have increased recently.[2,3] However, stress-induced cardiomyopathy occurs more frequently, especially in a veterinary hospital setting, when the patients are in an unfamiliar environment and frequent handling is needed. Stress-induced cardiomyopathy or catecholamine cardiomyopathy is characterized by a high level of catecholamines, which causes coronary vasoconstriction and myocardial ischemia in rabbits.[4] The endogenous release of catecholamines causes myocardial injury in a dose-dependent manner, which may have acute or delayed consequences.[5] Consequently, cardiac output is reduced, which adds to the severity of shock.

Stress is a physiologic response based on catecholamine and cortisol release by adrenal glands. It redistributes blood flow from visceral structures to skeletal muscle, which occurs by catecholamine-induced increase in arterial pressure, central venous pressure, and hindquarters blood flow with concurrent mesenteric and renal vasoconstriction.[6,7] Stress and epinephrine also have beneficial effects: stress increases glucose uptake from the small intestine and prevents hypotension in cases of severe blood loss.[7,8] Rabbits seem to have 2 types of cardiovascular response when exposed to stress.[6] In one study examining the effects of stress on rabbits, a model of acute threat was reproduced with an air jet. This study found a significant increase in heart rate and cardiac output. In the same study, rabbits were put in a box with oscillation reproducing an environmental stress, which noted a cardiac freezing response characterized by no increases in cardiac output or heart rate. In the hospital setting, both types of stimulus responses are expected and clinicians should try to minimize the stress.

Pet rabbits are expected to have better acceptance of handling than laboratory or wild rabbits. In laboratory animals, it has been shown that frequent contact increases compliance stress tolerance and reduces fear response.[9,10] When rabbits are healthy, rabbit owners should be encouraged to handle their pet whenever possible. Nevertheless, minimizing handling and stressors in the environment should be a constant goal of exotic clinicians, especially with rabbits that are not used to being handled.

Initial Assessment

History

A brief history may orientate clinicians at presentation of the sick pet, but a more thorough history should be obtained once the patient is stabilized.

Four keys points are evaluated:

- Signalment with breed, age, sex, neutered or entire.
- Record of recent trauma, outdoor exposure, potential toxin exposure.

- Previous medical records, including previous surgeries.
- Dietary history is also important because many conditions affect the gastrointestinal tract. Recent feeding and long-term diet should be reviewed critically.

Initial Clinical Assessment

Evaluation of mentation is a good indicator of shock whether the animal is stuporous or able to be aroused with noxious stimuli. Most rabbits in shock will not raise their heads from the ground (**Fig. 1**). A decreased level of consciousness implies brain injury or decreased cerebral perfusion.[11] Consistency of feces and urine are noted.

Initial clinical assessment focuses on a classic airway-breathing-circulation approach. It should be minimal until the rabbit is stabilized.

Because rabbits are obligate nasal breathers, making sure the airways are patent mainly involves examination of the upper respiratory tract. Observation is the first and most important step for breathing assessment. Normal respiratory rate is rapid; up to 30 to 60 breaths per minute. In cases of obvious respiratory distress, the patient is placed immediately in an oxygen cage before any further handling or other procedure is performed. Respiration is further evaluated by auscultation and ideally chest radiographs because many respiratory diseases are subclinical. Normal respiratory sounds are loud and harsh because the air is pulled through the narrow nasal turbinates.[12]

Circulation is evaluated by assessing heart rate, color of mucous membranes, capillary refill time, peripheral pulse, and body temperature. Normal heart rate in New Zealand white rabbits recorded without any restraint is approximately 220 beats per minute (bpm).[13] Resting heart rate of conscious healthy rabbits in other experiments varies from 140 bpm to 250 bpm.[6,14] Because there can be a high variability related to the level of stress induced by handling, it is important to record the normal heart range of your clients' healthy rabbits as a reference in case of emergency or other illness. Heart rate should increase in the early stage of compensatory hypovolemic shock but this stage is often not observed clinically.[11] It is postulated that vagal fibers are stimulated simultaneously with the sympathetic fibers making the heart rate normal or slow instead of increased as seen in dogs in shock.[15] The heart rate of rabbits in shock has been reported to be less than 180 bpm, which is categorized as bradycardia.[11] In the late decompensatory stage, the heart rate decreases with loss of sympathetic nervous system stimulation.

Skin tenting can help in determining the hydration status. Membrane moisture and luster of the cornea can be difficult to assess in rabbits. Abdominal palpation should

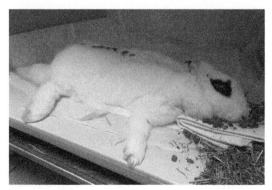

Fig. 1. Rabbit in shock with altered mentation and sternal recumbency. (*Courtesy of* Minh Huynh).

focus on the size of the stomach, the caecum, kidneys, and bladder. The stomach should be soft, compressible, and should not go past the last rib. Renal length is about 3 cm, the left kidney moving almost freely in the abdominal cavity. Abdominal auscultation is also helpful to assess gastrointestinal motility; lack of sound may indicate gastrointestinal stasis. Dental examination can be performed if the rabbit tolerates it well, but is not a priority.

Monitoring

Intensive care is time and cost consuming and can potentially raise ethical concerns for unnecessarily prolonging the life of a suffering animal. For those reasons, careful monitoring of the patient and of clinical and blood parameters must be performed throughout hospitalization (**Box 1**). Owners should be informed about the trends in recovery so that they can make informed decisions in cases of clinical deterioration.

Body Weight

Body weight and body score condition should be assessed. Body condition score is a subjective assessment focused on body fat. Rabbit body condition scales have been developed based on small mammal scales (in which 0 is emaciated and 5 is obese).[16] Other assessment methods for weight include the use of a zoometric index to assess body condition in rabbits based on measurement of the body weight and the distal forelimb length ratio.[17] This ratio was strongly correlated with body condition score and ranged from 0.16 to 0.21 in normal rabbits with optimum condition. Below those reference values, rabbits were considered underweight and above them rabbits were considered overweight.[17]

Body weight is fairly constant in healthy patients. However, critically ill patients often have a history of rapid weight fluctuation. Body weight should be checked once or twice a day during hospitalization, ideally with the same scale to avoid interscale variation.[18] Especially with dehydrated animals, weight gain can be an easy, if indirect, way to assess the efficiency of fluid therapy.

Body Temperature

Body temperature should be measured at admission in critically ill patients, then monitored closely during hospitalization. It allows vets to detect systemic disorders as soon as possible and to adapt treatment accordingly.[19]

Box 1
Goals of patient monitoring

- To know what treatment end points have been reached (eg, return to normovolemia)
- To know that safety limits have been reached (eg, efficiency of fluid therapy and signs of fluid overload)
- To obtain prognostic information (eg, data suggesting unlikely survival according to evidence-based medicine)
- To anticipate physiologic changes (eg, anorexia and gastrointestinal ileus)
- To aid in the diagnostic process (eg, to discover lung disease, intestinal obstruction)

Adapted from Boller E, Boller M. Assessment of fluid balance and the approach to fluid therapy in the perioperative patient. Vet Clin North Am Small Anim Pract 2015;45(5):896; with permission.

True fever should be differentiated from other causes of hyperthermia. Fever is a physiologic and beneficial response to endogenous pyrogen injury (eg, inflammation, infection, neoplasia). Fever can be triggered in rabbits by various infectious agents in a manner similar to that in other mammals.[20–22]

Hyperthermia caused by anything other than fever is caused by an inability of the animal to relieve excessive heat, which is often a result of an exogenous heat source (eg, external heat supplementation, oxygen cage, respiratory distress, seizures). Hyperthermia should be quickly treated by cooling measures in order to avoid irreversible complications.[19,23,24] Cooling the ears, which are physiologic heat dissipating structures, by placing ice packs or moisturizing with alcohol is usually effective in the author's experience. Conventional cooling measures, such as intravenous fluid or enema, are also efficient. Care must be taken to stop the cooling procedure when the temperature reaches normal values (38°C–39°C [100°F –102°F]).

Hypothermia, caused by an inability to maintain body temperature, is a common problem in critically ill patients and requires external heat supplementation. Recent studies have shown that rabbits that are hypothermic at admission have a risk of mortality that is 3 times higher than that of rabbits that are normothermic, with odds of death doubled for each 1°C decrease of rectal body temperature below the reference range (37.9°C–39.9°C [100.2°F–103.8°F]).[25] Like severe hyperthermia, hypothermia leads to altered coagulation, organ dysfunction, and electrolyte and acid-base abnormalities.[19,24,26]

Oxygen Saturation

Oxygen saturation (Spo_2) is indirectly measured by a spectrophotometric method: the pulse oximeter. Pulse oximetry is a noninvasive, easy-to-use, inexpensive, and safe tool for assessing hypoxemia. In conscious rabbits breathing room air, Spo_2 should be around 96%.[27] An Spo_2 measurement less than 94% is compatible with a hypoxemic state and requires oxygen supplementation. Values less than 90% are consistent with severe hypoxia. Waveform oscillations should be evaluated to make sure Spo_2 measurement is reliable. The sensor may be placed on shaved or hairless skin. In rabbits, the ear is the most accessible site.[27] In intact males, testicles are also an excellent site for probe placement (**Fig. 2**). Spo_2 may be underestimated by pigmented skin, vasoconstriction, hypothermia, hypoperfusion, severe anemia, and other conditions caused by poor perfusion. As in other mammals, pulse oximetry in rabbits evaluates hemoglobin saturation but does not evaluate the efficiency of gas exchange and cannot predict the real saturation of O_2.[27] Further analyses (arterial blood analysis) are needed.[24,28,29]

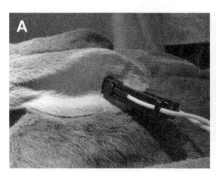 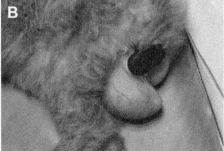

Fig. 2. Oximetry measurement in the ear (*A*) and on the testicle (*B*). (*Courtesy of* Minh Huynh).

Blood Pressure

Digital palpation

Pulse quality by digital palpation of aural, femoral, or dorsal pedal pulses can be performed (**Fig. 3**). Bounding, or hyperdynamic, pulses are a reflection of hyperdynamic state or diastolic disruption. Weak pulses may be secondary to decreased cardiac output, peripheral vasoconstriction, or decreased pulse pressure.[19]

Noninvasive blood pressure

Noninvasive, or indirect, methods of obtaining blood pressure are most commonly used in small animal medicine. There are several noninvasive blood pressure methods: Doppler, oscillometric, and plethysmographic methods. It is noteworthy that most methods have been investigated on anesthetized rabbits but not on conscious animals, in which stress and the repeatability of the measurement may be a concern.[30,31]

Because of its availability and ease of use, the Doppler method is the most commonly used (**Fig. 4**).[11] The front limb has been shown to be more reliable than the hind limb for obtaining blood pressure in rabbits.[32] There is a poor correlation between central arterial pressure measurement and Doppler measurement of the systolic arterial pressure in rabbits.[30] However, the Doppler method has been shown to be a reliable indicator of hypotension (<80 mm Hg) in this species, which makes this technique clinically relevant in case of shock.[31]

Oscillometric and plethysmographic methods are usually not used in a clinical context and are reported to be less reliable in small mammals.[11] Oscillometric measurements have been shown to have good correlation with central arterial pressure using the hind limb, especially in low-pressure measurement, whereas discrepancies become higher as the blood pressure increases.[32]

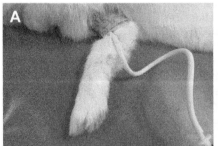
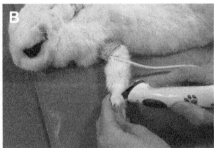
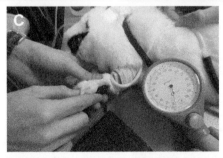

Fig. 3. Measurement of indirect blood pressure with a Doppler. A blood pressure cuff is placed above the elbow (*A*), the ventral aspect of the carpus is shaved (*B*), and the Doppler signal is applied with gel while the sphygmomanometer is inflated (*C*). (*Courtesy of* Minh Huynh).

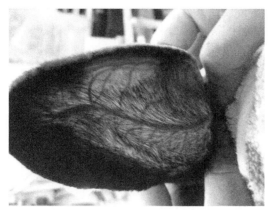

Fig. 4. The central aural artery is used for assessing pulse quality and for arterial blood sampling. (*Courtesy of* Minh Huynh).

Invasive blood pressure

Invasive, or direct, pressure measurement is not routinely performed in conscious rabbits. The central ear artery can be catheterized and provides direct blood pressure monitoring.[33] Because of the small size of most pet rabbits, a kink or a spasm of the artery is common, making the arterial catheter impractical. Furthermore, an ischemic injury to the pinnae is possible following catheterization. Recent studies have shown a discrepancy between auricular arterial blood pressure measurements compared with carotid arterial pressures, although other investigators have reported good reliability on readings of direct blood pressure between the two sites.[30,32]

Blood gas analysis and acid-base status

Blood gas analysis reflects gas exchange in the lungs. Most studies in pet rabbits have used a handheld blood gas machine, the i-STAT analyzer (Abbot Point of Care Inc, Abbott Park, IL), which uses disposable cartridges.[27,34,35] A summary of various measurements and reference intervals is presented in **Table 1**. However, a reference analyzer should be used whenever possible because significant discrepancies in blood gas values have been noted between the i-STAT device and a reference bench top analyzer, apart from the pH.[35]

Arterial samples are preferable for evaluating respiratory status. Reference intervals have been obtained from the central auricular artery.[27,34]

Blood gas analysis includes pH, partial arterial pressure of oxygen (Pa_{O_2}), and partial arterial pressure of carbon dioxide (Pa_{CO_2}). HCO_3- is extrapolated by the analyzer from the pH and P_{CO_2} levels.

Neutral pH is considered to be 7.4 in humans, dogs, and rabbits.[34] Nasal capnography is reported to have good correlation with Pa_{CO_2}, indicating that nasal capnography can be used in obligate nasal breathers such as rabbits.[36] There seems to be a poor agreement between venous P_{CO_2} measured with a point-of-care analyzer compared with a reference method using Severinghaus electrode.[35]

HCO_3- level reflects the metabolic component of acid-base balance. Low HCO_3- level indicates metabolic acidosis. High HCO_3- level indicates metabolic alkalosis and may be caused by pyloric obstruction, gastric stasis, or antacid treatment in rabbits.[34] HCO_3- follows a bimodal distribution in healthy rabbits.[34] HCO_3- level follows fluctuation of lactate levels in rabbits. A normal cause of lactate level increase occurs during the different stages of stool production; lactate level increases during the hard

Table 1
Summary of blood gas and electrolyte measurement in rabbits in 3 different studies using the i-STAT analyzer

	Ardiaca et al,[34] 2013	Eatwell et al,[27] 2013	Ardiaca et al,[34] 2013	Selleri & Girolamo,[35] 2014	Selleri & Girolamo,[35] 2014
Sample size	20 healthy rabbits	50 healthy rabbits	45 healthy rabbits	30 rabbits (13 healthy/17 ill)	30 rabbits (13 healthy/17 ill)
Sample type	Arterial sample	Arterial sample	Venous sample	Venous sample	Venous sample
Device used	i-STAT GC8+	i-STAT GC8+	i-STAT EC8+	i-STAT EC8+	Benchtop analyzer
pH	7.358–7.502	7.45 ± 0.04	7.389 ± 0.074	7.37 ± 0.114	7.378 ± 0.098
Pco_2 (mm Hg)	29.1–36.8	33.2 ± 3.19	40.9 ± 6.1	39.1 ± 8.4	29.4 ± 6.6
Po_2 (mm Hg)	75–101	78.52 ± 10.7	—	—	—
Sat O_2 (%)	93–96	95.98 ± 2	—	—	—
HCO_3- (mmol/L)	17.5–27.6	23.67 ± 2.82	—	—	—
Tco_2 (mmol/L)	18–29	24.72 ± 2.9	—	—	—
BE (mmol/L)	-12	-0.12 ± 3.2	—	—	—
Na (mmol/L)	136–142	141.38 ± 1.9	141 ± 2.6	142 ± 2.8	142.2 ± 2.9
K (mmol/L)	3.5–5.1	4.09 ± 0.4	4.7 ± 0.6	4.3 ± 0.9	4.5 ± 0.63
Cl (mmol/L)	—	—	93–113	105 ± 4	106.2 ± 3.3
iCa (mmol/L)	1.67–1.85	1.79 ± 0.07	—	—	—
BUN (mg/dL)	—	—	21 ± 6.2	17 ± 7.9	16.5 ± 8
Hematocrit (%)	23–42	31.78 ± 3.6	37 ± 4.3	35 ± 6	37 ± 3
Hemoglobin (g/dL)	7.8–14.3	10.8 ± 1.22	12.7 ± 1.5	12 ± 2	12 ± 1.2
Gly (mg/dL)	106–205	141.2 ± 16.9	93–251	162 ± 36	164 ± 45

Abbreviations: BE, base excess; BUN, blood urea nitrogen; iCa, ionized calcium; Sat O_2, O_2 saturation; Tco_2, total carbon dioxide.
   Data from Refs.[27,34,35]

feces phase and decreases during the production of soft feces.[37] During the lactate increase phase the bicarbonate level is therefore lower.

Acid-base status has been investigated in conscious pet rabbits.[27,34,35] Reference intervals have been obtained from arterial blood samples from the central auricular artery and from venous samples.[27,34,35] The most common abnormalities reported were acidemia in 40% of ill rabbits.[34] Acidemia can be classified as either metabolic or respiratory acidosis, which, according to the data from Ardiaca and colleagues,[34] are statistically equally represented in sick rabbits. Compensatory respiratory alkalosis is expected and diagnosed in 50% of metabolic acidosis cases. Loss of HCO_3- is frequently caused by renal and gastrointestinal disease. Dehydration and hypotension can also lead to production of lactic acid in the muscle and contribute to acidosis. In this same study, a respiratory acidosis was present in 30% of the animals with metabolic acidosis, suggesting that some rabbits in some cases are not able to compensate for the primary disorder. Signs of metabolic acidosis include the acidic odor of breath and urine, acidic urinary pH, fever, anorexia, and hypotension.[34]

Metabolic alkalosis is much less frequent (9% of cases) and respiratory alkalosis is uncommon in rabbits (0.5%). Hypochloremic alkalosis is seen in carnivores with pyloric obstruction and foreign body.[38] The gastric acid is trapped in the stomach and the alkaline secretion of the intestine is absorbed. Obstruction at a lower level can lead to HCO_3- leaking in the intestinal lumen, which can cause acidosis.

Electrolytes

Sodium

Sodium is the predominant cation in the body and accounts for the largest proportion of molecules and compounds determining osmolarity. Hypernatremia is often seen in cases of severe water deprivation (water bottle out of reach or neurologic signs preventing access). Hypotonic fluid loss causing hypernatremia may be renal or extrarenal in origin. Renal fluid loss is noted with renal failure, iatrogenic diuresis, persistent hyperglycemia, or postobstructive diuresis. Extrarenal hypotonic water loss with resulting hypernatremia can also be associated with diarrhea, intestinal obstruction, cutaneous loss, or peritonitis. The possibility of iatrogenic hypertonic fluid administration may need to be considered if applicable.

Special interest has developed for hyponatremia in rabbits.[39] Two types of hyponatremia can be seen in rabbits: true hyponatremia (hypotonic) and pseudohyponatremia (isotonic or hypertonic), which is based on osmolarity value. Approximation of the effective osmolality is made from the following formula[40]:

Plasma tonicity $= (2 \times Na)$ (mEq/L) $+$ (Glucose/18) (mg/dL)

Pseudohyponatremia in rabbits can be related to a high glucose value, or a sodium level decrease in response to high glucose level (related to fluid shift and dilution of the sodium). Prevalence of hyponatremia in general was 39% in a sample of 356 ill pet rabbits.[39] True hyponatremia was present in 71.9% of those cases. Severe hyponatremia (Na+ $\leq$ 129 mEq/L) was associated with 2.3 times higher risk of mortality than normonatremia in rabbits. Most of the severe cases were true hyponatremia.

Potassium

Major hyperkalemia can be seen with sampling artifact such as hemolysis, clotting, and improper sampling technique (ie, delayed analysis, excessive agitation, and inappropriate anticoagulant), and is especially common when needles less than 23 gauge are used for venipuncture. Furthermore, potassium level may be overestimated by point-of-care analyzers such as the i-STAT analyzer.[35] True hyperkalemia is seen in cases of oliguric or anuric acute kidney injury, urinary obstruction, or severe tissue necrosis or trauma.

Hypokalemia is seen in cases of dysorexia, loss of digestive fluid, renal failure, and stress-induced alkalosis. Use of loop diuretics is a common cause of iatrogenic hypokalemia, as is inadequate potassium supplementation when providing intravenous fluids containing dextrose.

Chloride
Chloride levels in rabbits are reported lower than other small mammal normal ranges.[34] In rabbits, hypochloremia was not associated with an increase in HCO_3- in two-thirds of the samples in a study by Ardiaca and colleagues,[34] who postulated that the alkalinizing effect of hypochloremia is less pronounced in rabbits.

Ionized calcium
Calcium metabolism is unique in rabbits and they normally have a high calcium level compared with other mammals. In an intensive care context, a truly increased ionized calcium level may indicate chronic or acute renal failure, granulomatous disease, and potentially neoplasia. Dietary disorders (excessive dietary calcium or vitamin D_3) are common but do not affect the health status of a rabbit in an intensive care unit. Hypocalcemia has been associated with lactation in rabbits. Other diseases reported to cause hypocalcemia in other small animals include pancreatitis, peritonitis, and gastrointestinal disease, but have not been shown to cause hypocalcemia in rabbits to the investigators' knowledge. In theory, severe acidosis can increase the ionized calcium (iCa) level because it enhances dissociation of the calcium bound to the protein.

Glucose
In a study by Harcourt-Brown and Harcourt-Brown,[41] normal values for blood glucose levels in healthy, nonstressed rabbits was 7.76 ± 2.4 mmol/L (1.4 ± 0.43 g/L) measured by a portable glucometer. The level of accuracy of different glucometer devices has not been investigated except for the i-STAT analyzer, which underestimates the value.[35] Blood glucose levels have been studied extensively as prognostic indicators, especially in critical pet rabbits with gastrointestinal obstruction.[41] Rabbits with gastrointestinal obstruction presented with glucose levels of more than 24.7 ± 3.9 mmol/L (4.45 ± 0.7 g/L). In this same study, rabbits with enterotoxemia and rabbits with ureteral stones also had increased glucose levels (19 ± 0.9 mmol/L and 18.9 ± 6.3 mmol/L, 3.42 ± 0.16 mmol/L and 3.4 ± 1.13 g/L, respectively) but the number of cases in this study was low in both of those groups. One investigator suggests that hyperglycemia elicits a concurrent decrease in sodium level, leading to a worsening of the condition.[39] Stress can also influence blood glucose level. In a study by Harcourt-Brown and Harcourt-Brown,[41] rabbits reported as being actively stressed had blood glucose levels around 13.7 ± 6.7 mmol/L (2.47 ± 1.21 g/L). Diabetes mellitus has not been reported in pet rabbits.[41] Laboratory animals with experimentally induced diabetes showed very high blood glucose values ranging from 30 to 33.4 mmol/L (5.4–6 g/L).[42] Hypoglycemia is reported in cases of starvation or sepsis.[41]

Lactate
Lactate is primarily produced by anaerobic reaction. A differentiation has been made because L-lactate (levorotatory) is produced by skeletal muscle, brain, red blood cells, and viscera, and D-lactate is produced by bacteria. L-Lactate measurements are used to determine peripheral perfusion in small mammals. D-Lactate levels are used to determine gastrointestinal ischemia in horses.[43]

Lactate measurement has been attempted in rabbits.[44,45] The reference range for D-lactate was 0.17 ± 0.08 mmol/L. D-Lactate levels can be influenced by diet, starvation, and gastrointestinal motility. Its clinical significance is still unknown in sick rabbits. Note that D-lactate level can be evaluated in peritoneal fluid as well as in plasma in horses and could be evaluated in rabbits with gastrointestinal stasis.[43] L-Lactate level is high in rabbits compared with other small mammals. The reference range for lactate levels in rabbits varies for example, 6.9 ± 2.7 mmol/L with the portable analyzer (Lactate Pro, Arkray KDK), 7.1 ± 1.6 mmol/L with a blood gas analyzer (NOVA stat profile M, Novamedical), and 5.1 ± 2.1 mmol/L by high-performance chromatography.[44] Another study found no correlation between D-lactate and L-lactate values when comparing healthy and sick rabbits.[45] To date, it has been difficult to evaluate lactate level as a prognostic indicator in rabbits. There are anecdotal reports of lactate monitoring in experimental design to assess tissue perfusion with a rabbit model.[46,47]

Coagulation

Coagulation parameters have been investigated in pet rabbits using 2 point-of-care analyzers (Idexx Coag Dx, Idexx Alfort, Alfortville, France; and MS QuickVet Coag Combo, Melet Schloesing Laboratory, Osny, France).[48] Prothrombin time (PT) was longer, and activated partial thromboplastin time (aPTT) was shorter using the MS QuickVet Coag Combo compared with the Idexx Coag Dx (**Table 2**).

In the past, coagulation parameters were useful in the detection of disseminated intravascular coagulation, hepatic disorders, and anticoagulant rodenticide intoxication in small mammals. Prolonged PT and aPTT time and disseminated intravascular coagulation have been shown in rabbits in cases of aflatoxin toxicity and rabbit hemorrhagic disease.[49,50] Prolonged PT and aPTT also are known to occur with sepsis, pancreatitis, and neoplasia in other small mammals.

Packed cell volume

Normal packed cell volume (PCV) ranges from 30% to 40% in pet rabbits.[51] Increase of PCV may indicate dehydration if total solids are also increased. Anemia is rare in rabbits.[51] Causes of nonregenerative anemia reported in rabbits include chronic inflammation, chronic bleeding, and benzimidazole intoxication.[51,52] Regenerative anemias can be caused by acute bleeding, such as endometrial aneurysm, liver lobe torsion, and lead toxicosis (**Fig. 5**).[51,53]

Urea

Urea level is commonly used to assess renal function in small mammals but it is not specific to renal function because many extrarenal parameters can also cause increases in blood urea level (blood urea nitrogen), such as circadian rhythm,

Table 2
Coagulation parameters in healthy rabbits using 2 different point-of-care analyzers

Parameter	PT (MS)	PT (Idexx)	aPTT (MS)	aPTT (Idexx)
Reference intervals	17.2–28.5	10.0–14.8	103.2–159.2	104.2–159.1
90% CI for lower limit	16.9–17.4	10.0–12.0	100.8–106.2	103.0–113.1
90% CI for upper limit	25.0–33.6	14.0–15.0	145.7–175.5	153.6–160

Abbreviation: CI, confidence interval.
Data from Mentre V, Bulliot C, Linsart A, et al. Reference intervals for coagulation times using two point-of-care analysers in healthy pet rabbits (Oryctolagus cuniculus). Vet Rec 2014;174(26):658.

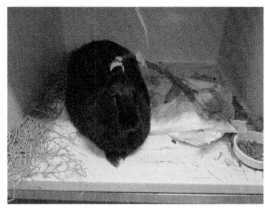

Fig. 5. Severe hemorrhage in rabbit with endometrial bleeding. (*Courtesy of* Minh Huynh).

alimentation, abnormalities in liver or intestinal function, and hydration status. Prerenal azotemia is secondary to decreased renal perfusion caused by dehydration, shock, or gastrointestinal hemorrhage, which leads to increased protein digestion. Renal azotemia is caused by parenchymal renal disease, whereas postrenal azotemia is caused by urinary tract obstruction or rupture. Azotemia has been investigated as a prognostic indicator in rabbits. Blood urea value more than 19.9 mmol/L was associated with a 3-fold higher risk of mortality compared with rabbits without azotemia.[54]

Protein
Total protein is the sum of globulin and albumin. Total serum protein level can be affected by physiologic status (eg, age, pregnancy, reproductive status) or pathologic events. Total protein is used in combination with PCV to evaluate hydration status. Increase of total protein level can also be related to chronic inflammation, such as that seen in abscesses.[55] Hypoproteinemia is commonly seen in cases of malnutrition. Extensive wounds, protein-losing nephropathies, and liver disease remain in the differential diagnosis.[55]

Urinalysis
Ideally, urinalysis is performed on a recently obtained urine sample and before provision of fluid therapy to the rabbit. Urine specific gravity notes the capacity of the kidneys to concentrate urine. Measurement of urine specific gravity is performed on the supernatant portion, after centrifugation, because rabbit urine is frequently rich in sediment.[55] Urine is usually dilute in rabbits compared with other mammals, with a reference range from 1.003 to 1.036. Prerenal azotemia is associated with values of more than 1.030, whereas renal failure is associated with urine specific gravity less than 1.013. Urinary pH is very high in rabbits normally (7.5–9) but rabbit urine can become acidic in cases of severe acidosis associated with hepatic lipidosis and anorexia.[55] Ketones from abnormal hepatic function can be observed. Monitoring of the urine output is useful in assessing the efficacy of fluid therapy, patency of the lower urinary tract, hydration, and renal function in general.[56,57] Normal urine output in rabbits ranges from 1 to 4 mL/kg/h, which is noticeably higher than that of a similar-sized carnivore. Influence of the diet is predominant, because an increased proportion of fresh vegetables enhances urine output.[56,57]

Fluid Therapy

Body water distribution

Rabbits are known to have a high water demand because of their digestive tract. Intraluminal gastrointestinal water accounts for 12% of total body water compared with 3% for a dog.[58]

The body of an adult rabbit consists of 58% of water with a loss of about 340 mL for a 3-kg rabbit per day.[59] Maintenance fluid therapy is 50 to 70 mL/kg/d.[60] Daily maintenance is estimated to be 3 to 4 mL/kg/h.[61] Intracellular fluid is approximatively two-thirds of total body water. Extracellular fluid is divided into the intravascular compartment (one-quarter) and the interstitial space (three-quarters). The definition of maintenance fluid rate is empirical so constant reassessment is needed to tailor the fluid rate to the needs of the patient.[62]

Routes of Administration

Oral fluids

Because a major portion of the total body water is in the digestive tract, oral administration can often be used for rehydration and can be part of the therapeutic plan for shock resuscitation.

Beneficial effects of sole oral fluid supplementation have been reported in cases of severe burn wounds.[63] In case of hypernatremia, oral supplementation may be safer than intravenous supplementation.[64] In the author's experience, when no venous access is available or poorly tolerated, oral rehydration via a nasogastric tube or esophagostomy tube may cause less discomfort and can be left in place for a fairly long period. Rabbits absorb water from the small intestine, the caecum, and also the descending colon.[1] Therefore this route cannot be used in cases of gastric impaction or obstruction. It is also postulated that fluid absorption from the digestive tract is slow and may not be indicated as a sole therapy in patients with extensive fluid loss.[62]

Subcutaneous fluids

Giving subcutaneous fluids to rabbits is easy to perform and they can be administered into the scruff of the neck or into the loose skin over the chest. Between 100 and 120 mL/kg/d are divided into several treatments.[60] Although 20 to 40 mL/kg can be given in 1 location, the author has experienced skin necrosis if a patient is given more than 20 mL/kg fluids subcutaneously. In shock, peripheral vasoconstriction reduces absorption and thus precludes the use of this route. Only isotonic fluids can be administered subcutaneously. Injection of 5% dextrose may shift fluid in the interstitial space and worsen the electrolyte imbalance.[62] The osmolality, although transient, of 5% dextrose in water can also lead to necrosis.

Intravenous fluids

Intravenous fluid therapy is the gold standard for fluid administration and rehydration. Several sites are accessible. The marginal ear vein is readily accessible and does not impair movement because the fluid line is held over the rabbit (**Fig. 6**). Complications include marginal ear necrosis or cartilaginous fracture in nonlop breeds.[60] The cephalic vein and the lateral saphenous vein can be used as they are in dogs and cats.[60] When a fluid line is placed, the rabbit's movement can be impaired and the animal can chew the line. A custom-made protection can be applied to prevent this complication (see **Fig. 6**). Use of a vascular access port in the jugular vein is uncommon, although this technique is promising especially in critical care patients.[65]

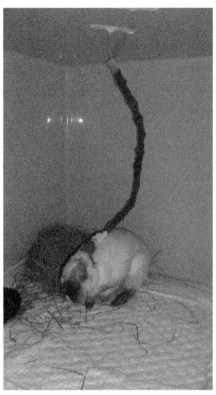

Fig. 6. Intravenous catheter placed in the marginal vein in a rabbit. The intravenous line is held over the head of the rabbit and the line is protected with a custom-made device made of Vetrap and plastic syringe. (*Courtesy of* Charly Pignon).

Intraosseous fluids

Intraosseous fluid administration is comparable with intravenous access.[66] Complications include extravasation, which can occur around the catheter placement site because the insertion of the needle may progressively loosen with time. The proximal humerus, greater trochanter of the femur, and tibial crest are commonly used.[60]

Peritoneal dialysis

Intraperitoneal fluid administration has been used extensively in rabbits as a model of peritoneal dialysis.[67–69] The principle is to use the peritoneal membrane as a surface of exchange for fluid and solute. Use in pet rabbits is anecdotal.[70] Peritoneal dialysis is very time consuming and labor intensive. Percutaneous placement of the catheter is preferred, although surgical placement avoids accidental cecal perforation. A commercial peritoneal dialysis catheter (15-Fr 35-cm Cook Spiral Acute Peritoneal Dialysis Catheter; Cook Veterinary Products, Spencer, IN) or a similar peritoneal dialysis catheter can be used. Complications include peritonitis, pain, infection of the subcutaneous tract, protein loss, and overhydration. This technique is mainly used in case of oliguric or anuric renal failure but success of the therapy is limited. Peritoneal dialysis is considered as a last option strategy in rabbits with renal failure and carries a poor prognosis.

Intrarectal fluid therapy

Intrarectal fluid therapy can be used in rabbits and in the author's experience is remarkably well tolerated. An infusion of isotonic saline over a 15-minute period has been proved to be efficient in a model of hypovolemic shock.[71] The fluid is warmed and administered into the colon over 15 minutes. This technique is easy to perform and can be a rapid technique for an early rehydration plan. Although this technique can help to warm the patient, the rectal temperature can no longer be used for monitoring body temperature because it is inaccurate.

Fluid Choice

Crystalloids

Crystalloid fluid can be balanced or nonbalanced, isotonic, hypertonic, or hypotonic. Isotonic solutions have tonicity similar to the extracellular fluid. Lactated Ringer solution, Plasmalyte-148, and Normosol-R are balanced crystalloid fluids commonly used in veterinary medicine. NaCl 0.9% is an unbalanced isotonic fluid. Crystalloid fluids are the basis of fluid therapy because they contribute to hydrostatic pressure but effects on oncotic pressure are poor. They rapidly disseminate to the extracellular space. Only 20% to 40% of isotonic fluids administered intravenously remain in the vascular space after 30 to 60 minutes. Indications for use include reestablishment of effective circulating volume and restoration of organ perfusion.

Hypertonic crystalloids are hyperosmolar solutions containing high concentrations of sodium and chloride typically marked as 7.5% to 10% NaCl. The hyperosmolarity leads to rapid intravascular volume expansion with a minimal volume of hypertonic solution provided compared with colloids and isotonic crystalloids. The effect is transient and must be replaced with colloid or isotonic crystalloids for longer term effect. Hypertonic solutions should be used with caution in dehydrated patients because the extravascular fluid is depleted and cannot easily be shifted back into the intravascular space. Because of the risk of hypernatremia, sodium levels should be checked before and after administration.

In studies examining rabbits with cerebral edema, hypertonic saline has been proved to be equivalent or superior to mannitol in decreasing intracranial hypertension, improving cerebral perfusion, and reducing cerebral edema.[72] This result was not consistently repeatable.[73,74] However this information could be useful in cases of acute vestibular syndrome when rabbits are likely to have brain trauma and cerebral edema.

Potassium supplementation

Potassium supplementation of isotonic crystalloids is recommended according to the guidelines used in small mammal medicine. Alternatively, oral potassium gluconate can be administered at 5 to 8 mEq per day divided in 3 doses (**Table 3**).

Bicarbonate supplementation

Administration of $NaHCO_3$ is reserved for clinical situations in which the blood pH is less than 7.1 to 7.2 despite fluid therapy. Correction can be challenging.

The dose of bicarbonate is calculated to increase to the desire level and is multiplied by the body weight. One-third is administered and the pH is reassessed.

Dose of bicarbonate to administer = (target bicarbonate level − serum bicarbonate level) × body weight (kg) × 0.3

Colloid

Colloidal fluids contain macromolecules. They convey strong oncotic pressure across the vascular barrier and confer benefits to correct hypotension in patients with shock.

Table 3
Potassium supplementation table

Serum Potassium Concentration (mEq/L)	mEq KCl to Add to 1 L of Fluid	Maximum Fluid Rate Infusion (mL/kg/h)
<2.0	20	6
2.1–2.5	15	8
2.6–3	10	12
3.1–3.5	7	18
3.6–5	5	25

Data from DiBartola SP, Bateman S. Introduction to fluid therapy. In: DiBartola SP, editor. Fluid, electrolyte, and acid base disorders in small animal practice. 3rd edition. Saint Louis (MO): Saunders Elsevier; 2006. p. 325–44.

Colloids have been studied in a rabbit model of shock and remain one of the most valuable adjuncts to compensate for severe hemorrhage.[75,76] Dextran has been proved superior to hydroxyethyl starch in the first hour of resuscitation to maintain mean arterial pressure.[76] Hydroxyethyl starch is also a valid option.[75] Recent studies in human medicine have not proved a superior efficacy in colloids compared with crystalloids in fluid resuscitation; therefore, use in veterinary medicine for resuscitation is debatable.[77,78]

Transfusion

Transfusion is rarely reported in pet rabbit medicine.[61,79,80] It is reasonable to assume that a rabbit with a PCV of 15% or less may benefit from red blood cell transfusion, as would a rabbit patient with acute blood loss exceeding 20% of its blood volume. Rabbits do not seem to have blood groups and transfusion reactions are hypothetical.[79] It is reasonable to perform a simplified cross match before the procedure to check for potential agglutination (2 drops of plasma from the recipient are mixed with 1 drop of blood from the donor), although simplified cross match is no longer recommended in small animal medicine because of numerous false-positives. Donor rabbits need to be in good health, ideally a medium to large breed, and have an initial PCV of more than 35%. One percent of body weight is considered safe to collect.

The blood is collected in an anticoagulant citrate dextrose solution and infused to the recipient at a rate of 0.5 mL/kg in the first 20 minutes, then decreased to a maintenance fluid rate and given over 2 to 4 hours. Use of a micropore filter (Hemo-Nate) can be recommended.[79]

Intralipid

Intralipid solutions have been evaluated in various experimental models of toxicity in rabbits.[81–83] Their clinical use has not been reported yet in pet rabbits. Administration is potentially beneficial in cases of toxicosis of lipophilic molecules such as fipronil or high concentrations of permethrin.

Fluid volume replacement

The first goal of fluid therapy is to restore the intravascular volume and increase the blood pressure. Several strategies are possible (**Box 2**). Clinical situations and fluid choice suggestions are provided in **Table 4**.

If the animal is still not responsive, causes must be investigated (eg, excessive vasoconstriction, hypoglycemia, electrolyte imbalance, acid-base disorder, cardiac dysfunction). In cases of hemorrhagic shock, hypotensive resuscitation (14–18 mL/kg/h)

Box 2
Protocol suggested by Lichtenberger and Lennox

1. A bolus of 7.5% hypertonic saline (3 mL/kg over 10 minutes)

2. A bolus of hetastarch (3 mL/kg over 5–10 minutes)

3. Assessment of systolic blood pressure until it is greater than 40 mm Hg

4. Correction of fluid deficit

5. Aggressive warming (**Fig. 7**)

6. Isotonic crystalloid 10 mL/kg with hetastarch (5 mL/kg) given over 15 minutes until blood pressure increases to more than 90 mm Hg

Adapted from Lichtenberger M, Lennox A. Updates and advanced therapies for gastrointestinal stasis in rabbits. Vet Clin North Am Exot Anim Pract 2010;13(3):534; with permission.

---

was more beneficial than normotensive resuscitation (27–37 mL/kg/h), suggesting that a lower fluid rate should be recommended in hemorrhagic shock.[47]

Hypoglycemia must be treated with a bolus of dextrose 50% at dose of 0.25 mL/kg using a 1:1 dilution with normal saline. If hypoglycemia persists, a constant-rate infusion (CRI) of low-concentration dextrose (1.25%) is recommended. A CRI of hetastarch at 0.8 mL/kg/h combined with crystalloid can be used in case of hypoproteinemia, although there is no current evidence that colloid maintains oncotic pressure.

Fluid Deficit Correction

Dehydration is estimated based on body weight loss, mucous membrane dryness, decreased skin turgor, sunken eyes, and altered mentation. In cases that are difficult to assess clinically, PCV and protein level can be useful. However, in small animal medicine, clinician estimation, PCV, and TS cannot predict change in body weight following fluid therapy.[84]

Fluid requirements are estimated as follows:

$$\% \text{ Dehydration} \times \text{body weight (kg)} \times 1000 \text{ mL/L} = \text{fluid deficit (mL)}$$

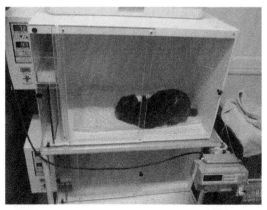

Fig. 7. Warming, as in this brooder, is necessary during the fluid resuscitation procedure. (*Courtesy of* Charly Pignon).

Table 4
Fluid choice suggested in various clinical situations encountered with rabbits in critical care

Clinical Situation	Risks	Type of Fluid	Rate	Route of Administration
Starvation	Hypoproteinemia	Colloid	0.8 mL/kg/h	IV or IO
	Hypoglycemia	Dextrose 50%	0.25 mL/kg bolus + 1 mL/kg/h diluted	IV or IO or PO
	Hypovolemia	Crystalloid[a]	First day: 6–8 mL/kg/h	IV or IO or SC
			Second day: 3–4 mL/kg/h	
	Hypernatremia	Oral water[a]	First day: 5–10 mL/kg/4 h	PO mixed food
			Second day: 10–15 mL/kg/4 h	
Gastrointestinal stasis	Hypovolemia	Colloid	3 mL/kg bolus	IV or IO
		Crystalloid[a]	3–4 mL/kg/h	IV or IO or SC
		Oral water[a]	10–15 mL/kg/4 h	PO with or without food
Gastrointestinal obstruction	Hypovolemia	Colloid	3 mL/kg bolus	IV or IO
	Hyperglycemia	Crystalloid	10–15 mL/kg bolus then 6–8 mL/kg/h	IV or IO
	Hyponatremia			
Diarrhea	Hypovolemia	Colloid	3 mL/kg bolus	IV or IO when possible
	Hypoglycemia	Dextrose 50%	0.25 mL/kg bolus + 1 mL/kg/h diluted	IV or IO when possible
	Hypokalemia	Crystalloid	3–4 mL/kg/h + potassium supplementation	IV or IO or SC
		Oral water	10–15 mL/kg/4 h	PO with or without food
Endometrial aneurysm	Hypovolemia	Hypertonic	3 mL/kg bolus	IV or IO
	Anemia	Colloid	3 mL/kg bolus	IV or IO
		Crystalloid	10–15 mL/kg bolus	IV or IO
			3–4 mL/kg/h	
		Whole blood	3–4 mL/kg/h	IV or IO
Oliguric renal failure	Hypovolemia	Crystalloid + dextrose/insulin	3–4 mL/kg/h	IV or IO or consider peritoneal dialysis
	Hyperkalemia	Mannitol	0.25–1 g/kg bolus	IV or IO
Vestibular syndrome	Hypovolemia	Hypertonic	3 mL/kg bolus	IV or IO
	Potential increased intracranial pressure	Crystalloid	3–4 mL/h	IV or IO or SC

Abbreviations: IO, intraosseous; IV, intravenous; PO, by mouth.
[a] Assuming 5% dehydration.

Dehydration requirements are added to fluid volume for maintenance (3–4 mL/kg/h). If fluid losses occurred within the last 24 hours, replacement should be done within 6 to 8 hours. If losses occurred over 24 to 72 hours, then dehydration deficits are replaced over 24 hours.

For example:
 A 1.2-kg rabbit is estimated with a 5% dehydration. He has not eaten over the past 2 days.
 Fluid maintenance: $1.2 \times 4 \times 24 = 115$ mL
 Fluid deficit: $5/100 \times 1.2 \times 1000 = 60$ mL deficit
The suggested fluid therapy would be:
 Fluid deficit + maintenance over 24 hours: $(115 + 60)/24$ h $= 7.2$ mL/h over 24 hours
Eventually this volume can be shared by the oral and intravenous routes.
 Oral: 50 mL shared in 5 administrations with or without nutritional fiber over 24 hours
 Intravenous: $(115 + 60) - 50 = 125/24$ h $= 5.2$ mL/h over 24 hours

Therapeutics

Sedation
As mentioned previously, stress and catecholamine peaks can have detrimental effects on the cardiovascular dynamics of the rabbit and may alter the distribution of drugs, especially alpha 2 agonists.[85] Several drugs can be used (**Table 5**) for mild sedation. Use of a therapeutic agent for sedation must not preclude environmental measures such as noise reduction and minimal handling.

Positive inotropes
Various drugs are used to maintain blood pressure and increase the cardiac output in small animal medicine. Dopamine as well as phenylephrine have been evaluated in rabbits.[46] Dopamine at 5 to 30 µg/kg/min was found to have no effect on isoflurane-induced hypotension and phenylephrine at 2 µg/kg/min was also found to be minimally effective. From a clinical point of view, inotropic drugs do not seem useful in rabbits at the doses used for cats and dogs.

Anticholinergics In cases of bradycardia, fluid therapy, supplemental warming, and treatment of potential pain must be initiated. However, anticholinergic drugs may be useful in cases of severe bradycardia that are not responsive to standard resuscitation measures. Atropine is the most commonly used anticholinergic drug. However, 60% of domestic rabbits possess atropine esterases, which can rapidly break down atropine to reduce its efficacy and duration of action. Atropine can still be administered to domestic rabbits and has an effect using a dose range of 0.1 to 0.5 mg/kg as an intravenous/intraosseous bolus.[88]

Table 5 Sedative drugs used in rabbits		
Drugs	**Dose (mg/kg)**	**Reference**
Midazolam	0.25–1	86
Butorphanol	0.1–0.5	86
Dexmedetomidine	0.05–0.2	86
Alfaxalone	4–6	87

Glycopyrrolate is a quaternary ammonium anticholinergic, twice as potent and with a longer duration of action than atropine. In rabbits, the use of glycopyrrolate at a dose of 0.01 to 0.02 mg/kg is recommended instead of atropine; however, its slower onset of action and shorter half-life may be of concern in an emergency situation.[89]

Pain Management

Pain management is crucial and presenting pain management options is beyond the scope of this article (See Allweiler SI: How to Improve Anesthesia and Analgesia in Small Mammals, in this issue.) Severe visceral pain is noted in many cases of shock, such as gastrointestinal obstruction or renal urolithiasis. Constant reassessment of pain is needed to address the patient's analgesia requirements. Pain scoring systems usually include assessment of movement and activity, both of which are usually impaired during shock.[90] A novel method of pain scoring using facial observation may be helpful in a critical care context.[91]

Opioids

Pure mu agonists are effective and provide rapid onset and dose-dependent analgesia. Hydromorphone and morphine have been used successfully for analgesia in rabbits.[92] Methadone has recently been investigated at a dose of 2 mg/kg. It provided quicker onset and longer duration of analgesia than morphine.[93]

Fentanyl is a potent mu agonist with short duration of action, which makes it convenient in an intensive care context. Pain level can be reassessed on an hourly basis. Fentanyl is most commonly administered as a CRI but can also be provided with transdermal patch.[94] Side effects include respiratory depression and gastrointestinal stasis. Fentanyl injection bolus induces a decrease in mean arterial pressure, heart rate, and body pressure.[95] Repeated boluses have a cumulative effect.[95] It has been shown to decrease the isoflurane minimum alveolar concentration (MAC) and improve mean arterial pressure and cardiac output under anesthetic conditions.[96,97]

Lidocaine

Lidocaine potentially has multiple benefits, including analgesia, promotion of gastrointestinal motility, and increased visceral perfusion. It has been used successfully in equine medicine to prevent postoperative ileus, to alleviate ischemic injury, and for its antiinflammatory effect, although the mechanism is not known and visceral analgesia has not been shown.[98–100]

Lidocaine infusions have been used in a rabbit model of endotoxemia, in which it reduced the inflammatory response and improved the mean arterial pressure.[101] It has been proved to decrease the isoflurane MAC under anesthetic conditions.[101]

Ketamine

Ketamine is a dissociative used commonly in rabbit anesthesia. In small mammal medicine, low-dose ketamine used by CRI shows beneficial effect in postoperative analgesia.[102] Combination of fentanyl and ketamine infusion has been recommended for use in rabbits.[61] Use of the combination may be beneficial but more studies are warranted to assess the safety and the efficacy of this combination in rabbits.

Oxygen

Because shock is in essence a lack of oxygen delivery to the tissue, oxygen supplementation is never detrimental in a first approach. In various models of experimental shock, such as hemorrhagic, hypovolemic, endotoxinic shock, inflammatory lung injury is often present, making subclinical ventilatory dysfunction common.[103,104]

Clinicians need to assess whether oxygen therapy is useful and whether it needs to be continued after initial stabilization. If the rabbit is able to maintain an oxygen saturation greater than 93% on room air, oxygen supplementation is generally not necessary. The stress induced by the oxygen cage or overheating may outweigh the benefit of the oxygen therapy.

Antibiotics

Antibiotics can be administrated whenever an infectious process causes shock. Experimental septic shock has been successfully induced with *Escherichia coli*, *Staphylococcus* sp, *Pseudomonas* sp, and *Pasteurella multocida*.[105–108] Anaerobic sepsis has also been experimentally induced.[109]

Bactericidal antibiotics should be preferred in an emergency context. Intravenous antibiotics used in this situation include fluoroquinolones, trimethoprim-sulfamide, and aminoglycosides, with caution for aminoglycosides being potentially nephrotoxic. Marbofloxacin pharmacokinetics have been recently published (oral only) and enrofloxacin is widely used.[110,111] Metronidazole has been shown to reduce formation of intra-abdominal abscesses.[109] Oral use of clindamycin, erythromycin, lincomycin, penicillins, amoxicillin-clavulanic acid, and cephalosporins is toxic in rabbits, and should be avoided.

Steroids

Use of steroids is controversial in rabbits and does not seem beneficial in clinical shock, because there is the risk of immunosuppression, increased risk for infection, and gastric ulceration. The use of steroids in shock in rabbits is not recommended until further studies show their efficacy.

A summary of drugs used in critical care is presented (**Table 6**).

Nutrition

Energy needs

Early nutrition is especially important in herbivore species. The rabbit stomach is virtually never empty. Nutrition provides glucose, protein, and water, which are all basic requirements.

Table 6
Selected drugs used in rabbit critical care

Molecule	Dose	Intervals (h)	Reference
Oxymorphone	0.1–0.3 mg/kg	3–4	92
Morphine	1–2 mg/kg	3–4	92
Methadone	2 mg/kg	3–4	—
Fentanyl	5–10 μg/kg/h	CRI	97
Fentanyl patch	12.5 μg/kg	48	94
Lidocaine	3–5 mg/kg/h	CRI	112
Ketamine	1-2 mg/kg/h	CRI	61
Marbofloxacin	2–5 mg/kg	24	110
Enrofloxacin	5 mg/kg	12	111
Sulfamide trimethoprim	30 mg/kg	12	113
Metronidazole	15–30 mg/kg	12	109

Several methods have been recommended to determine the rabbit energy requirements. One estimation of the resting energy requirement (RER) can be calculated with the following formula:

$$RER = K \times 70 \times (body\ weight\ [kg])0.75$$

K is the coefficient factor needed to adjust the daily needs. Ill rabbits may have a factor from 1.2 to 2 but starvation may decrease the metabolic rate. With this formula, a 1.2-kg rabbit needs 80 kcal per day. Fiber content should comprise between 13.6% and 20% dry matter, and protein should be around 16.1% to 26%.[12]

Three products are licensed for rabbit critical care nutrition (**Table 7**). They are designed as liquid to semiliquid formulas to allow syringe feeding. Only the Critical Care Fine Grind (Oxbow product) and the Emeraid herbivore (Lafeber Company) are fluid enough to be given through a 10-F or 8-F nasogastric tube. For further information about nutritional content, refer to the article by Proenca and colleagues.[114]

Nutritional support is given gradually. In the absence of spontaneous ingestion, rabbits can receive 75% to 100% of their daily needs by assisted feedings. In patients that are debilitated, it is reasonable to start with 25% to 50% of their daily requirements. In rabbits that have been anorectic for a long period, blood glucose level should be checked and glycemia level should be increased before enteral nutrition.

The quantity of food is divided into 4 to 5 administrations per day. For slower administration (trickle feeding), the liquid formula can be further diluted and administered via syringe pump connected to a nasogastric tube or esophagostomy tube with a rate of 3 to 4 mL/kg/h.

Addition of fructo-oligosaccharides provides substrate for fermentation activity in the caecum,[115] and has been shown to decrease morbidity in rabbits in cases of diarrhea. It also improves growth, performance, and weight gain in growing rabbits.[116] Oligosaccharides can be added safely in the diet of the rabbit, whereas gluco-oligosaccharides do not seem to have the same beneficial effect and seem to cause diarrhea in young rabbits.[117]

Nasogastric tube In some situations, syringe feeding is poorly tolerated. Patients can be very stressed, dyspneic, have oropharyngeal injury, or can be debilitated and unable to swallow. In these cases, the placement of a nasogastric tube is recommended.[118] It can stay in place up to 5 days, but rhinitis may occur after a longer period (**Fig. 8**). Unlike domestic carnivores, the placement of an Elizabeth collar is not

Table 7
Composition of 3 commercial diets licensed for critical care in rabbits

	Emeraid Herbivore (Lafeber)	Critical Care Formula Fine Grind (Oxbow Product)	Recovery (Supreme Petfood)
Energy density, dry (kcal/g)	2.95	2.6[a]	NA
Energy density, mixed[b] (kcal/mL)	1.32	1.3	NA
Crude protein (%)	19	16	17
Crude fiber (%)	32	21–26	19
Fat (%)	9.5	3	2

Abbreviation: NA, not available
[a] Manufacturer indicates 24 kcal/teaspoon, with 1 teaspoon calculated as 9 g.
[b] Following recommendation of the manufacturer.

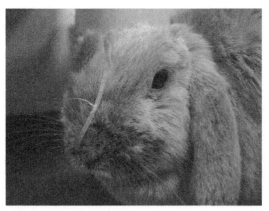

Fig. 8. Nasogastric tube in a dwarf lop rabbit. (*Courtesy of* Minh Huynh).

recommended in rabbits. The collar can induce significant stress leading to anorexia and does not allow ingestion of the caecotrophs necessary for the functioning of the digestive system.[61] Ideally, if caecotrophs are not eaten or in cases of enterotoxemia, caecotrophs can be supplemented too.

Esophagostomy tube An esophagostomy tube should be considered if syringe feeding, or if nasogastric tube placement is not possible because of the patient's clinical status (eg, maxillofacial fracture, significant obstruction of nasal cavities secondary to severe nasal discharge).[119] The introduction of the esophagostomy tube requires general anesthesia and follows the same principles as in dogs and cats (**Fig. 9**). Unlike the nasogastric tube, the esophagostomy tube can remain in place for several weeks or months and allow coarser feeding formula.

Parenteral Nutrition

Parenteral nutrition can be administered in rabbits.[120,121] The basic principle of parenteral nutrition is using intravenous solutions for nutritional support. Total parenteral nutrition is limited in rabbits because of cost and limited knowledge of exact nutritional requirements. Another limitation of the technique is the need for a central line because of the macromolecules used. However, if the intravenous solution has an osmolarity

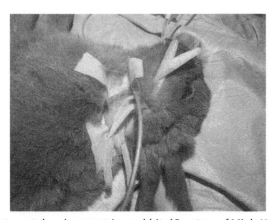

Fig. 9. Esophagostomy tube placement in a rabbit. (*Courtesy of* Minh Huynh).

less than 550 mOsm/L it can still be used in a peripheral catheter.[120] The intraperitoneal route has been used experimentally for total parenteral nutrition with success in rabbits.[122]

Decision-making criteria for parenteral nutrition have been defined by Orcutt[121] as follows:

- Corrections of electrolyte and acid-base abnormalities have been made
- Nutritional intake is anticipated to be less than the energy requirements for 3 days
- Enteral route cannot be safely accessed
- Hospitalization is likely to continue over the next 3 days

Parenteral nutrition requires compounding to produce a total nutrient admixture (TNA). Once the bag is reconstituted it should not be used for more than 24 hours; however, some investigators have used a single bag for 3 days with no reported side effects.[121] A combination of dextrose and lipid is the main source of energy. It is recommended to administer high-fat TNA solutions. Fat solution decreases the osmolarity of the TNA and matches the patient's need for neoglucogenesis. There are reports of rabbits tolerating up to 80% fats covering the RERs, although solutions with more than 60% lipids are usually not recommended.[121] Examples of TNA formulation are provided by Orcutt.[121] Complications include thrombophlebitis and infection. Strict aseptic techniques are mandatory. Staff members should be trained to work aseptically when connecting lines and the line should not be disconnected.

Cardiopulmonary Resuscitation

Cardiopulmonary arrest is a lethal condition in veterinary medicine, with only 6% to 7% of small animals surviving to hospital discharge.[123] Although few clinical data are available in the literature concerning rabbits, the Reassessment Campaign on Veterinary Resuscitation (RECOVER) completed in 2012 generated a set of evidence-based, consensus guidelines to provide a clear basis for cardiopulmonary resuscitation in canine and feline practice.[124] In rabbits, one retrospective study included 15 animals that experienced cardiopulmonary arrest.[125] Return of spontaneous circulation occurred in 7 animals. Two of the rabbit patients experienced only transient return of spontaneous circulation, 5 had longer survival (up to 26 hours), 1 was later euthanized, and 3 died. In this study, only 1 rabbit survived to discharge. Return of spontaneous circulation rate and survival rate were similar to those reported in canine or feline studies.[125]

SUMMARY

Intensive care in rabbits requires a thorough knowledge of rabbit physiology along with knowledge of clinical techniques as well as experimental laboratory data. Even without extensive clinical data regarding shock in rabbits, using experimental laboratory data and extrapolating from treatment of shock in other small mammals (or dogs and cats), treatment of critically ill rabbits can be successful.

ACKNOWLEDGMENTS

Many thanks to Liz Guieu who kindly reviewed this article.

REFERENCES

1. Campbell-Ward ML. Gastrointestinal physiology and nutrition. In: Quesenberry KE, Carpenter JW, editors. Ferrets, rabbits and rodents: clinical medicine and surgery. Saint Louis (MO): Elsevier Saunders; 2012. p. 183–92.

2. Huston SM, Ming-Show Lee P, Quesenberry KE, et al. Cardiovascular disease, lymphoproliferative disorders and thymomas. In: Quesenberry KE, Carpenter JW, editors. Ferrets, rabbits and rodents: clinical medicine and surgery. Saint Louis (MO): Elsevier Saunders; 2012. p. 257–68.

3. Pariaut R. Cardiovascular physiology and diseases of the rabbit. Vet Clin North Am Exot Anim Pract 2009;12(1):135–44, vii.

4. Simons M, Downing SE. Coronary vasoconstriction and catecholamine cardiomyopathy. Am Heart J 1985;109(2):297–304.

5. Downing SE, Chen V. Myocardial injury following endogenous catecholamine release in rabbits. J Mol Cell Cardiol 1985;17(4):377–87.

6. Schadt JC, Hasser EM. Hemodynamic effects of acute stressors in the conscious rabbit. Am J Physiol 1998;274(3 Pt 2):R814–21.

7. Schadt JC, Hasser EM. Hemodynamic effects of blood loss during a passive response to a stressor in the conscious rabbit. Am J Physiol Regul Integr Comp Physiol 2004;286(2):R373–80.

8. Oyebola DD, Taiwo EO, Idolor GO, et al. Effect of adrenaline on glucose uptake in the rabbit small intestine. Afr J Med Sci 2011;40(3):225–33.

9. Swennes AG, Alworth LC, Harvey SB, et al. Human handling promotes compliant behavior in adult laboratory rabbits. J Am Assoc Lab Anim Sci 2011;50(1):41–5.

10. Burhans LB, Smith-Bell C, Schreurs BG. Effects of extinction on classical conditioning and conditioning-specific reflex modification of rabbit heart rate. Behav Brain Res 2010;206(1):127–34.

11. Lichtenberger M, Ko J. Critical care monitoring. Vet Clin North Am Exot Anim Pract 2007;10(2):317–44.

12. Paul-Murphy J. Critical care of the rabbit. Vet Clin North Am Exot Anim Pract 2007;10(2):437–61.

13. Marano G, Grigioni M, Tiburzi F, et al. Effects of isoflurane on cardiovascular system and sympathovagal balance in New Zealand white rabbits. J Cardiovasc Pharmacol 1996;28(4):513–8.

14. Turner Giannico A, Ayres Garcia DA, Lima L, et al. Determination of normal echocardiographic, electrocardiographic, and radiographic cardiac parameters in the conscious New Zealand white rabbit. J Exotic Pet Med 2015;24(2):223–34.

15. Lichtenberger M. Principles of shock and fluid therapy in special species. Semin Av Ex Pet Med 2004;13(3):142–53.

16. Mullan SM, Main DC. Survey of the husbandry, health and welfare of 102 pet rabbits. Vet Rec 2006;159(4):103–9.

17. Sweet H, Pearson AJ, Watson PJ, et al. A novel zoometric index for assessing body composition in adult rabbits. Vet Rec 2013;173(15):369.

18. Eliott DA. Nutritional assessment. In: Silverstein DC, Hopper K, editors. Small animal critical care medicine. Saint Louis (MO): Saunders Elsevier; 2009. p. 856–9.

19. Hackett B. Physical examination. In: Silverstein DC, Hopper K, editors. Small animal critical care medicine. 1st edition. Saint Louis (MO): Saunders Elsevier; 2009. p. 2–5.

20. Comer JE, Ray BD, Henning LN, et al. Characterization of a therapeutic model of inhalational anthrax using an increase in body temperature in New Zealand white rabbits as a trigger for treatment. Clin Vaccine Immunol 2012;19(9):1517–25.

21. Parsonnet J, Gillis ZA, Richter AG, et al. A rabbit model of toxic shock syndrome that uses a constant, subcutaneous infusion of toxic shock syndrome toxin 1. Infect Immun 1987;55(5):1070–6.

22. Panda A, Tatarov I, Masek BJ, et al. A rabbit model of non-typhoidal salmonella bacteremia. Comp Immunol Microbiol Infect Dis 2014;37(4):211–20.

23. Miller JB. Hyperthermia and fever. In: Silverstein DC, Hopper K, editors. Small animal critical care medicine. 1st edition. Saint Louis (MO): Saunders Elsevier; 2009. p. 21–6.

24. Pachtinger G. Monitoring of the emergent small animal patient. Vet Clin North Am Small Anim Pract 2013;43(4):705–20.

25. Di Girolamo N, Toth G, Selleri P. Prognostic value of rectal temperature at hospital admission in client-owned rabbits. J Am Vet Med Assoc 2016;248(3): 288–97.

26. Todd J, Powell LL. Hypothermia. In: Silverstein DC, Hopper K, editors. Small animal critical care medicine. Saint Louis (MO): Saunders Elsevier; 2009. p. 720–2.

27. Eatwell K, Mancinelli E, Hedley J, et al. Use of arterial blood gas analysis as a superior method for evaluating respiratory function in pet rabbits (*Oryctolagus cuniculus*). Vet Rec 2013;173(7):166.

28. Sorell-Raschi L. Sedation monitoring. In: Silverstein DC, Hopper K, editors. Small animal critical care medicine. 1st edition. Saint Louis (MO): Saunders Elsevier; 2009. p. 887–90.

29. Sorell-Raschi L. Blood gas and oximetry monitoring. In: Silverstein DC, Hopper K, editors. Small animal critical care medicine. 1st edition. Saint Louis (MO): Saunders Elsevier; 2009. p. 878–82.

30. Barter LS, Epstein SE. Comparison of Doppler, oscillometric, auricular and carotid arterial blood pressure measurements in isoflurane anesthetized New Zealand white rabbits. Vet Anaesth Analg 2014;41(4):393–7.

31. Harvey L, Knowles T, Murison PJ. Comparison of direct and Doppler arterial blood pressure measurements in rabbits during isoflurane anaesthesia. Vet Anaesth Analg 2012;39(2):174–84.

32. Ypsilantis P, Didilis VN, Politou M, et al. A comparative study of invasive and oscillometric methods of arterial blood pressure measurement in the anesthetized rabbit. Res Vet Sci 2005;78(3):269–75.

33. Wesslau C, Bottger S, Schonert G, et al. A simple method of blood pressure measurement in nonanesthesized rabbits. Z Exp Chir Transplant Kunstliche Organe 1984;17(5):298–302 [in German].

34. Ardiaca M, Bonvehi C, Montesinos A. Point-of-care blood gas and electrolyte analysis in rabbits. Vet Clin North Am Exot Anim Pract 2013;16(1):175–95.

35. Selleri P, Girolamo ND. Point-of-care blood gases, electrolytes, chemistries, hemoglobin, and hematocrit measurement in venous samples from pet rabbits. J Am Anim Hosp Assoc 2014;50(5):305–14.

36. Evans JM, Hogg MI, Rosen M. Correlation of alveolar PCO2 estimated by infrared analysis and arterial PCO2 in the human neonate and the rabbit. Br J Anaesth 1977;49(8):761–4.

37. Vernay M. Origin and utilization of volatile fatty acids and lactate in the rabbit: influence of the faecal excretion pattern. Br J Nutr 1987;57(3):371–81.

38. Boag AK, Coe RJ, Martinez TA, et al. Acid-base and electrolyte abnormalities in dogs with gastrointestinal foreign bodies. J Vet Intern Med 2005;19(6):816–21.

39. Bonvehi C, Ardiaca M, Barrera S, et al. Prevalence and types of hyponatraemia, its relationship with hyperglycaemia and mortality in ill pet rabbits. Vet Rec 2014; 174(22):554.

40. Rose BD. Clinical physiology of acid-base and electrolytes. New York: McGraw-Hill; 1984.

41. Harcourt-Brown FM, Harcourt-Brown SF. Clinical value of blood glucose measurement in pet rabbits. Vet Rec 2012;170(26):674.

42. Roth SI, Conaway HH. Animal model of human disease. Spontaneous diabetes mellitus in the New Zealand white rabbit. Am J Pathol 1982;109(3):359–63.

43. Yamout SZ, Nieto JE, Beldomenico PM, et al. Peritoneal and plasma D-lactate concentrations in horses with colic. Vet Surg 2011;40(7):817–24.

44. Langlois I, Planche A, Boysen SR, et al. Blood concentrations of D- and L-lactate in healthy rabbits. J Small Anim Pract 2014;55(9):451–6.

45. Hupfeld C. Lactate concentration in blood of healthy and ill rabbits. Tierärztliche Praxis. Ausgabe K, Kleintiere/Heimtiere 2009;37(4):244–9.

46. Gosliga JM, Barter LS. Cardiovascular effects of dopamine hydrochloride and phenylephrine hydrochloride in healthy isoflurane-anesthetized New Zealand white rabbits (*Oryctolagus cuniculus*). Am J Vet Res 2015;76(2):116–21.

47. Zhang YM, Gao B, Wang JJ, et al. Effect of hypotensive resuscitation with a novel combination of fluids in a rabbit model of uncontrolled hemorrhagic shock. PLoS One 2013;8(6):e66916.

48. Mentre V, Bulliot C, Linsart A, et al. Reference intervals for coagulation times using two point-of-care analysers in healthy pet rabbits (Oryctolagus cuniculus). Vet Rec 2014;174(26):658.

49. Baker DC, Green RA. Coagulation defects of aflatoxin intoxicated rabbits. Vet Pathol 1987;24(1):62–70.

50. Abrantes J, van der Loo W, Le Pendu J, et al. Rabbit haemorrhagic disease (RHD) and rabbit haemorrhagic disease virus (RHDV): a review. Vet Res 2012;43:12.

51. Fudge A. Rabbit hematology. In: Fudge A, editor. Laboratory medicine: avian and exotic pets. Philadelphia: WB Saunders; 2000. p. 273–5.

52. Graham JE, Garner MM, Reavill DR. Benzimidazole toxicosis in rabbits: 13 cases (2003 to 2011). J Exotic Pet Med 2014;23(2):188–95.

53. Stanke NJ, Graham JE, Orcutt CJ, et al. Successful outcome of hepatectomy as treatment for liver lobe torsion in four domestic rabbits. J Am Vet Med Assoc 2011;238(9):1176–83.

54. Zoller G, di Girolamo N, Huynh M. Biochemical predictor of short-term outcome in rabbits with urologic disorders. Paper presented at: ExoticsCon. San Antonio, TX, August 31 - September 2, 2015.

55. Melillo A. Rabbit clinical pathology. J Exotic Pet Med 2007;16(3):135–45.

56. Tschudin A, Clauss M, Codron D, et al. Water intake in domestic rabbits (*Oryctolagus cuniculus*) from open dishes and nipple drinkers under different water and feeding regimes. J Anim Physiol Anim Nutr (Berl) 2011;95(4):499–511.

57. Clauss M, Burger B, Liesegang A, et al. Influence of diet on calcium metabolism, tissue calcification and urinary sludge in rabbits (*Oryctolagus cuniculus*). J Anim Physiol Anim Nutr (Berl) 2012;96(5):798–807.

58. Cizek LJ. Total water content of laboratory animals with special reference to volume of fluid within the lumen of the gastrointestinal tract. Am J Physiol 1954;179(1):104–10.

59. Suckow MA, Brammer DW, Rush HG, et al. Biology and diseases of rabbits. In: Fox JG, Anderson LC, Loew FM, et al, editors. Laboratory animal medicine. 2nd edition. Toronto: Academic press; 2002. p. 329–64.

60. Graham J, Mader DR. Basic approach to veterinary care. In: Quesenberry KE, Carpenter JW, editors. Ferrets, rabbits and rodents: clinical medicine and surgery. 3rd edition. Saint Louis (MO): Elsevier Saunders; 2012. p. 174–82.

61. Lichtenberger M, Lennox A. Updates and advanced therapies for gastrointestinal stasis in rabbits. Vet Clin North Am Exot Anim Pract 2010;13(3):525–41.

62. DiBartola SP, Bateman S. Introduction to fluid therapy. In: DiBartola SP, editor. Fluid, electrolyte, and acid base disorders in small animal practice. 3rd edition. Saint Louis (MO): Saunders Elsevier; 2006. p. 325–44.

63. Ruan J, Zhang BQ, Wang G, et al. Improving myocardial mechanics parameters of severe burn rabbits with oral fluid resuscitation. Zhonghua Shao Shang Za Zhi 2008;24(4):254–7 [in Chinese].

64. Hogan GR, Dodge PR, Gill SR, et al. The incidence of seizures after rehydration of hypernatremic rabbits with intravenous or ad libitum oral fluids. Pediatr Res 1984;18(4):340–5.

65. Perry-Clark LM, Meunier LD. Vascular access ports for chronic serial infusion and blood sampling in New Zealand white rabbits. Lab Anim Sci 1991;41(5):495–7.

66. Morris RE, Schonfeld N, Haftel AJ. Treatment of hemorrhagic shock with intraosseous administration of crystalloid fluid in the rabbit model. Ann Emerg Med 1987;16(12):1321–4.

67. Dziuk E, Siekierzynski M. Experimental model of peritoneal dialysis. Acta Physiol Pol 1973;24(3):465–72.

68. Gotloib L, Crassweller P, Rodella H, et al. Experimental model for studies of continuous peritoneal' dialysis in uremic rabbits. Nephron 1982;31(3):254–9.

69. Zunic-Bozinovski S, Lausevic Z, Krstic S, et al. An experimental, non-uremic rabbit model of peritoneal dialysis. Physiol Res 2008;57(2):253–60.

70. Wojick K, Berube D, Barr Iii J. Clinical technique: peritoneal dialysis and percutaneous peritoneal dialysis catheter placement in small mammals. Journal of Exotic Pet Medicine 2008;17(3):181–8.

71. Girisgin AS, Acar F, Cander B, et al. Fluid replacement via the rectum for treatment of hypovolaemic shock in an animal model. Emerg Med J 2006;23(11):862–4.

72. Liu S, Li L, Luo Z, et al. Superior effect of hypertonic saline over mannitol to attenuate cerebral edema in a rabbit bacterial meningitis model. Crit Care Med 2011;39(6):1467–73.

73. da Silva JC, de Lima Fde M, Valenca MM, et al. Hypertonic saline more efficacious than mannitol in lethal intracranial hypertension model. Neurol Res 2010;32(2):139–43.

74. Liu SQ, Zhang KN, Zheng HX, et al. Comparison of mannitol and hypertonic saline in treatment of intracranial hypertension of rabbits. Zhejiang Da Xue Bao Yi Xue Ban 2012;41(2):166–70 [in Chinese].

75. Komori M, Takada K, Tomizawa Y, et al. Effects of colloid resuscitation on peripheral microcirculation, hemodynamics, and colloidal osmotic pressure during acute severe hemorrhage in rabbits. Shock 2005;23(4):377–82.

76. Strecker U, Dick W, Madjidi A, et al. The effect of the type of colloid on the efficacy of hypertonic saline colloid mixtures in hemorrhagic shock: dextran versus hydroxyethyl starch. Resuscitation 1993;25(1):41–57.

77. Annane D, Siami S, Jaber S, et al. Effects of fluid resuscitation with colloids vs crystalloids on mortality in critically ill patients presenting with hypovolemic shock: the CRISTAL randomized trial. JAMA 2013;310(17):1809–17.

78. Cazzolli D, Prittie J. The crystalloid-colloid debate: Consequences of resuscitation fluid selection in veterinary critical care. J Vet Emerg Crit Care (San Antonio) 2015;25(1):6–19.
79. Lichtenberger M. Transfusion medicine in exotic pets. Clin Tech Small Anim Pract 2004;19(2):88–95.
80. Lichtenberger M. Shock and cardiopulmonary-cerebral resuscitation in small mammals and birds. Vet Clin North Am Exot Anim Pract 2007;10(2):275–91.
81. Harvey MG, Cave GR. Intralipid infusion ameliorates propranolol-induced hypotension in rabbits. J Med Toxicol 2008;4(2):71–6.
82. Harvey M, Cave G, Ong B. Intravenous lipid emulsion-augmented plasma exchange in a rabbit model of clomipramine toxicity; survival, but no sink. Clin Toxicol (Phila) 2014;52(1):13–9.
83. Karcioglu M, Tuzcu K, Sefil F, et al. Efficacy of resuscitation with intralipid in a levobupivacaine-induced cardiac arrest model. Turk J Med Sci 2014;44(2): 330–6.
84. Hansen B, DeFrancesco T. Relationship between hydration estimate and body weight change after fluid therapy in critically ill dogs and cats. J Vet Emerg Crit Care (San Antonio) 2002;12(4):235–43.
85. Raekallio M, Ansah OB, Kuusela E, et al. Some factors influencing the level of clinical sedation induced by medetomidine in rabbits. J Vet Pharmacol Ther 2002;25(1):39–42.
86. Santangelo B, Micieli F, Mozzillo T, et al. Transnasal administration of a combination of dexmedetomidine, midazolam and butorphanol produces deep sedation in New Zealand White rabbits. Vet Anaesth Analg 2016;43(2):209–14.
87. Huynh M, Poumeyrol S, Pignon C, et al. Intramuscular administration of alfaxalone for sedation in rabbits. Vet Rec 2015;176(10):255.
88. Harrison PK, Tattersall JE, Gosden E. The presence of atropinesterase activity in animal plasma. Naunyn Schmiedebergs Arch Pharmacol 2006;373(3):230–6.
89. Olson ME, Vizzutti D, Morck DW, et al. The parasympatholytic effects of atropine sulfate and glycopyrrolate in rats and rabbits. Can J Vet Res 1994;58(4):254–8.
90. Leach MC, Allweiler S, Richardson C, et al. Behavioural effects of ovariohysterectomy and oral administration of meloxicam in laboratory housed rabbits. Res Vet Sci 2009;87(2):336–47.
91. Keating SCJ, Thomas AA, Flecknell PA, et al. Evaluation of EMLA cream for preventing pain during tattooing of rabbits: changes in physiological, behavioural and facial expression responses. PLoS One 2012;7(9):e44437.
92. Barter LS. Rabbit analgesia. Vet Clin North Am Exot Anim Pract 2011;14(1): 93–104.
93. Touzot-Jourde G, Nino V, Holopherne-Doran D. Oral communications. J Vet Pharmacol Ther 2015;38:1–81.
94. Foley PL, Henderson AL, Bissonette EA, et al. Evaluation of fentanyl transdermal patches in rabbits: blood concentrations and physiologic response. Comp Med 2001;51(3):239–44.
95. Baumgartner CM, Koenighaus H, Ebner JK, et al. Cardiovascular effects of fentanyl and propofol on hemodynamic function in rabbits. Am J Vet Res 2009; 70(3):409–17.
96. Tearney CC, Barter LS, Pypendop BH. Cardiovascular effects of equipotent doses of isoflurane alone and isoflurane plus fentanyl in New Zealand white rabbits (*Oryctolagus cuniculus*). Am J Vet Res 2015;76(7):591–8.

97. Barter LS, Hawkins MG, Pypendop BH. Effects of fentanyl on isoflurane minimum alveolar concentration in New Zealand white rabbits (*Oryctolagus cuniculus*). Am J Vet Res 2015;76(2):111–5.

98. Cook VL, Jones Shults J, McDowell M, et al. Attenuation of ischaemic injury in the equine jejunum by administration of systemic lidocaine. Equine Vet J 2008;40(4):353–7.

99. Cook VL, Jones Shults J, McDowell MR, et al. Anti-inflammatory effects of intravenously administered lidocaine hydrochloride on ischemia-injured jejunum in horses. Am J Vet Res 2009;70(10):1259–68.

100. Torfs S, Delesalle C, Dewulf J, et al. Risk factors for equine postoperative ileus and effectiveness of prophylactic lidocaine. J Vet Intern Med 2009;23(3):606–11.

101. Taniguchi T, Shibata K, Yamamoto K, et al. Lidocaine attenuates the hypotensive and inflammatory responses to endotoxemia in rabbits. Crit Care Med 1996;24(4):642–6.

102. Wagner AE, Walton JA, Hellyer PW, et al. Use of low doses of ketamine administered by constant rate infusion as an adjunct for postoperative analgesia in dogs. J Am Vet Med Assoc 2002;221(1):72–5.

103. Engelbrecht FM, Mouton WL, van Schalkwyk LJ. Shock lung–experimental studies on a haemorrhagic hypovolaemic rabbit model. S Afr Med J 1983;64(11):400–4.

104. Cuevas P, De la Maza LM, Gilbert J, et al. The lung lesion in four different types of shock in rabbits. Arch Surg 1972;104(3):319–22.

105. Elmas M, Yazar E, Uney K, et al. Influence of *Escherichia coli* endotoxin-induced endotoxaemia on the pharmacokinetics of enrofloxacin after intravenous administration in rabbits. J Vet Med A Physiol Pathol Clin Med 2006;53(8):410–4.

106. Arko RJ, Rasheed JK, Broome CV, et al. A rabbit model of toxic shock syndrome: clinicopathological features. J Infect 1984;8(3):205–11.

107. Kurahashi K, Kajikawa O, Sawa T, et al. Pathogenesis of septic shock in *Pseudomonas aeruginosa* pneumonia. J Clin Invest 1999;104(6):743–50.

108. Jaglic Z, Jeklova E, Christensen H, et al. Host response in rabbits to infection with *Pasteurella multocida* serogroup F strains originating from fowl cholera. Can J Vet Res 2011;75(3):200–8.

109. Simopoulos C, Kouskoukis C, Polychronides A, et al. Effect of different combinations of antibiotics on experimental septic peritonitis in rabbits. Int J Clin Lab Res 1994;24(3):167–70.

110. Marin P, Alamo LF, Escudero E, et al. Pharmacokinetics of marbofloxacin in rabbit after intravenous, intramuscular, and subcutaneous administration. Res Vet Sci 2013;94(3):698–700.

111. Elmas M, Uney K, Yazar E, et al. Pharmacokinetics of enrofloxacin following intravenous and intramuscular administration in angora rabbits. Res Vet Sci 2007;82(2):242–5.

112. Schnellbacher RW, Carpenter JW, Mason DE, et al. Effects of lidocaine administration via continuous rate infusion on the minimum alveolar concentration of isoflurane in New Zealand white rabbits (*Oryctolagus cuniculus*). Am J Vet Res 2013;74(11):1377–84.

113. Jenkins JR. Gastrointestinal disease. In: Quesenberry KE, Carpenter JW, editors. Ferrets, rabbits and rodents: clinical medicine and surgery. 2nd edition. Saint Louis (MO): Saunders Elsevier; 2004. p. 169.

114. Proenca LM, Mayer J. Prescription diets for rabbits. Vet Clin North Am Exot Anim Pract 2014;17(3):485–502.

115. Bovera F, Marono S, Di Meo C, et al. Effect of mannanoligosaccharides supplementation on caecal microbial activity of rabbits. Animal 2010;4(9):1522–7.
116. Bovera F, Lestingi A, Iannaccone F, et al. Use of dietary mannanoligosaccharides during rabbit fattening period: effects on growth performance, feed nutrient digestibility, carcass traits, and meat quality. J Anim Sci 2012;90(11):3858–66.
117. De Blas C, Wiseman J. The nutrition of the rabbit. Oxon (United Kingdom): CABI Publishing; 2003.
118. Rosen LB. Nasogastric tube placement in rabbits. J Exotic Pet Med 2011;20(1): 27–31.
119. Makidon P. Esophagostomy tube placement in the anorectic rabbit. Lab Anim (NY) 2005;34(8):33–6.
120. Remillard RL. Parenteral nutrition support in rabbits and ferrets. J Exotic Pet Med 2006;15(4):248–54.
121. Orcutt CJ. Parenteral nutrition for small exotic herbivores. Exot DVM 2000;2(3): 39–43.
122. Kalfarentzos F, Spiliotis J, Christopoulos D, et al. Total parenteral nutrition by intraperitoneal feeding in rabbits. Eur Surg Res 1988;20(5–6):352–7.
123. Hofmeister EH, Brainard BM, Egger CM, et al. Prognostic indicators for dogs and cats with cardiopulmonary arrest treated by cardiopulmonary cerebral resuscitation at a university teaching hospital. J Am Vet Med Assoc 2009; 235(1):50–7.
124. Fletcher DJ, Boller M, Brainard BM, et al. RECOVER evidence and knowledge gap analysis on veterinary CPR. Part 7: clinical guidelines. J Vet Emerg Crit Care (San Antonio) 2012;22(Suppl 1):S102–31.
125. Buckley GJ, DeCubellis J, Sharp CR, et al. Cardiopulmonary resuscitation in hospitalized rabbits: 15 cases. J Exotic Pet Med 2011;20(1):46–50.

Common Emergencies in Rabbits, Guinea Pigs, and Chinchillas

Julie DeCubellis, DVM, MS

KEYWORDS

• Rabbits • Chinchillas • Guinea pigs • Emergency

KEY POINTS

• Many illnesses seen in small hindgut fermenting herbivore exotic pets are the result of suboptimal diets and husbandry.
• Diets lacking sufficient coarse, high-fiber hays can lead to dental disease and abnormal cecal fermentation, resulting in dysbiosis, enteritis, stasis, and/or life-threatening obstruction or volvulus.
• Rabbits and rodents are exceptionally sensitive to antibiotics and corticosteroids, and care must be taken to choose an appropriate therapy for each species.

INTRODUCTION

Rabbits, guinea pigs, and chinchillas are small hindgut fermenting herbivores that are popular exotic pets. Although they share many physiologic features, they have each developed unique adaptive differences to survive in often-harsh environments on grass-based diets. The illnesses seen in them as pets are frequently related to suboptimal diets and husbandry (small enclosures, poor ventilation, low-fiber and less-abrasive diets) but also to the relative longevity of captive animals (chronic disease, immunosuppression, infection). As prey species, they attempt to mask their illness, and can present with an acute problem (anorexia) that is often the result of several chronic (poor diet, dental disease) and subacute (dysbiosis, enteritis) problems. This article discusses some of the more common diseases seen in rabbits, guinea pigs, and chinchillas presenting for emergent evaluation, highlighting differences. Management of acute trauma and shock is covered in the adjoining article (See Huynh M: Rabbit Physiology and Treatment for Shock, in this issue).

Disclosure Statement: The author has nothing to disclose.
Calgary Avian & Exotic Pet Clinic, Bay 1, 2308-24th Street Southwest, Calgary, Alberta T2T 5H8, Canada
E-mail address: j_decubellis@yahoo.com

Vet Clin Exot Anim 19 (2016) 411–429
http://dx.doi.org/10.1016/j.cvex.2016.01.003   vetexotic.theclinics.com
1094-9194/16/$ – see front matter © 2016 Elsevier Inc. All rights reserved.

ORAL AND GASTROINTESTINAL DISEASE
Anorexia and Dysbiosis

Anorexia in small hindgut fermenting herbivores results from many different ailments, ranging from dental disease and malocclusion, chronic gastrointestinal tract disturbances, and deficiencies from inappropriate diets, antibiotic use, painful conditions, environmental stressors, and acute traumatic events, such as gastrointestinal stasis (ileus), distension, obstruction, and volvulus. The onset of anorexia, even if it is the result of a chronic process, is a medical emergency in these animals, as gastrointestinal stasis, fluid and electrolyte imbalances, and hepatic lipidosis can develop rapidly following cessation of eating.[1]

The intestinal tracts of rabbits, guinea pigs, and chinchillas are adapted to perform hindgut (cecal) fermentation of coarse, high-fiber grass hays. Although all are slightly different, the cecal intestinal flora contains abundant gram-positive organisms, and a mixture of anaerobic bacteria and low levels of commensal fungi and protozoa. Fermentation supplies glucose and lactose and serves as a significant source of volatile fatty acids. In addition to abundant dry fecal pellets, nutrient-rich cecotrophs are intermittently excreted and are usually promptly reingested. Shifts in the intestinal flora, from inappropriate diets containing low fiber and high carbohydrates, inability to eat coarse grains due to dental disease, or from antibiotic-associated losses (eg, penicillins, bacitracin), allows for proliferation of opportunistic pathogens (*Encephalitozoon coli, Pseudomonas aeruginosa, Clostridium* spp.), or dysbiosis. These pathogenic organisms can cause a secondary bacterial enteritis or enterotoxemia illness, especially in young and immunocompromised animals.[2,3]

The dysbiotic intestinal microenvironment is less efficient at fermentation, leading to gastrointestinal stasis/ileus and increased gas production. Because rabbits, guinea pigs, and chinchillas are unable to vomit or eructate due a prominent limiting ridge at the gastroesophageal junction, this gas accumulates in the stomach causing gastric dilation. Rabbits normally have retained ingesta and fur within their stomachs that are regulated by continuous gastric fluid production and intestinal motility. With hypomotility and subsequent dehydration of gastric and intestinal contents, the retained ingesta and fur pellets coalesce into a firm mass that can cause obstruction. Obstruction is most frequent at the T-shaped junction of the ileum and cecum: the sacculus rotundus. In guinea pigs, gastric distension can be complicated by a life-threatening volvulus.[2,3]

Dental Disease

Rabbits, guinea pigs, and chinchillas have continuously growing (elodont) teeth with long crowns (hypsodont) and no anatomic roots (aradicular).[4] In part due to their increased longevity and less-abrasive diets as pets, their teeth (especially the molars and premolars, or cheek teeth) are not effectively ground, and large enamel points and spurs can form, leading to maladjustment of the occlusal angle with impaired mastication, lingual and buccal mucosal trauma, and even tongue entrapment. Apical crown extension into the maxilla can cause significant bony remodeling and sinonasal complications. Secondary infections and abscess formation are common, and can be difficult to detect in long-haired breeds. In guinea pigs, inadequate vitamin C will accelerate progression of dental disease due to friability of the gingiva and periodontal ligaments. Animals with dental disease develop a preference for softer, low-fiber foods that can exacerbate gastrointestinal stasis and dysbiosis. In addition, incompletely chewed food can form an esophageal obstruction, or choke, especially in chinchillas.[2,4]

Evaluation of Anorexia

Assessment of anorexia requires a detailed clinical history, including husbandry, contacts, diet, and elimination. Initial triage should identify animals that are severely ill (depressed, immobile, recumbent) and might require aggressive resuscitation or surgical intervention. Most anorexic animals will appear lethargic, thin, and with a poor conditioned coat (**Fig. 1**). Of note, sick guinea pigs are generally intolerant of examination, and can even progress rapidly to cardiopulmonary arrest with procedural intervention (refer to **Fig. 2** for handling and venipuncture techniques).[5]

Following vital measurements (see **Table 1** for reference values),[6,7] a detailed examination should include an oral examination with an otoscope and cone or nasal speculum as tolerated. Because of their small size, examination on a nonsedated animal is difficult, and a negative examination cannot exclude underlying dental disease. In rabbits, dental overgrowth causes points on the lateral edges of the upper cheek teeth and on the medial edges of the lower teeth, with corresponding buccal and lingual mucosal ulcerations, respectively (**Fig. 3**B). Incisor malocclusion is also common in rabbits, and more readily apparent to owners (**Fig. 3**A). In guinea pigs, large buccal skin folds and often-abundant food debris (not indicative of impaction) make examination difficult. Evidence of incisor malocclusion usually reflects severe cheek teeth disease that may be more difficult to visualize. Friable mucosa with increased tooth mobility should prompt further assessment of hypovitaminosis C (lameness, joint and soft tissue hematomas, diarrhea). Periapical abscesses often have evidence of facial swelling or even exophthalmos (**Fig. 3**C). Unlike rabbits and other rodents, apical reserve extension can be significant and disproportionate to crown growth in chinchillas, leading to maxillary bone damage and sinonasal and lacrimal disease, even with minimal malocclusion.[4] Genetic predisposition to the development of dental disease is well documented in some chinchillas.[8] Complete assessment of dental disease requires multiple view radiographs and/or computed tomography scan, which can be performed on referral.

Abdominal examination and imaging are essential to help differentiate mild stasis-associated disease from significant gastric dilation requiring decompression, or acute obstruction. Before palpating the abdomen, examine for the presence and consistency of fecal pellets (**Fig. 4**). With stasis, pellets will be reduced in number and are often small, firm, and irregular. With an acute obstruction, pellets may be significantly

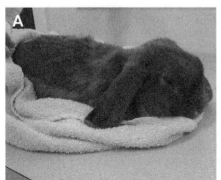
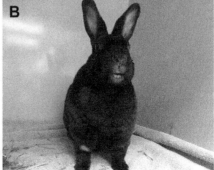

Fig. 1. Presentations of seriously ill rabbits. (*A*) Rabbit with a foreign body obstruction is immobile, minimally interactive, and has a dull coat. (*B*) Rabbit with respiratory distress breathing with an open mouth and flared nostrils.

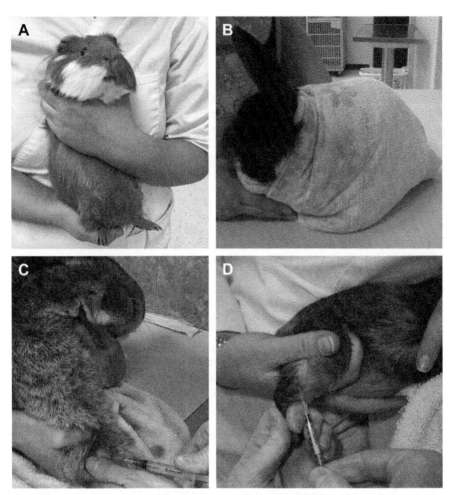

Fig. 2. Handling, restraint, and venipuncture techniques. Rabbits, guinea pigs, and chinchillas are easily stressed with examination and procedures, and care is needed to reduce stress and prioritize examination and procedures. Their hindlimbs are powerful and muscular, yet their skeleton is relatively fragile, making them subject to limb and back fractures with improper restraint and hindlimb support. (*A*) Restraint of guinea pig by supporting its weight with one hand under the thorax and cupping its dorsum and hindquarter with the other. (*B*) Towel restraint in a rabbit (bunny burrito) is useful for facial and dental examination, drug administration, and syringe feeding. (*C*) Rabbit venipuncture using the cephalic vein. (*D*) Guinea pig venipuncture using the lateral saphenous veins. Common accessible sites include the lateral saphenous, cephalic, femoral, jugular, and lateral ear veins.

reduced or even absent. Rectal prolapse may be seen with stasis, especially in chinchillas. In rabbits, abdominal palpation will usually reveal a doughy mass in the cranial abdomen, consistent with a mat of hair and fiber in the stomach (not evidence of obstruction). The stomach may be full, but should be soft and compressible. A small amount of intestinal gas may be normally palpated. A dilated (often below the rib cage), firm, and noncompressible stomach suggests significant dilation and possible obstruction. Fluid-filled and gas-filled intestines also may be palpated in these cases.

Table 1
Normal biologic and physiologic measurements

Parameter	Rabbit	Guinea Pig	Chinchilla
Adult body weight	Male: 1.5–5.0 kg Female: 1.5–6.0 kg	Male: 900–1200 g Female: 700–900 g	Male: 450–600 g Female: 550–800 g
Birth weight, g	30–80	60–100	30–50
Rectal temperature	38.5–40°C (101.3–104°F)	37.2–39.5°C (99–103.1°F)	36.1–37.8°C (97–100°F)
Heart rate, beats per minute	130–325	230–380	100–150
Respiratory rate, breaths per minute	30–60	40–100	40–80
Life span, y	5–6 (up to 15)	4–5	8–10
Breeding onset, male	6–10 mo	90–120 d	240–540 d
Breeding onset, female	4–9 mo	60–90 d	240–540 d
Reproductive cycle	Induced ovulation	—	—
Gestation period, d	29–35	59–72	105–115
Litter size	4–10	2–5	2–3
Weaning age	4–6 wk	14–28 d	36–48 d

Hepatic enlargement may be present from lipidosis, although liver lobe torsion also is a more rare cause of acute anorexia and stasis in rabbits.[9]

Abdominal radiographs are performed to assess for stasis and obstruction. In rabbits, the stomach and cecum normally contain ingesta and a small amount of gas, but a large ingesta-filled stomach or a stomach with a crescent of air surrounding the ingesta is suggestive of stasis (**Fig. 5**). The intestines are often diffusely dilated with generalized stasis, although as a reference remain less than twice the width of L2 in the spine. With isolated gastric dilation, the intestinal gas pattern may be normal. In acute obstruction, the air-filled stomach can extend well below the rib cage (**Fig. 6**). There is often significant intestinal dilation proximal to the obstruction, with absence of air distally, although this can be less noticeable at the ileocecocolic junction. In guinea pigs, massive gastric dilation (especially if there is caudal or right-sided rotation) with minimal intestinal gas is concerning for gastric distension–associated volvulus (**Fig. 7**).[2,3] Although examination and imaging are most often helpful to distinguish stasis from obstruction, the diagnosis can be challenging, and one should remember that true obstruction is a more rare event and surgical intervention is a potentially morbid procedure in these ill patients.

Additional diagnostic evaluations (see **Table 2** for reference values)[6,7] also should be performed to help determine the etiology of stasis and severity of disease. These include a complete blood count (anemia, thrombocytopenia, infection), biochemistry panels (azotemia, renal insufficiency, hepatic lipidosis, ketosis), and urinalysis. Fecal examination and culture for opportunistic pathogens also should be performed, although culture interpretation is often difficult, as opportunistic organisms are normal colonizers.

Treatment of Stasis and Obstruction

Treatment of acute obstruction or gastric dilatation-volvulus (GDV) is aimed at emergent stabilization, correcting fluid losses, providing analgesia, and performing decompression. Carefully monitor vital signs (systolic blood pressure) and place an intravenous (IV) or intraosseous (IO) catheter and administer isotonic crystalloids (up to 100 mL/kg

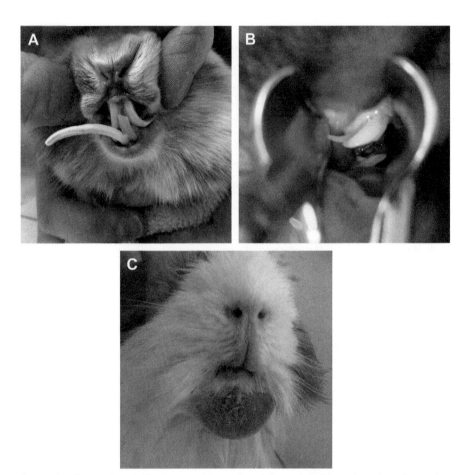

Fig. 3. Significant dental disease requiring referral for sedated imaging, dental examination, and surgical intervention. (*A*) Incisor malocclusion in a rabbit. The presence of incisor malocclusion is often indicative of significant malocclusive disease in the cheek teeth. (*B*) Oral examination in a rabbit with malocclusive disease of the cheek teeth showing abnormal lingual (*bottom*) and buccal (*top*) elongation. (*C*) Periapical (molar tooth reserve crown) abscess in a guinea pig.

per hour to stabilize; refer to rabbit and rodent formularies in **Table 3**) to correct hypovolemia, oxygen, and opioids provided for analgesia (buprenorphine, 0.03–0.05 mg/kg every 6–8 hours; or hydromorphone, 0.1 mg/kg every 8 hours).[10] Antifoaming agents, such as simethicone (70 mg/kg every 1 hour, repeating up to three times), are sometimes used, although their efficacy is controversial. Gastric decompression is attempted using an orogastric tube under light sedation (midazolam, 0.2–1 mg/kg intramuscularly [IM]/IV), as percutaneous trocarization carries a significant risk of gastric rupture. Surgical intervention is generally not successful for GDV, and the overall prognosis is poor. Exploratory surgery may be necessary for obstructed rabbits with evidence of prolonged ileus and/or compacted gastric contents.[2,3,11]

Treatment of unobstructed stasis depends on the severity and duration of the presenting condition. If the appetite is decreased but the animal is stable without evidence of obstruction, outpatient treatment can be done. Administer subcutaneous fluids to correct

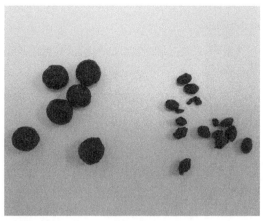

Fig. 4. Normal (left) versus abnormal (right) rabbit feces. Gastrointestinal hypomotility results in passage of fewer fecal pellets that are often small, firm, dry, and irregular in shape.

losses, give a prokinetic (metoclopramide, 0.5 mg/kg subcutaneously [SC]/orally [PO] every 6–12 hours; or cisapride, 0.5 mg/kg PO every 8–12 hours), and supply an easily consumed fiber-rich food (eg, Critical Care, Oxbow Animal Health, Murdock, NE) in addition to their normal diet. If anorexia is more prolonged, but the animal is stable, admission to the hospital is necessary for more careful monitoring of vital signs, more aggressive supportive care, and quiet rest. In addition, provide maintenance fluid therapy (100–120 mL/kg per day IV, or divided every 8 hours SC), analgesia (buprenorphine, 0.01–0.05 mg/kg SC/IV/IM, every 6–12 hours),[12] and treatment for possible gastric ulceration (ranitidine, 2–5 mg/kg PO/SC every 12 hours; or omeprazole, 0.5–1.0 mg/kg PO/IV every 24 hours).[13,14] Supplemental nutrition is given with a critical care diet for herbivores

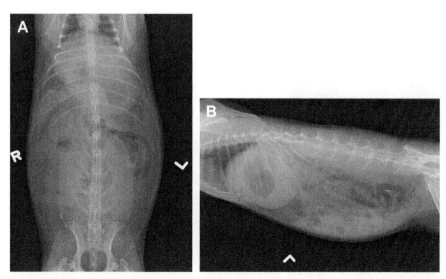

Fig. 5. Survey ventrodorsal (*A*) and lateral (*B*) radiographs of a rabbit with gastrointestinal stasis secondary to dental disease. Note the stomach distention with ingesta and gas pocket and gas within the intestinal tract.

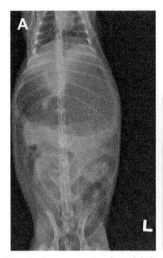
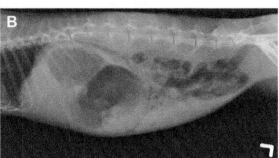

Fig. 6. Survey ventrodorsal (*A*) and lateral (*B*) radiographs of a rabbit with acute gastrointestinal obstruction due to hairball impaction. Note the severely distended gas-filled and fluid-filled stomach with large amounts of gas within the intestines.

(Oxbow Critical Care for Herbivores, Oxbow Animal Health, Murdock, NE; 15 mL/kg every 8 hours syringe feeds; see **Fig. 8**), or if the animal will not accept syringe feeds, a nasogastric tube can be placed and an enteral nutrition formula provided for up to several days ($\sim$ 175 kcal/d for an adult, diluted 50% with water, 20 mL every 6 hours).[15–17] Antibiotics are generally reserved for ill animals with significant dysbiosis/enteritis from gram-negative pathogens. Empiric therapy can be initiated before culture results (trimethoprim sulfa, 30 mg/kg every 12 hours; metronidazole, 20–30 mg/kg every 12 hours; or enrofloxacin, 10–20 mg/kg every 12–24 hours). In our experience, penicillin should not be administered to guinea pigs OR chinchillas. For parasitic enteritis, environmental disinfecting is needed as well as treatment (metronidazole, 20–30 mg/kg PO every 12–24 hours for 5 days; fenbendazole, 20–50 mg/kg PO every 24 hours for 5 days; trimethoprim sulfa, 30 mg/kg PO every 12–24 hours for 5–10 days). Vitamin C supplementation

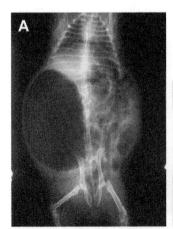
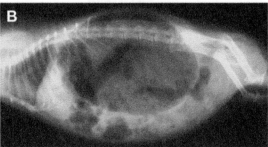

Fig. 7. Survey ventrodorsal (*A*) and lateral (*B*) radiographs of a guinea pig with GDV showing massive gastric distension occupying the entire right hemiabdomen.

Table 2
Hematologic and serum biochemical values of rabbits and rodents

Measurement	Rabbits	Guinea Pig	Chinchillas
Packed cell volume, %	30–50	35–45	27–54
Red blood cells, $10^6/\mu L$	4–8	4–7	5.6–8.4
Hemoglobin, g/dL	8–17.5	11–17	11.8–14.6
White blood cells, $10^3/\mu L$	5–12	7–14	5.4–15.6
Neutrophils, %	35–55	20–60	39–54
Lymphocytes, %	25–60	30–80	45–60
Monocytes, %	2–10	2–20	0–5
Eosinophils, %	0–5	0–5	0–5
Basophils, %	2–8	0–1	0–1
Alkaline phosphatase, U/L	4–70	—	6–72
Alanine transaminase, U/L	14–80	10–25	10–35
Amylase, U/L	200–500	—	—
Aspartate aminotransferase, U/L	14–113	—	96
Bicarbonate, mEq/L	16.2–31.8	—	—
Bile acids, $\mu mol/L$	<40	—	—
Bilirubin, total, mg/dL	0–0.75	0.3–0.9	0.6–1.3
Calcium, mg/dL	8–14.8	7.8–10.5	5.6–12.1
Chloride, mEq/L	92–112	98–115	108–129
Cholesterol, mg/dL	12–116	20–43	50–302
Creatinine, mg/dL	0.5–2.6	0.6–2.2	0.4–1.3
Glucose, mg/dL	75–150	60–125	109–193
Phosphorus, mg/dL	2.3–6.9	5.3	4–8
Potassium, mEq/L	3.5–7	6.8–8.9	3.3–5.7
Protein, total, g/dL	5.4–7.5	4.6–6.2	3.8–5.6
Albumin, g/dL	2.5–5	2.1–3.9	2.3–4.1
Globulin, g/dL	1.5–3.5	1.7–2.6	0.9–2.2
Sodium, mEq/L	138–155	146–152	142–166
Triglycerides, mg/dL	124–156	0–145	—
Urea nitrogen, mg/dL	15–50	9–32	17–45

(50–100 mg/kg daily) is provided if clinically indicated in guinea pigs.[2] Animals treated for unobstructed stasis should begin to show some clinical improvement and increased fecal pellets within 12 to 24 hours, although significant improvement may not be evident for several days.

RESPIRATORY DISEASE

Rabbits are obligate nasal breathers, so even upper respiratory infections can cause severe respiratory compromise. Infections commonly result from direct extension of dental infections into the nasal cavity, nasal foreign bodies (food), and from opportunistic overgrowth of commensal organisms, most notably *Pasteurella multocida* and *Bordetella bronchiseptica*.[18,19] Opportunistic infections occur in rabbits with suboptimal husbandry (overcrowding, exposure to high levels of ammonia and particulates), as well as in young rabbits and those with immune suppression. Both upper and lower disease present with dyspnea, and stridor or open mouth breathing can be observed, the latter being a poor

Table 3
Rabbit and rodent formulary

Agent	Rabbit Dosage	Rodent Dosage
Antimicrobial		
Enrofloxacin (Baytril, Bayer)	5–10 mg/kg PO, SC, IM q12h Limit or dilute SC, IM injections (necrosis)	5–20 mg/kg PO, SC, IM q12h Limit or dilute SC, IM injections (necrosis)
Penicillin G (Benzathine form)	42,000–84,000 IU/kg SC q7d Do not give oral penicillins to rabbits	22,000 IU/kg IM q24h Do not give penicillins to guinea pigs, avoid or use with caution in chinchillas
Metronidazole	20 mg/kg PO q12h 40 mg/kg PO q24h	10–20 mg/kg PO q12h Loss of appetite in chinchillas
Trimethoprim sulfa	15–30 mg/kg PO q12h 30 mg/kg SC, IM q12h SC may cause necrosis	15–30 mg/kg PO, SC, IM q12h SC may cause necrosis
Antiparasitic		
Fenbendazole	20 mg/kg PO q24h × 28d (*Encephalitozoon cuniculi* dosing) Rare aplastic anemia and arteritis reported	20–50 mg/kg PO q24h × 5d (antiprotozoal dosing)
Ivermectin	0.2–0.4 mg/kg SC q10–14d 0.4 mg/kg for ectoparasites	0.2–0.4 mg/kg SC q7–14d 0.4 mg/kg for ectoparasites
Metronidazole	20 mg/kg PO q12h (antiprotozoal dosing)	25 mg/kg PO q12h Loss of appetite in chinchillas
Selamectin (Revolution, Pfizer)	12 mg/kg topically apply at base of neck	6 mg/kg (chinchillas) 20–30 mg/kg (guinea pigs)
Analgesic		
Buprenorphine	0.01–0.05 mg/kg SC, IV, IM q6–12h	0.05–0.1 mg/kg SC q6–12h
Meloxicam (Metacam, Boehringer Ingelheim Vetmedica)	0.3 mg/kg PO q24h × 10d	≥0.5 mg/kg PO, SC q24h
Ophthalmologic		
Ciprofloxacin, 0.3% (Ciloxan, Alcon)	Topical to eyes q8–12h	Topical to eyes q8–12h
Ketorolac tromethamine 0.1% (NSAID)	Topical to eyes q8–12h	Topical to eyes q8–12h
Gastrointestinal		
Activated charcoal (1 g/5 mL water)	1 g/kg PO q4–6h	1 g/kg PO q4–6h
Simethicone	65–130 mg q1h × 2–3 prn	70 mg/kg q1h × 2–3 prn
Cimetidine	5–10 mg/kg PO, SC, IM, IV q6–12h	5–10 mg/kg PO, SC, IM, IV q6–12h
Ranitidine	2–5 mg/kg PO, SC q12h	2–5 mg/kg PO, SC q12h
Metoclopramide	0.2–1 mg/kg PO, SC q6–8h	0.2–1 mg/kg PO, SC, IM q12h
Cisapride (Propulsid, Janssen)	0.5 mg/kg PO q8–12h	0.5 mg/kg PO q8–12h
Lactated Ringer solution	100–150 mL/kg/d constant rate infusion or divided SC q6–12h (maintenance fluids)	50–100 mL/kg/d constant rate infusion or divided SC q6–12h (maintenance fluids)

Abbreviations: IM, intramuscular; IV, intravenous; NSAID, nonsteroidal anti-inflammatory drug; PO, oral; prn, as needed; q, every; SC, subcutaneous.

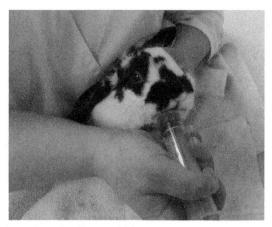

Fig. 8. Technique for syringe feeding a rabbit.

prognostic sign (see **Fig. 1**B). Rabbits with upper respiratory disease have clear to muco-purulent nasal and/or ocular discharge. On physical examination, there may be audible harsh breathing and inspiratory rales with upper airway disease; and crackles, wheezes, or diminished sounds with lower airway disease and pneumonia. Culture and sensitivity can be performed from nasal aspirate and lavage samples. Radiographs can be helpful to determine the etiology and extent of upper respiratory disease, and to confirm broncho-pneumonia or consolidation in the thorax. Complete blood count is helpful, and neutro-philia, leukopenia, anemia of chronic disease may be seen. Treatment is aimed at resolving dyspnea with oxygen therapy, supportive care, and antibiotics (enrofloxacin, 5–10 mg/kg PO every 12 hours; or trimethoprim sulfa 30 mg/kg PO every 12 hours) for 14 days, providing an extended course if needed.[18]

Pneumonia is a common infection in pet guinea pigs. Most cases result from oppor-tunistic infections with *Streptococcus pneumoniae* and *B bronchiseptica*, both of which are asymptomatically carried in many guinea pigs. Infection arises during conditions of stress, inappropriate housing and ventilation, introduction of new animals, hypovitami-nosis C, and cohousing with rabbits, which are normally colonized with *B bronchisep-tica*. Mild respiratory disease also may be associated with guinea pig adenovirus.[20] Clinical presentation is variable, and can include dyspnea, nasal discharge, sneezing, lethargy, and anorexia. Concomitant middle ear infections are not uncommon and can present as torticollis and/or nystagmus. In addition to physical examination findings of respiratory infection, radiographs should demonstrate bronchopneumonia or consolidation and possible pleural effusion. Complete blood count and biochemistry panel are helpful to document infection and possible dehydration or early sepsis. Cul-ture and sensitivity from exudate or aspirates can be performed, knowing that both spe-cies can normally be cultured from asymptomatic pigs. Therapy is aimed at stabilizing the acutely ill patient, and providing supportive care, including supplemental oxygen, fluid therapy, nutritional support (necessary with antibiotic administration) with vitamin C, and antibiotic therapy (trimethoprim sulfa, 30 mg/kg PO/SC every 12 hours; or enrofloxacin, 10–20 mg/kg every 24 hours) for several weeks.[20]

GENITOURINARY DISEASE
Urolithiasis and Sediment

Stranguria and hematuria from urolithiasis is a common emergency presentation in guinea pigs (**Fig. 9**A). Calculi are typically radiopaque calcium salts, and

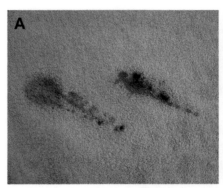
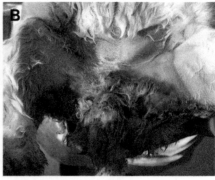

Fig. 9. Complications of urolithiasis and cystitis. (*A*) Hematuria spotting on a cage towel from a guinea pig. (*B*) Severe urine scalding and superficial ulcerations in a rabbit.

hypercalcemia from an alfalfa-based diet is a known risk factor.[21] Cystitis is a common complication. Animals may have a hunched posture and can vocalize during urination. On physical examination, cystic calculi can be palpated, and an enlarged nonexpressible urinary bladder is present with urethral obstruction. Urinalysis, urine culture, complete blood count, and calcium levels can document hypercalcemia, urinary calculi, and possible azotemia from obstruction, or potential infection. Abdominal radiographs should be taken with the hind limbs stretched away from the body to visualize possible urethral calculi. Ultrasound is also helpful to localize calculi. Minimally invasive, catheter-based stone removal can be attempted for small urethral sediment, but cystotomy is required to remove cystic calculi. Fluid therapy should be initiated and nutritional support and pain management provided. Empiric treatment for concurrent cystitis can also be started (trimethoprim sulfa, 30 mg/kg PO every 12 hours) before culture results. Following surgery and diuresis, dietary modifications to reduce calcium intake can be helpful, including using timothy hay and pellets instead of alfalfa, and avoiding fresh greens. Potassium citrate (47 mg/kg PO every 24 hours) may be useful in preventing urinary calcium precipitation, but uroliths in guinea pigs frequently recur.[22]

Although rabbits normally excrete porphyrin pigments giving the urine a rust color, true hematuria most commonly occurs due to cystitis, calcium sediment, and in older female rabbits, uterine adenocarcinoma. Calciuria, presumed from excessive intake of calcium-rich foods like alfalfa, is seen in many rabbits. Urinary retention and chronic cystitis are believed to precipitate the formation of calcium carbonate micro-urinary calculi, or bladder sludge. These are smaller than uroliths seen in guinea pigs, but can still produce urethral obstruction.[23] On physical examination, the obstructed bladder will be firm and distended. Urine scalding may be present (**Fig. 9**B). Laboratory assessment includes a complete blood count (leukocytosis), biochemistry panel (renal insufficiency, dehydration, azotemia), and urinalysis and culture (hematuria, proteinuria, infection, sediment). Radiographs can detect calcium calculi, but a small amount of sludge is normal. Treat underlying infections with appropriate antibiotics (trimethoprim sulfa 30 mg/kg PO every 12 hours; or enrofloxacin, 5–10 mg/kg PO every 12 hours), and supply diuresis to aid in flushing sediment gradually. If needed, sediment is removed by manual expression of the bladder with or without sedation (midazolam, 0.5–2 mg/kg IM/IV; or diazepam, 0.5 mg/kg IM) or general anesthesia,[12] followed by catheterization and abundant flushing with saline. Larger calculi and ureteroliths require cystotomy for removal. High-calcium foods, alfalfa, and vitamin and mineral supplements should be minimized postoperatively and diuresis maintained by adequate hydration.[24] Urinary calculi are also seen in chinchillas, although less commonly than in guinea pigs and rabbits. Diagnosis and treatment are essentially the same as in those species.[25]

Paraphimosis

Adult male chinchillas can present with paraphimosis due to a restrictive ring of fur and smegma at the base of the penis (fur ring). This is most common in breeding males, but also seen in pets, and can present with stranguria, excessive grooming of the area, lethargy, and anorexia. On identification of fur ring, the penis can be lubricated and the material removed. In cases of paraphimosis, a hypertonic solution (50% dextrose) can be applied to reduce edema. Fur rings can lead to infection of the prepuce and glans penis (balanoposthitis), most commonly from *P aeruginosa*, and antibiotic therapy can be considered if there is evidence of more systemic infection.[25,26]

NEUROLOGIC DISEASE
Vestibular Disease: Torticollis

Head tilt from vestibular disease is one of the more dramatic presentations in rabbits (**Fig. 10**A). There are thought to be 2 primary infectious causes. Peripheral vestibular disease can result from otitis interna infections with *P multocida* that damage the inner ear labyrinth, petrous bone, and vestibular nerve. Central disease can result from central nervous system infections with *Encephalitozoon cuniculi* that damage the vestibular nuclei and pathways. Vestibular damage also can result from toxins (lead), trauma (vertebral fracture, petrous or tympanic bulla fracture), degenerative joint disease or spondylosis, metabolic disease (hepatic encephalopathy), cerebrovascular disease, and neoplasia. Affected rabbits present with acute-onset head tilt, and can also have nystagmus, ataxia, circling (toward the lesion), rolling, lateral recumbency, and rarely seizures.[27] On examination, assess cranial nerve and general neurologic function.[28] Evidence of respiratory compromise, mucopurulent discharge, or otitis can suggest pasteurellosis. Examine and stain for traumatic corneal ulcerations. Complete blood count may show regenerative anemia with basophilic stippling with lead toxicity, and a level can be obtained. Biochemistry panel can show dehydration, evidence of renal insufficiency with encephalitozoonosis, or hepatic dysfunction. *E cuniculi* titers should be obtained and nasal and/or otic discharge should be cultured. Radiographic

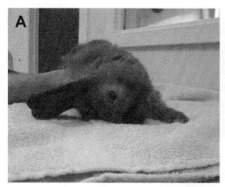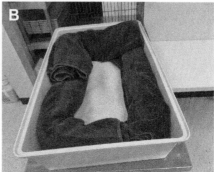

Fig. 10. (*A*) Torticollis in a rabbit. The head deviates toward the affected side. (*B*) Padding cages is helpful to protect vestibular rabbits from injury.

analysis is useful to examine for fractures and bony abnormalities, although many studies are normal. Accurate antemortem diagnosis is difficult, and postmortem histopathologic analysis is often required for a definitive diagnosis.[27]

Treatment is aimed at supportive care and antibiotics for infectious causes. The cage should be padded (**Fig. 10**B) and the rabbit propped in a sternal position to avoid further injury. Subcutaneous fluid therapy and supplemental nutritional support are provided (food, syringe feeds, or nasogastric feeds depending on ability). Disorientation and rolling can be abated with meclizine HCl (12.5–25 mg/kg PO every 8–12 hours). In the absence of a noninfectious etiology, start treatment for empiric *P multocida* infection with enrofloxacin (10 mg/kg every 12 hours) or trimethoprim sulfa (30 mg/kg every 12 hours), pending culture and *E cuniculi* titers. Empiric treatment for encephalitozoonosis (fenbendazole, 20 mg/kg every 24 hours for 28 days) is controversial and generally not recommended, as it has been associated with cases of potentially lethal aplastic anemia.[29] Seizures are a rare complication, and can be treated with diazepam or midazolam (1–2 mg/kg). Corticosteroids are contraindicated in the treatment of vestibular disease due to the immunosuppressive and gastrointestinal side effects in rabbits.[27,30]

CUTANEOUS DISEASE
Sarcoptic Mange

Ectoparasitic infections are seen in all species, but are particularly severe in guinea pigs, often prompting emergency presentation. Ectoparasitic infection with *Trixacarus caviae* is transmitted by direct infection, and is most commonly seen following introduction of a new infected animal or in older guinea pigs with compromised immune systems.[25] The sarcoptid mite lives in the outer layers of the skin, causing intense pruritus, scaling and crusting, and alopecia (**Fig. 11**). Self-inflicted wounds from scratching and biting are common, as are neurologic behaviors such as circling. Intense pruritus can produce short episodes of seizurelike activity requiring emergent evaluation and antiepileptic therapy. Treatment (all in-contact animals) is with selamectin (15–30 mg/kg topically every 2–3 weeks) or ivermectin (0.2–0.5 mg/kg SC/PO every 7–14 days), as well as environmental decontamination. We have found ivermectin to be superior for treating severe infestations. Infections are also contagious to humans.[22,25]

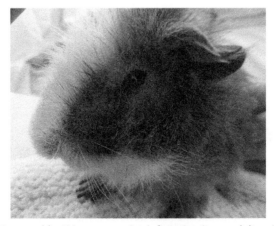

Fig. 11. Dermatitis caused by *Trixacarus caviae* infestation in an adult guinea pig.

Urine Scalding

Perineal scalding from urine can be severe in rabbits (see **Fig. 9B**). In addition to urinary obstruction and cystitis, other causes include urinary incontinence (neurologic disease, spinal trauma, encephalitozoonosis), incorrect posturing (obesity, arthritis, cramped housing, pododermatitis), prominent perineal skin folds (obesity), and reproductive disease (*Treponema* infection).[24] Initial assessment includes examination for possible urinary obstruction and neurologic disease, as well as other biomechanical and infectious causes. The skin of the perineum, inner thighs, tail, and rump should be carefully examined to look for evidence of secondary infection. Scalded and devitalized areas are prone to infestation with fly maggots, especially when housed outdoors in the summer months, which may be concealed in matted fur. Following initiation of supportive care and sedation if needed (midazolam, 0.5–2 mg/kg IM/IV; diazepam, 0.5–2 mg/kg IM), the scalded areas should be carefully clipped to remove all residual fur, and cleaned with a chlorhexidine-based shampoo. Maggots should be thoroughly removed and devitalized skin debrided, if required. The site should be gently cleaned daily and treated with topical silver sulfadiazine (avoid topical antibiotics that can be ingested). Rabbits also should be discharged with an analgesic (meloxicam, 0.3–0.5 mg/kg PO every 24 hours), antibiotics for secondary infection (trimethoprim sulfa, 30 mg/kg PO every 12 hours), and/or an antiparasitic agent for myiasis (ivermectin, 0.4 mg/kg SC, with second dose at follow-up in 14 days), in addition to any treatments required for the underlying cause of urinary dysfunction.[24,31]

Fur Slip

As a prey species, chinchillas have developed a method to epilate large patches of fur when grabbed under stress, including improper handling of pets. It is important to recognize fur slip, a harmless physiologic response, and differentiate it from infectious and nutritional causes of alopecia. On examination, fur slip results in a well-demarcated area of alopecia with exposure of smooth, healthy skin. The back of the neck and hindquarters are common sites. Patchy alopecia with thick and flaky skin may be evidence of an underlying nutritional deficiency (fatty acids, zinc) or dermatophytosis; and patchy alopecia in the shoulders, flanks, and paws may be due to fur chewing from environmental stressors, systemic illness, or dental disease. Treatment of alopecia is dependent on the underlying etiology. No treatment is necessary for fur slip aside from counseling on proper handling, and the fur is generally replaced within 4 to 6 months.[25]

REPRODUCTIVE DISEASE
Pregnancy Toxemia

Pregnancy toxemia, more common in guinea pigs, is a complication of late gestation or peripartum that is caused by the increased metabolic demands of late pregnancy and early lactation, particularly in obese animals with fatty livers. Another type can also result from uteroplacental ischemia and obstruction of central venous return due to compression by the gravid uterus (preeclampsia type, mostly in guinea pigs). Pregnant animals presenting with anorexia, depression, and collapse should be emergently evaluated for pregnancy toxemia, as death can occur within days. Hypertension is present with preeclampsia. Abdominal ultrasound is helpful to assess fetal number and viability. Laboratory assessment (complete blood count, biochemistry panel, urinalysis) is necessary to assess for metabolic dysregulation/ketosis, or infection. Treatment is with aggressive supportive care, including IV/IO fluid rehydration, dextrose, nutritional support, analgesia, and emergency cesarean delivery if hypertension or other evidence of uteroplacental insufficiency is present. The prognosis is often grave.[22,32]

Dystocia

In older, often obese guinea pigs bred for the first time after 7 to 8 months of age, there is a marked increase in dystocia and stillbirths due to inadequate separation of the pubic symphysis. During normal parturition, pups are delivered within a 30-minute period, with a 5-minute rest period between pups.[22,32] Dystocia should be considered when a gravid female strains for more than 20 minutes, or fails to produce any pups after 2 hours of intermittent straining. On examination, the pubic symphysis should have at least a finger width of separation to permit passage of pups. Ultrasound is needed to assess the number and viability of pups. Laboratory assessment should be performed to look for evidence of toxemia, metabolic complications, or infection. Initial treatment is with supportive care, including fluid therapy, nutritional support, and analgesia as detailed previously. If the pubic symphysis has separated, oxytocin (1–2 units IM) can be given and the vagina lubricated to assist parturition. If this fails to resolve the dystocia, or if the symphysis fails to separate, cesarean delivery is necessary.[22,32]

TRAUMA AND SHOCK
Heat Stroke

Because guinea pigs and chinchillas are adapted to higher elevation and mountain environments, they are relatively heat intolerant, and can develop heat stroke with prolonged exposure to temperatures above 80°F (28°C) and in high humidity. Animals housed in poorly ventilated enclosures next to radiators or sunny windows are at risk throughout the year. Heat stroke is most common in chinchillas. Affected animals can present with hyperthermia, lethargy progressing to recumbency, ptyalism, panting, and/or poor peripheral perfusion.[25] Animals should be gradually cooled with water baths, avoiding rapid cooling that can cause fatal hypothermia. Alcohol can be applied to the feet and ears. Aggressive parenteral fluid therapy is also needed to improve perfusion and replace evaporative losses. Nonsteroidal anti-inflammatory agents or corticosteroids have been used to minimize toxemia, but the latter is not recommended. The prognosis is generally guarded.[26]

Limb Fractures

Limb fractures are not an uncommon presentation to emergency clinics, particularly in the elongated delicate limbs of chinchillas. Housing in cages with wire mesh that permits feet and/or limbs to become entrapped and rough handling are the most common causes of limb fractures. Fractures are not always apparent at rest, but should be detected on ambulation, prompting owners to seek attention. Recent fractures can be set with a splint or cast, and stabilized with an internal pin as needed. For severe fractures with excessive tissue trauma, amputation may be necessary. Fracture callous formation is quick (1–2 weeks) facilitating an acceptable recovery in most.[33]

Traumatic Wounds

Conspecific bite wounds are common in small exotics, either from dominant females attacking males, or from existing animals attacking a newly introduced animal (**Fig. 12**). Bite wounds from other household pets, particularly dogs, are also common. Diagnosis is based on history of attack, and clinical evidence of puncture wounds, lacerations, contusions, or if trauma was more remote, skin necrosis and/or abscess. The patient should be quickly assessed, stabilized, and given fluids, analgesics, and

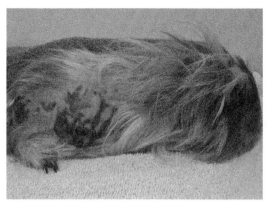

Fig. 12. Trauma caused by cage mate attack in an adult guinea pig.

antibiotics as previously mentioned. Wound care is similar to that for other species. A more detailed examination can be performed under sedation or general anesthesia, wherein penetrating open wounds should be explored to rule out internal injury, and aerobic and anaerobic cultures obtained. Surgical debridement and thorough lavage with warm saline is performed, and open wounds left to attempt healing by secondary intention. The animal should be discharged with analgesics and antibiotics with scheduled follow-up.[33]

Ocular Trauma

Chinchillas (and to a lesser degree rabbits and guinea pigs) have large eyes, predisposing them to ocular trauma and infections. Excessive sand bathing, inappropriate sand, poor housing (sharp edges), or even sharp hay can cause corneal ulceration. Secondary colonization of defects may lead to conjunctivitis, most commonly from *P aeruginosa* in chinchillas and *Chlamydophila caviae* in guinea pigs.[25,26] Bone remodeling and abscessation from maxillary dental disease, or inflammatory sinonasal disease can obliterate the nasolacrimal duct and cause ocular discharge, or epiphora. Animals will present with serous-milky (epiphora) or purulent (abscess, conjunctivitis) ocular discharge; with painful red (conjunctivitis) or cloudy (corneal ulceration) eye(s); and/or with possible blepharospasm. Findings of dental disease or respiratory or systemic infection may be present. Conjunctival or corneal culture samples should be obtained before detailed ocular examination. Palpation of the maxilla may reveal a mass from bony remodeling or abscess. Assess cranial nerve, corneal, and pupillary reflexes to determine extent of involvement. Fluorescein dye should be applied to the corneal surface to look for ulceration.[33]

Epiphora is commonly treated with a broad approach, including topical nonsteroidal anti-inflammatory drugs (flurbiprofen, 0.03% solution, or diclofenac, 0.1% solution, every 6–12 hours for 10–14 days), systemic anti-inflammatory agents (meloxicam, 0.3–0.5 mg/kg PO every 12–24 hours for 10–14 days), and topical broad-spectrum antibiotics (tobramycin, gentamycin, ciprofloxacin, or oxytetracycline/polymyxin B for 7–10 days). In rabbits, the lacrimal duct is catheterized and flushed with saline, but this is not possible in smaller animals. Epiphora often recurs and is irreversible if long-standing damage has obliterated the lacrimal duct. For localized conjunctivitis, culture is followed by thorough lavage with saline. Topical broad-spectrum antibiotics are used, and if there is evidence of systemic infection, empirical therapy can be started (enrofloxacin, 10–20 mg/kg SC/IM/IV every 12–24 hours; or ceftazidime,

25 mg/kg SC/IM/IV every 8 hours). Corneal ulcerations also should be treated with topical antibiotics, and atropine (1% solution or ointment) and systemic anti-inflammatory agents (meloxicam) also have been used. Chinchilla sand baths should be restricted until the ocular disease resolves.[25,26]

ACKNOWLEDGMENTS

The author thanks Dr Kerry Korber and Dr Leticia Materi and the staff of Calgary Avian and Exotic Pet Clinic for providing many of the radiographic and clinical images for this article.

REFERENCES

1. Harcourt-Brown F. Anorexia in rabbits. Causes and effects. Practice 2002;24: 358–67.
2. DeCubellis J, Graham J. Gastrointestinal disease in guinea pigs and rabbits. Vet Clin North Am Exot Anim Pract 2013;16:421–35.
3. Huynh M, Pignon C. Gastrointestinal disease in exotic small mammals. J Exo Pet Med 2013;22:118–31.
4. Capello V. Dental diseases. In: Capello V, Gracis M, Lennox AM, editors. Rabbit and rodent dentistry handbook. 1st edition. Ames (IA): Wiley-Blackwell; 2005. p. 113–63.
5. Joslin JO. Blood collection techniques in exotic small mammals. J Exo Pet Med 2009;18(2):117–39.
6. Mayer J. Rodents. In: Carpenter JW, Marion CR, editors. Exotic animal formulary. 4th edition. St Louis (MO): Elsevier Saunders; 2013. p. 477–516.
7. Fiorello CV, Divers SJ. Rabbits. In: Carpenter JW, Marion CR, editors. Exotic animal formulary. 4th edition. St Louis: Elsevier Saunders; 2013. p. 518–59.
8. Jekl V, Hauptman K, Knotek Z. Quantitative and qualitative assessments of intraoral lesions in 180 small herbivorous mammals. Vet Rec 2008;162:442–9.
9. Graham J, Basseches J. Liver lobe torsion in pet rabbits clinical consequences, diagnosis, and treatment. Vet Clin North Am Exot Anim Pract 2014;17:195–202.
10. Lichtenberger M, Lennox AM. Critical care of the exotic companion mammal (with a focus on herbivorous species): the first twenty-four hours. J Exo Pet Med 2012; 21:284–92.
11. Harcourt-Brown TR. Management of acute gastric dilation in rabbits. J Exo Pet Med 2007;16(3):168–74.
12. Hawkins MG. Advances in exotic mammal clinical therapeutics. J Exo Pet Med 2014;23:39–49.
13. Hedley J. Critical care of the rabbit. Practice 2011;33:386–91.
14. Remillard RL. Parenteral nutrition support in rabbits and ferrets. J Exo Pet Med 2006;15(4):248–54.
15. Whittington JK. Esophagostomy feeding tube use and placement in exotic pets. J Exo Pet Med 2013;22:178–91.
16. Rosen LB. Nasogastric tube placement in rabbits. J Exo Pet Med 2011;20(1): 27–31.
17. Orosz SE. Critical care nutrition for exotic animals. J Exo Pet Med 2013;22: 163–77.
18. Lennox AM. Respiratory diseases and pasteurellosis. In: Quesenberry KE, Carpenter JW, editors. Ferrets, rabbits and rodents. Clinical medicine and surgery. 3rd edition. St Louis (MO): Elsevier Saunders; 2012. p. 205–16.

19. Rougier S, Galland D, Boucher S, et al. Epidemiology and susceptibility of pathogenic bacteria responsible for upper respiratory tract infections in pet rabbits. Vet Microbiol 2006;115(1–3):192–8.
20. Yarto-Jaramillo E. Respiratory system anatomy, physiology, and disease: guinea pigs and chinchillas. Vet Clin North Am Exot Anim Pract 2011;14:339–55.
21. Hawkins MG, Ruby AL, Drazenovich TL, et al. Composition and characteristics of urinary calculi from guinea pigs. J Am Vet Med Assoc 2009;234:214–20.
22. Hawkins MG, Bishop CR. Disease problems of guinea pigs. In: Quesenberry KE, Carpenter JW, editors. Ferrets, rabbits and rodents. Clinical medicine and surgery. 3rd edition. St Louis (MO): Elsevier Saunders; 2012. p. 295–310.
23. Jenkins JR. Rabbit diagnostic testing. J Exo Pet Med 2008;17(1):4–15.
24. Richardson V. Urogenital diseases in rabbits. Practice 2012;34:554–63.
25. Riggs SM, Mitchell MA. Chinchillas. In: Mitchel MA, Tully TN, editors. Manual of exotic pet practice. 1st edition. St Louis (MO): WB Saunders; 2009. p. 474–91.
26. Mains C, Donnelly TM. Disease problems of chinchillas. In: Quesenberry KE, Carpenter JW, editors. Ferrets, rabbits and rodents. Clinical medicine and surgery. 3rd edition. St Louis (MO): Elsevier Saunders; 2012. p. 311–25.
27. Meredith AL, Richardson J. Neurological diseases of rabbits and rodents. J Exo Pet Med 2015;24:21–33.
28. Mancinelli E. Neurologic examination and diagnostic testing in rabbits, ferrets, and rodents. J Exo Pet Med 2015;24:52–64.
29. Graham JE, Garner MM, Reavill DR. Benzimidazole toxicosis in rabbits: 13 cases (2003-2001). J Exo Pet Med 2014;23:188–95.
30. Fisher PG, Carpenter JW. Neurologic and musculoskeletal diseases. In: Quesenberry KE, Carpenter JW, editors. Ferrets, rabbits and rodents. Clinical medicine and surgery. 3rd edition. St Louis (MO): Elsevier Saunders; 2012. p. 245–56.
31. Harcourt-Brown F. Skin diseases. In: Textbook of rabbit medicine. London: Butterworth; 2002. p. 229–32.
32. Bishop CR. Reproductive medicine of rabbits and rodents. Vet Clin North Am Exot Anim Pract 2002;5:507–35.
33. Johnson DH. Emergency presentations of the exotic small mammalian herbivore trauma patient. J Exo Pet Med 2012;21:300–15.

Medical and Surgical Emergencies in Ferrets

Nicola Di Girolamo, DMV, GPCert(ExAP), MSc(EBHC)*,
Paolo Selleri, DMV, PhD, DECZM (Herpetology & Small Mammals)

KEYWORDS

- Small mammals • Seizures • Hypoglycemia • Critical care • Congestive heart failure
- Trauma • Intoxication • Chylothorax

KEY POINTS

- Hypoglycemic seizure is one of the most common emergencies in ferrets.
- Primary hypoparathyroidism needs to be considered in seizuring ferrets with low calcium, high phosphorus, and maintained renal function.
- Anemia is a common consequence of hyperestrogenism, which typically results from uncontrolled estrus in female ferrets or adrenal disease; currently, medical alternatives to gonadectomy and adrenalectomy should be considered.
- Gastrointestinal foreign bodies and biliary disorders are both common causes of acute abdomen in ferrets.
- Congestive heart failure is usually secondary to valvular disorder, atrioventricular block, dilated and restrictive cardiomyopathies, and hypertension and requires immediate medical treatment (eg, diuretics, thoracentesis).

 Video content accompanies this article at http://www.vetexotic.theclinics.com

INTRODUCTION

Ferrets presented for an emergency should be immediately triaged. The cardiovascular (mucous membrane color, capillary refill time, and pulse rate and quality), respiratory (rate and effort), and central nervous (consciousness) systems should be assessed early.[1] If the ferret is considered unstable, further evaluation of vital physiologic parameters (blood pressure, rectal temperature, oxygen saturation of hemoglobin [SpO_2], electrocardiogram [ECG], and blood glucose) is required together with a prompt institution of treatment (**Fig. 1**). If the ferret is considered stable, further historical questioning and a complete physical examination may proceed.

The author has nothing to disclose.
Clinica per Animali Esotici, Centro Veterinario Specialistico, Via Sandro Giovannini 53, Roma 00137, Italy
* Corresponding author.
E-mail address: nicoladiggi@gmail.com

Vet Clin Exot Anim 19 (2016) 431–464
http://dx.doi.org/10.1016/j.cvex.2016.01.006
1094-9194/16/$ – see front matter © 2016 Elsevier Inc. All rights reserved.

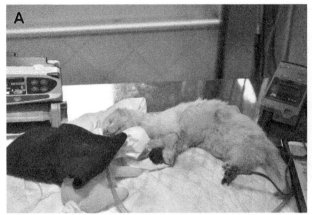
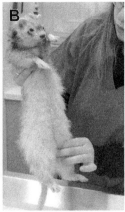

Fig. 1. Preliminary hospitalization approach to an instable ferret (*A*). Notice SpO$_2$ measurement, oxygen, and IV fluid therapy from the cephalic vein. During triage, pulse is easily obtained by palpation of the femoral arteries (*B*).

SEIZURES

Seizures commonly occur in ferrets and may be consequent to a wide variety of causes. However, true spontaneous epileptic seizures have never been described in ferrets, and seizures are usually reactive, that is, caused by metabolic or toxic conditions.[2] Hypoglycemia is considered the most common condition causing seizures in ferrets; however, other conditions, including electrolyte disorders, intoxication, hepatic encephalopathy, hypothyroidism, uremic encephalopathy, hypoxia, and hyperglycemia, may also be the cause.[3]

Hypoglycemia

Hypoglycemic seizures are an extremely common emergency presentation in ferrets. Typically, hypoglycemia in ferrets is the consequence of hyperinsulinemia caused by pancreatic β-cell tumors (ie, insulinomas).[4–6] Other causes that should be included in the differentials for hypoglycemia include anorexia, liver disorders, and hypoadrenocorticism.[7] Ferrets with severe hypoglycemic crises are usually stuporous and may present with opisthotonus (Video 1) and nystagmus (Video 2). Often the crises are accompanied by vocalizations (Video 3).

Diagnosis of hypoglycemia is based on detection of a blood glucose level lower than 60 to 70 mg/dL.[8,9] Although tempting for its easiness, diagnosis of hypoglycemia should never be based only on the use of portable blood glucose meters (PBGM). PBGM for use in humans unpredictably underestimate blood glucose in ferrets[10] and have specificity for diagnosis of hypoglycemia in ferrets of 50%,[9] which means that half of the ferrets in which the PBGM detect hypoglycemia are actually normoglycemic (false positives).[9] PBGM developed for canine and feline patients (Alphatrak, Abbott, Abbott Park, IL) provide results that are more in agreement with laboratory analyzers.[10] However, given the clinical importance of the diagnosis, these methods should be mainly used for screening and monitoring instead of for diagnosing. Instead, the diagnosis on presentation should be based on a hexokinase-based laboratory analyzer whenever possible. An empirical approach to the ferret presented with suspected hypoglycemic seizures is as follows:

- Placement of an intravenous (IV) catheter preferably in the cephalic vein (**Fig. 2**) under manual restraint. Alternatively, catheterize the saphenous or jugular vein (**Fig. 3**).

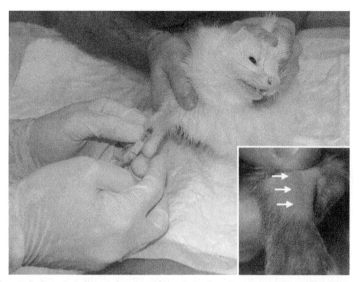

Fig. 2. The cephalic vein is the author's preferred site for placement of IV catheters in conscious ferrets. Inset: notice the straight course of the vein (*arrows*). (*Courtesy of* Nicola Di Girolamo, Rome, Italy.)

Intraosseous catheterization should be avoided, because with proper technique, IV catheterization is almost always feasible.

- Collect an adequate amount of blood from the catheter itself in a lithium-heparin–coated tube. Alternatively, obtain a blood sample to be placed in the collection tube under manual restraint (**Figs. 4** and **5**).
- Immediate measurement of glucose with a point-of-care device that uses the hexokinase method (eg, VetScan VS2, Abaxis, Darmstadt, Germany).
- Ideally, concurrently measure other electrolytes, including ionized calcium.
- If hypoglycemia is confirmed, slow administration of a bolus of 33% glucose solution or 50% dextrose solution (2–3 mL) followed by constant-rate infusion (CRI) of 5% glucose (10 mL/kg/h). Notice that there is potential risk of phlebitis by using high osmotic solutions.

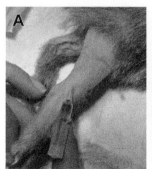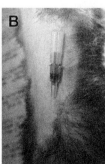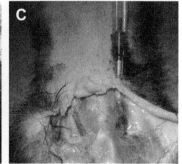

Fig. 3. Alternative sites for IV catheter placement: saphenous (*A*) and jugular vein (*B*). The anatomy of the jugular veins is showed in a ferret cadaver (*C*). Intraosseous catheters are avoidable in ferrets if proper technique for IV catheterization is used. (*Courtesy of* Nicola Di Girolamo, Rome, Italy.)

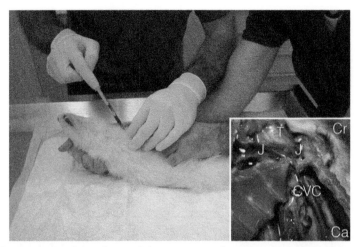

Fig. 4. Blood sampling from the cranial vena cava under manual restraint. Although it is a blind technique, the anatomic landmarks are well established. The needle should be inserted cranial to the first rib and lateral to the manubrium of the sternum. Inset: anatomy of the site in a ferret cadaver. Notice that the jugular veins merge into the cranial vena cava just below the first rib. Ca, caudal; Cr, cranial; CVC, cranial vena cava; J, jugular vein; T, trachea. (*Courtesy of* Nicola Di Girolamo, Rome, Italy.)

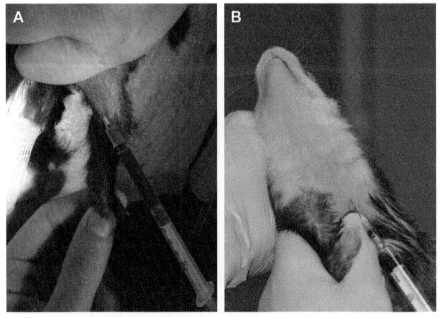

Fig. 5. Blood sampling from the saphenous (*A*) and the jugular (*B*) veins under manual restraint. (*Courtesy of* Nicola Di Girolamo, Rome, Italy.)

- If the seizures persist, a second bolus of glucose/dextrose solution and administration of diazepam (rectally or IV, 0.5 mg/kg; CRI, 0.5–1.5 mg/kg/h) or midazolam (rectally or IV, 0.5 mg/kg; CRI, 0.3 mg/kg/h) may be administered.
- If available, a CRI of glucagon may be administered at a rate of 15 ng/kg/min (6.8 ng/lb/min).[11]
- Serial monitoring (ie, every 4–8 hours) of glucose concentration with a hexokinase method.

After management of hypoglycemic crisis and stabilization of the ferret, ultrasound of the pancreas assists in the identification of neoplasia (**Fig. 6**). Surgery, especially when partial pancreatectomy is performed, has a good prognosis (**Fig. 7**).[6] However, recurrences do occur, and in such cases, medical treatment may palliate the symptoms.[4] Medical treatment for long-term management of insulinomic ferrets may include corticosteroids, diazoxide, and octreotide, among other drugs.

Hypocalcemia

A less common cause of seizures in ferrets is severe hypocalcemia.[12] For the diagnosis, complete blood work, including ionized calcium, is indicated. Although no proper reference ranges for ionized calcium in ferrets are established, values higher than 1.1 mmol/L may be considered normal based on dogs' and cats' reference ranges (reference needed and unpublished data). Currently, there are point-of-care devices that evaluate ionized calcium along with the other electrolytes requiring only 0.2 mLs of whole blood (eg, CG8+ Cartridge, i-STAT, Abaxis, Darmstadt, Germany); however, their validity in ferrets has not been assessed. Differential diagnoses for hypocalcemia should include hypoparathyroidism, pseudohypoparathyroidism, hypomagnesemia, renal failure, acute pancreatitis, hypoalbuminemia, puerperal tetany, ethylene glycol intoxication, intestinal malabsorption, nutritional secondary hyperparathyroidism, and tumor lysis syndrome.[12,13] Among these causes, primary hypoparathyroidism has been recently diagnosed in 2 ferrets and pseudohypoparathyroidism in another ferret.[12–14] Diagnosis of these conditions is based on a combination of low-serum ionized calcium concentration, high-serum phosphorus concentration,

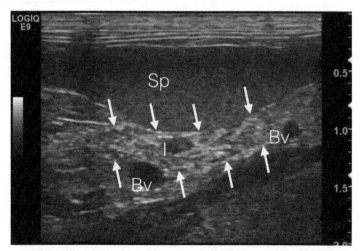

Fig. 6. Visualization of a hypoechoic mass in the left branch of the pancreas (*arrows*) of a ferret presented with hypoglycemic seizures, consistent with an insulinoma. Bv, blood vessel; I, insulinoma; Sp, spleen. (*Courtesy of* Annalisa Nicoletti, DMV, Rome, Italy.)

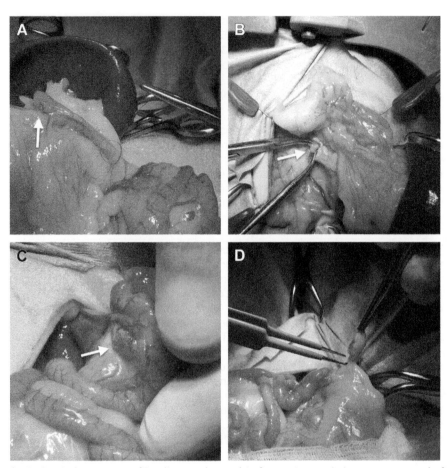

Fig. 7. Surgical treatment of insulinomas (*arrows*) in ferrets. In certain instances, removal of the neoplasm may be required to resolve the hypoglycemic crisis. Care needs to be paid to avoid the pancreatic duct. (*A*) Left pancreatectomy for multiple insulinomas on the left pancreatic limb. Given the free nature of the left limb, partial pancreatectomy is easily performed after placement of a monofilament ligature at the base of the limb. (*B*) Partial pancreatectomy for insulinoma on the body of the pancreas. The tissue enclosed in the 2 hemostatic forceps is removed. (*C*) Insulinoma on the right pancreatic limb. Notice the close relationship with the duodenum, which makes a radical pancreatectomy often unfeasible in these cases. (*D*) Nodulectomy of the previous insulinoma. This technique should be limited to insulinomas that cannot be removed with surrounding pancreatic tissue. (*Courtesy of Nicola Di Girolamo, Rome, Italy.*)

and appropriate renal function (based on serum chemistry values of serum urea nitrogen and creatinine) in the face of low parathyroid hormone (PTH) concentrations (hypoparathyroidism)[12] or high PTH concentrations (pseudohypoparathyroidism).[14]

Emergency treatment of hypocalcemic seizures is managed by CRI administration of calcium gluconate at 2 to 3 mg/kg/h, with continuous ECG monitoring controlling for bradycardia, ventricular premature complexes/contractions, or shortening of the QT interval (**Fig. 8**).[12,13] In case of spontaneous primary hypoparathyroidism, long-term maintenance therapy with dihydrotachysterol (orally, 12–20 μg/kg/d) and calcium monitoring is indicated to control clinical signs.[12,13]

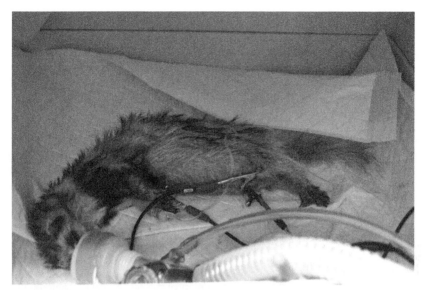

Fig. 8. Emergency treatment of hypocalcemic seizures managed by administration of calcium gluconate (2–3 mg/kg/h) with ECG monitoring. (*Courtesy of* Nicola Di Girolamo, Rome, Italy.)

Other Causes of Seizures

Other disorders that occasionally cause central neurologic signs and seizures in ferrets include brain tumors, intoxication, and infectious diseases (viral, fungal, and protozoan infections), including distemper, rabies, Aleutian disease, systemic corona-virus, *Cryptococcus*, and *Toxoplasma gondii* infection (**Fig. 9**).[2,15–18]

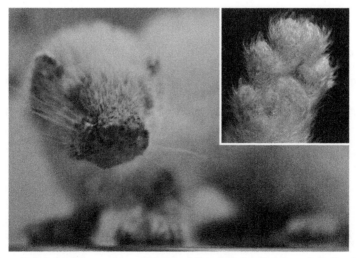

Fig. 9. Hyperkeratosis of the muzzle and foot pad (*inset*) during distemper infection in ferrets. Other presenting complaints include naso-ocular discharge, respiratory distress, and neuro-logic signs. (*Courtesy of* Nicola Di Girolamo, Rome, Italy.)

ANEMIA

Anemia in ferrets should be worked up as in other domestic animals. A preliminary diagnosis of anemia is formulated based on clinical features (**Fig. 10**) and hematology (hematocrit <45%). Most causes of anemia in other animals also occur in ferrets, including immune-mediated forms.[19] Typical causes of anemia in ferrets are lymphoma and hyperestrogenism.

Hyperestrogenism-Related Anemia

Hyperestrogenism may be secondary to prolonged estrus in female ferrets (either intact or neutered with ovarian remnant), adrenal disorders, or, rarely, estrogen-producing tumors (**Fig. 11**).[20–24] The mechanism behind anemia in intact female ferrets is from the lack of spontaneous ovulation. In the absence of copulation, ovulation does not occur, and the maintained production of estrogens by the follicles may result in bone marrow aplasia, with consequent pancytopenia.[20,21]

Clinical signs of hyperestrogenism in female ferrets include swelling of the vulva, alopecia, and pruritus, among others (**Fig. 12**). In male ferrets, gynecomastia and dysuria as a consequence of prostatic cysts are occasionally observed during hyperestrogenism.

Emergency treatment includes (1) stabilization of the ferret and (2) removal of the source of endogenous estrogen production.[25]

Transfusions

Transfusions are anecdotally indicated for hematocrit values lower than 25%.[26] Ferrets do not have clinically significant blood groups[27]; therefore, any healthy adult male ferret is an appropriate donor. As a clinical guide, avoid sampling more than 1% of the ferret body weight (ie, in a 1.5-kg ferret, 15 mL of blood). Some investigators suggest drawing blood with cardiac puncture to permit a rapid, clot-free collection.[27] However, in the author's clinical experience, transfusion is safely performed even with blood samples obtained from the cranial vena cava with a 23-G needle and use of a 170-μm clot filter (**Fig. 13**). Rate of administration of blood for the recipient depends on the underlying disorder (ie, acute vs chronic loss) and ranges from 20 minutes to a maximum of 4 hours.[28] Ferret blood stored using citrate-phosphate-dextrose-adenine should not be used for transfusion after 7 days of storage at 4°C.[29]

Removal of estrogen source

Hyperestrogenism from persistent-estrus Currently, gonadectomy in ferrets is discouraged given the consequent increase in risk of developing adrenal disease.[30]

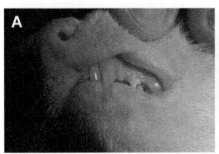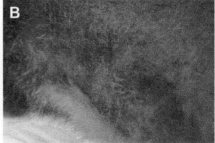

Fig. 10. Pallor of the oral mucous membrane (A) and subdermal hemorrhagic effusion (B) in a ferret with anemia and thrombocytopenia. (*Courtesy of* Nicola Di Girolamo, Rome, Italy.)

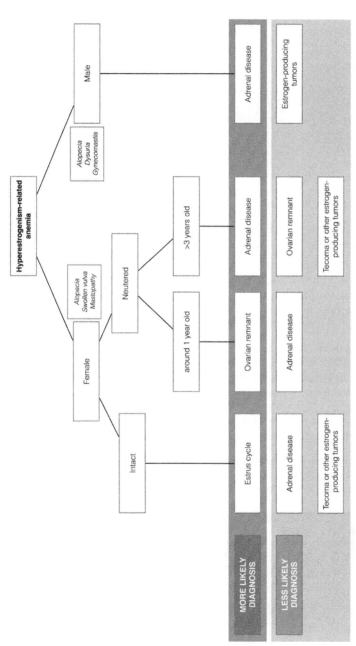

Fig. 11. Suggested differential diagnoses to consider during hyperestrogenism-related anemia.

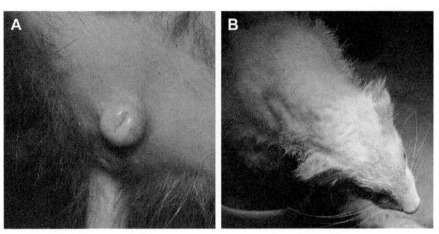

Fig. 12. Clinical signs of hyperestrogenism, swollen vulva (*A*), and alopecia (*B*). (*Courtesy of* Nicola Di Girolamo, Rome, Italy.)

Therefore, alternative medical treatments should be elected. In ferrets, ovulation may be induced with the following[26,31,32]:

- Human chorionic gonadotropin (100 IU)
- Medroxyprogesterone (15 mg)
- Proligestone (40 mg)
- Gonadotropin-releasing hormone (GnRH; 20 μg/kg)
- Long-term depot GnRH agonists (4.7 mg deslorelin acetate [Suprelorin, Virbac])

Hyperestrogenism from adrenal hyperplasia or neoplasia Current therapies for adrenal disease in ferrets include medical and/or surgical treatment. The GnRH agonist, deslorelin acetate, 4.7-mg dose proved to be an interesting alternative to surgical adrenalectomy.[33] However, in ferrets that do not respond to medical treatment (ie, persistence of symptoms, evidence of increase in size of the adrenal gland[34]) (**Fig. 14**), surgery is indicated (**Fig. 15**). Percutaneous ultrasound-guided alcoholization of the adrenal gland may be a palliative alternative (**Fig. 16**).

Hyperestrogenism from estrogen-producing tumors The treatment of choice depends on type of tumor, location, and so on. Ideally, as soon as the ferret is stabilized, prompt surgical removal is indicated to discontinue estrogen production.[24]

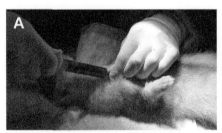
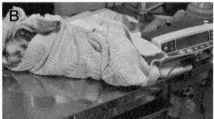

Fig. 13. Transfusions in ferrets are empirically indicated for hematocrit values lower than 25%. Any healthy adult male ferret is an appropriate donor because ferrets do not have clinically significant blood. In the author's clinical experience, transfusion is safely performed even with blood samples obtained from the cranial vena cava with a 23-G needle (*A*). Blood is then perfused in the receiver (*B*).

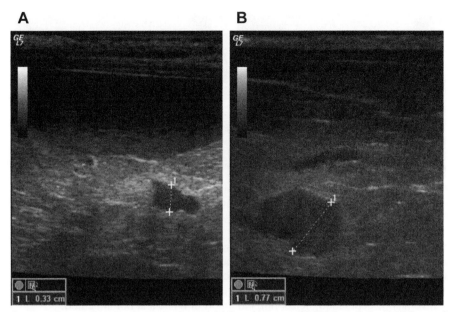

Fig. 14. Echographic visualization of normal (*A*) and increased left adrenal gland (*B*) (normal thickness <3.9 mm). (*Courtesy of* Annalisa Nicoletti, DMV, Rome, Italy.)

INTOXICATION

Because of their curious nature and strong jaws that allow them to open pill vials and sealed containers, ferrets are prone to toxin exposure. Because of their small size, even small ingestions of a toxicant can lead to a large exposure on a milligram per kilogram basis.[35] Furthermore, intoxication in ferrets may occur as a consequence of inherited defects, as in the case of copper toxicosis.[36] The treatment of toxicity in ferrets should be approached the same as in any other species.[35] General treatments should be started and, when available, specific therapy for a toxicant should be instituted. If there is substantial evidence of recent intoxication (ie, within 2 hours), when indicated, emesis can be achieved with oral administration

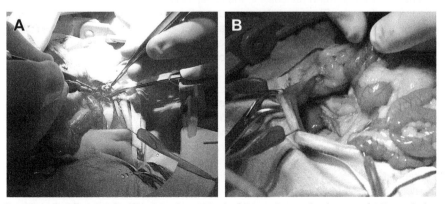

Fig. 15. Left (*A*) and right (*B*) adrenalectomies in ferrets. Currently, the use of 4.7-mg deslorelin acetate depot is a medical alternative to surgery, which remains required in certain cases. (*Courtesy of* Nicola Di Girolamo, Rome, Italy.)

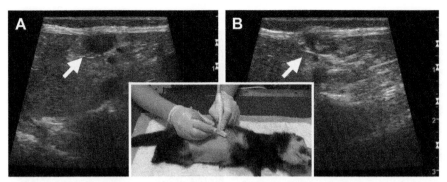

Fig. 16. Ultrasound-assisted alcoholization of an enlarged adrenal gland (*arrow*) in a ferret. (*A*) Adrenal gland before the procedure. (*B*) Adrenal gland after percutaneous injection of 0.05 mL of 95% ethanol with a 25-G needle. (*Courtesy of* Annalisa Nicoletti, DMV, Rome, Italy.)

of 3% hydrogen peroxide (0.45 mL/kg), syrup of ipecac (0.25–1 mL/kg, orally), or apomorphine (0.04 mg/kg, IV, subcutaneously, or intramuscularly [IM]).[35,37] Emesis should not be induced for ingestion of corrosives such as alkalis, acids, cationic detergents, and petroleum distillates.[35] Finally, if the animal is already symptomatic (eg, vomiting, depressed, seizuring), induction of emesis is not indicated.[37]

Ibuprofen Toxicosis

A single tablet of common size ibuprofen (200 mg) could be fatal to an average-sized ferret.

Common presenting complaints include the following[38]

- Neurologic signs (93.1% of ferrets with presumed toxicosis): depression, coma, ataxia, recumbency, tremors, and weakness
- Gastrointestinal (GI) signs (55.2%): anorexia, vomiting, retching or gagging, diarrhea, and melena
- Renal signs: polydipsia, polyuria, dysuria, renal failure
- Other findings: shallow breathing, metabolic acidosis, dehydration, and hypothermia.

Treatment for ibuprofen toxicosis in the ferret includes stabilization, GI decontamination, fluid diuresis, GI protection, and supportive care. The ingestion of ibuprofen has an unfavorable prognosis unless the animal is decontaminated early and given aggressive treatment. However, in a retrospective study of suspect ibuprofen toxicosis, death was reported in only 14% of cases (4/29 cases).[38]

Anticoagulant Rodenticide

Anticoagulant rodenticides interfere with the liver's production of clotting factors II, VII, IX, and X. Signs of hemorrhage are not evident right after intoxication, typically taking 1 to 3 days after ingestion to occur. Hemorrhages may occur anywhere, including thorax, abdomen, subcutis, and central nervous system (**Fig. 17**).[39] Emergency treatment should be aimed at stopping hemorrhage, correcting anemia, and supplementing vitamin K1. Although there is a lack of clinical research data on ferrets, vitamin K1 is empirically indicated at a dose of 5 mg/kg divided every 8 to 12 hours.[35] Oral vitamin K1 should be given with a fatty meal because bile acids are needed for its absorption, while injections are generally discouraged for the risk of anaphylactic reactions.[39] Plasma or whole blood may be given in symptomatic ferrets to provide clotting factors.

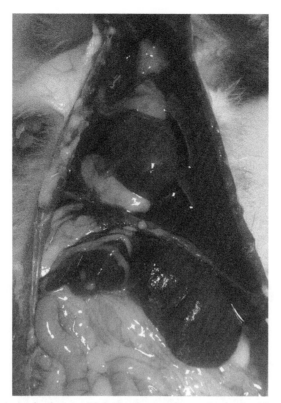

Fig. 17. Post-mortem of a ferret with hemothorax after anticoagulant intoxication.

In case of anemia, whole blood transfusions are indicated. Course of treatment depends on the rodenticide (around 2–4 weeks) during which coagulation parameters should be monitored (**Table 1**).[35,40]

ACUTE ABDOMEN

Ferrets presented with an acute onset of abdominal pain should be closely evaluated, because the underlying cause of acute abdomen in the ferret may be minor and transient

Table 1 Coagulation times, fibrinogen concentration, and antithrombin activity in 18 clinically healthy ferrets using an ACL 3000 Analyzer		
Coagulation Parameter	**Mean**	**Range**
PT (s)	10.9	(10.6–11.6)
PTT	20.0	(18.6–22.1)
PTT + ellagic acid	18.1	(16.5–20.5)
Fibrinogen	107.4	(90.0–163.5)
Antithrombin (%)	96	(69.3–115.3)

Abbreviations: PT, prothrombin time; PTT, partial thromboplastin time.
Adapted from Benson KG, Paul-Murphy J, Hart AP, et al. Coagulation values in normal ferrets (Mustela putorius furo) using selected methods and reagents. Vet Clin Pathol 2008;37:288.

or an immediately life-threatening process. Acute abdomen may result from specific injury or disease of the peritoneal or retroperitoneal structures, diaphragm, or body wall constituents,[1] with pain from the spine also frequently referred as abdominal pain.

Gastrointestinal Obstruction

GI foreign bodies are particularly common in ferrets, especially in young individuals.[41] Ferrets seem to be attracted to plastic and latex objects. Vomiting and/or diarrhea are frequent presenting complaints. Occasionally, gastric dilatation-volvulus may occur.[42] Radiography and ultrasonography are usually sufficient for diagnosis (**Fig. 18A**), although in some instances, other diagnostic techniques are required (**Fig. 18B**). Obstructing intestinal foreign bodies should be considered a surgical emergency, and exploratory laparotomy should be performed as soon as the ferret is able to withstand general anesthesia (**Fig. 19**).

Intestinal Perforation

Intestinal perforation may occur as a consequence of GI foreign bodies or neoplasia of the intestinal tract and should be considered a surgical emergency. Treatment

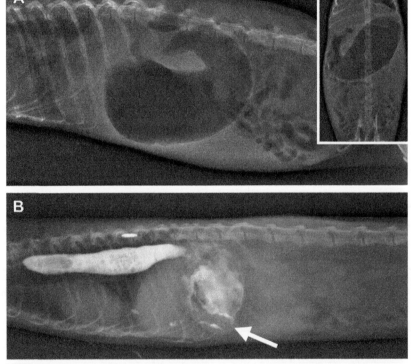

Fig. 18. Radiographic findings in ferrets with GI foreign bodies. (*A*) Lateral radiograph of a gas-dilated stomach. Inset: ventrodorsal view. (*B*) Ferret presented with regurgitation; ultrasound was not diagnostic. Contrast radiograph shows a filling defect in the stomach (*arrow*) consistent with a large foreign body (trichobezoar). Notice the subsequent dilated esophagus, which should not be confused with an idiopathic megaesophagus. Barium should be never administered in cases of possible GI perforation. (*Courtesy of* Nicola Di Girolamo, Rome, Italy.)

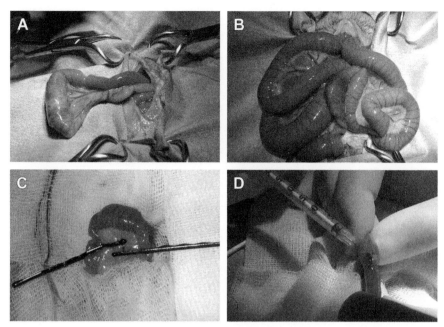

Fig. 19. Urgency of enterotomy for foreign body removal depends on several factors. (*A*) Enterotomy in a ferret presented for anorexia. (*B*) Enterotomy in a ferret that was force-fed for 2 days by the referring veterinarian. Notice extreme dilation of the intestinal tract before the obstruction. These cases should be considered surgical emergencies. (*C*) Use of hair clip to avoid surgical field contamination. (*D*) Injection of saline by use of a 0.3-mL syringe with a 31-G needle to assess absence of leaking from the enterotomy site. (*Courtesy of* Nicola Di Girolamo, Rome, Italy.)

consists of stabilization of the patient and resection of the affected tract of the intestine (**Fig. 20**). In cases of perforating foreign bodies, excision of a small area of intestine around the perforation (after foreign body removal) may be a valid alternative to end-to-end anastomosis. In the author's experience, the prognosis is generally guarded.

Biliary Disorders

Biliary disorders are increasingly being diagnosed in ferrets.[43,44] Ferrets with biliary disorders may present with discolored (acholic) feces (**Fig. 21**), icteric mucus membranes, vomiting, anorexia, and lethargy. Alanine aminotransferase (ALT) and total bilirubin are usually elevated (reference ranges, ALT: 70–100 U/L; total bilirubin: 0.2–0.5).[45] Ultrasonography of the gallbladder may identify surgical emergencies (ie, obstruction and rupture; **Fig. 22**A).

- Cholelithiasis and obstruction
  - Usually requires immediate surgical treatment, with removal of the cholelith (**Fig. 22**B).[43]
- Cholecystitis
  - Depending on the severity of the disorder, it may be appropriate to attempt medical treatment, such as antibiotics, gastroprotectants, and ursodeoxycholic acid (**Fig. 23**A, B). In severe cases, cholecystectomy is indicated (**Fig. 23**C).

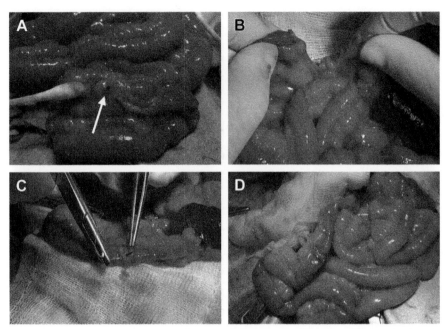

Fig. 20. Emergency enterectomy in a ferret with intestinal perforation. (*A*) Intestinal perforation (*arrow*). Notice the altered surrounding tissue and peritonitis. (*B*) Enterectomy. (*C*, *D*) Anastomosis of the 2 cut ends in a simple interrupted pattern with monofilament absorbable suture. (*Courtesy of* Nicola Di Girolamo, Rome, Italy.)

- Rupture of the gallbladder
  - Requires immediate surgical treatment, consisting of cholecystectomy and peritoneal lavage (**Fig. 24**).[44]

Spleen Disorders

Conditions requiring immediate surgical treatment include splenic torsion and rupture. Both are quite uncommon in ferrets.[42] Splenomegaly is a more common condition but usually does not require emergency treatment. However, in some cases, generalized

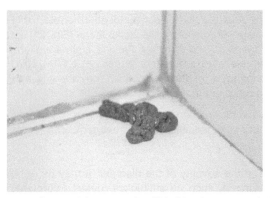

Fig. 21. Acholic feces in a ferret with ruptured gallbladder. (*Courtesy of* Nicola Di Girolamo, Rome, Italy.)

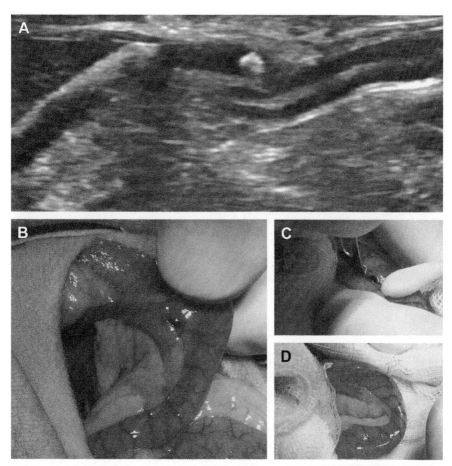

Fig. 22. Cholelithiasis in ferrets may be a surgical emergency. (*A*) Ultrasonographic visualization of a cholelith in the common bile duct. Notice the dilation of the duct. (*B–D*) Surgical removal of the cholelith from the common bile duct. (*Courtesy of* Nicola Di Girolamo, Rome, Italy.)

splenomegaly (hypersplenism) or large splenic masses may result in weakness, lethargy, anorexia, and even vomiting from mechanical compression of the stomach (**Fig. 25**A). In these cases, splenectomy may resolve the symptoms (**Fig. 25**B).[46,47] Histology should always be performed on the removed spleen for diagnosis of subtle lymphomas.

Intervertebral Disk Prolapse

Intervertebral disk prolapse in ferrets generally occurs at the level of the lumbar vertebrae and results in ambulatory deficits of the hind limbs (Video 4).[48,49] Vertebral trauma can lead to a similar clinical presentation. Such alteration should not be confused with the common hind limb weakness that affects ferrets in a variety of conditions, including hypoglycemia and congestive heart failure (CHF), or with paresis related to neuromuscular disease, as in a course of myasthenia gravis or disseminated idiopathic myositis.[50,51] A preliminary indication during emergency consultation may be provided by radiographs of the lumbar vertebrae. Definitive diagnosis requires

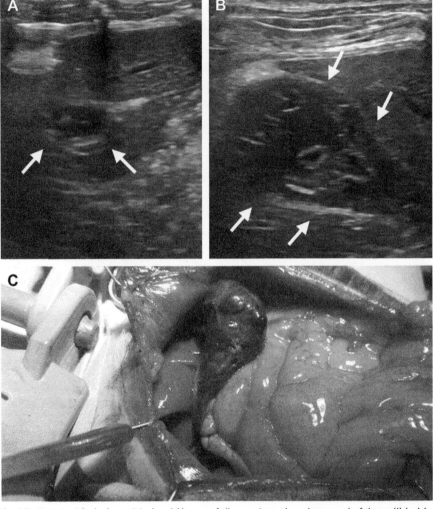

Fig. 23. Ferret with cholecystitis should be carefully monitored, and removal of the gallbladder should be performed if required. (*A*) Gallbladder presenting a thickened wall but normal content (*arrows*). The ferret was successfully managed medically. (*B*) Necrotizing cholecystitis in a ferret. Notice thickened wall and structured content of the gallbladder (*arrows*). (*C*) Surgical removal of the gallbladder in (*B*). After blunt isolation of the gallbladder, the cystic duct is ligated and the gallbladder excised. (*Courtesy of* Nicola Di Girolamo, Rome, Italy.)

myelography, computed tomography (CT), or MRI, although the latter 2 techniques are preferred. Treatment options include hemilaminectomy and/or conservative physiotherapy, hydrotherapy, and low-level laser therapy.[48,49,52]

ACUTE KIDNEY INJURY

In ferrets, acute kidney injury (AKI) (acute renal failure) may result from prostatic disease, urolithiasis, ureteral obstruction (stenotic and retrocaval ureters), toxic exposure, and infectious disease (**Fig. 26**).[38,53–55]

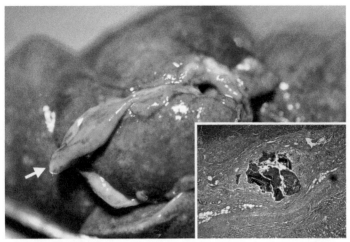

Fig. 24. Post-mortem appearance of a ruptured gallbladder (*arrow*) in a ferret resulting in bile peritonitis. Inset: presence of bile plug within bile duct. (*Courtesy of* Raffaele Melidone, Boston, MA.)

Initial laboratory evaluation should include a complete blood count, serum biochemistry profile, assessment of acid-base status, urinalysis, and urine culture. Hyperkalemia occurs primarily in oliguric or anuric ferrets. Radiography and ultrasonography may serve as a diagnostic imaging step to aid in the assessment of a ferret with suspected AKI (**Fig. 27**). CT and excretory urography may be required to characterize

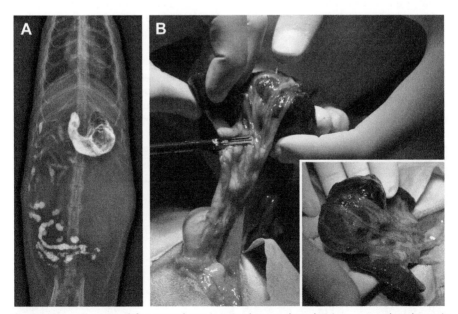

Fig. 25. Ferret presented for several vomit episodes per days despite a normal endoscopic aspect of the stomach. (*A*) Contrast radiography shows the compression caused by a splenic mass in the GI tract. (*B*) Removal of the spleen by use of a tissue-sealing device (Enseal, Ethicon). Inset: Notice the large splenic mass. (*Courtesy of* Nicola Di Girolamo, Rome, Italy.)

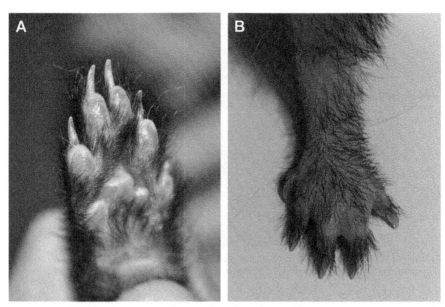

Fig. 26. Dermatologic lesions in ferrets with kidney failure. (*A*) Skin ulcers presumed to be secondary to uremia in a ferret with kidney failure. (*B*) Edema of the extremities in a ferret with nephrotic syndrome. (*Courtesy of* Nicola Di Girolamo, Rome, Italy.)

some disorders (**Fig. 28**), for example, focal dilation of the ureters (**Fig. 29**). The primary treatment should be aimed at the underlying cause of AKI (eg, ureteral bypass, antidotes for toxins); however, correction and maintenance of the animal's hydration, acid-base, and electrolyte status are the mainstays of management for AKI.

Urethral Obstruction

Urethral obstruction is a condition that requires immediate care and may be secondary to prostate enlargement (frequently secondary to adrenal disease), urethrolithiasis, and urethral masses. In male ferrets, even small uroliths may cause a life-threatening post-renal obstruction because of the narrow diameter of the urethra and the os penis. The

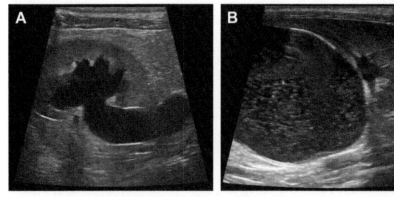

Fig. 27. Common ultrasonographic findings in ferrets with kidney failure. (*A*) Segmental ureteral dilation and hydronephrosis. (*B*) Large cyst in the renal parenchyma.

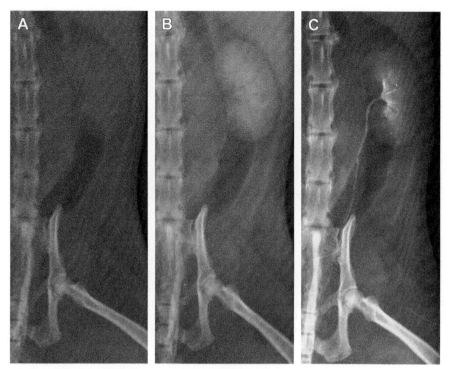

Fig. 28. Different phases of left renal enhancement during excretory urography in a ferret. (*A*) Plain radiograph, before administration of IV contrast medium. (*B*) Nephrographic phase. The nephrographic opacity should decrease progressively with time after injection. (*C*) Pyelographic phase. The width of pelvic recesses, renal pelvis, and proximal ureter may be measured in this phase. (*Courtesy of* Nicola Di Girolamo, Rome, Italy.)

urethrolith may be dislodged by means of urethral catheterization and retrograde urohydropulsion to the bladder (**Fig. 30**). If retrograde urohydropulsion is unsuccessful, perineal urethrostomy or temporary tube cystostomy permits urine voidance (**Fig. 31**). Temporary tube cystostomy may be performed as follows[56]:

- During laparotomy, a cystostomy tube (5- or 8-French Foley catheter) is passed in a paramedian incision in the ventral body wall.
- A Foley catheter is passed into the urinary bladder, inflated, and fixated with a purse-string suture.
- The bladder is tacked to the body wall with simple interrupted sutures.
- The abdomen is closed routinely, and the skin around the exiting Foley catheter is closed with a purse-string suture. A finger-trap connected to the purse-string suture is placed around the Foley catheter.

DIABETIC KETOACIDOSIS

Diabetic ketoacidosis is a severe, life-threatening complication of diabetes mellitus, characterized by the biochemical triad of hyperglycemia, acidosis, and ketosis. As compared with dogs and cats, ferrets rarely suffer diabetes mellitus. Diabetes

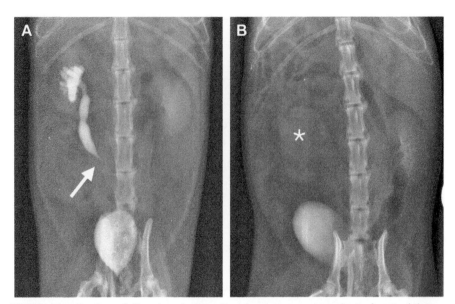

Fig. 29. Visualization of disorders during altered excretory urography in ferrets. (*A*) Presence of a segmental ureteral stenosis (*arrow*) and subsequent hydronephrosis of the right kidney. (*B*) Lack of contrast enhancement of the right kidney (*asterisk*). (*Courtesy of* Nicola Di Girolamo, Rome, Italy.)

mellitus in ferrets may be spontaneous, iatrogenic, or as a postoperative sequela to pancreatectomy.[57–59] Treatment of diabetes ketoacidosis consists of fluid therapy, electrolyte corrections, and insulin therapy.[57,59] Previous experience suggests using initially short-acting insulin to gain glycemic control (0.25 U/kg, IM, every 4 hours),[57]

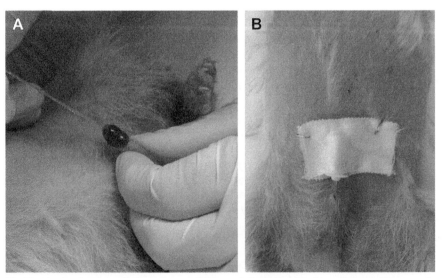

Fig. 30. Urethral catheterization in a male ferret (*A*). Notice fixation of the catheter to the skin (*B*). (*Courtesy of* Daniele Petrini, Pisa, Italy.)

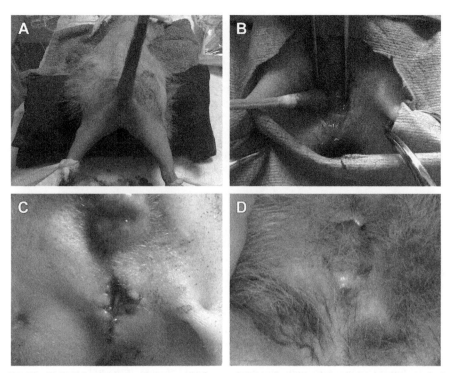

Fig. 31. Perineal urethrostomy in a male ferret. (*A*) Preparation of the ferret on the surgical table. (*B*) Incision of the skin, retraction of the perineal muscles, and exposure of the urethra. The localization of the urethra is favored by the previous positioning of a urinary catheter. (*C*) Placement of monofilament sutures from the urethral wall to the perineal skin. (*D*) Appearance of the surgical site 6 months after treatment. (*Courtesy of* Nicola Di Girolamo, Rome, Italy.)

after which switching to long-acting insulin (insulin glargine) for maintenance glycemic control (0.5 U, subcutaneously, every 12 hours).[58]

CONGESTIVE HEART FAILURE

Cardiac disease in ferrets is far more common than previously thought,[60] and CHF is a common emergency condition in ferrets requiring immediate care. Ferrets with CHF may present to the emergency department with cough, respiratory distress, syncope, ascites, and/or generalized or hind limb weakness. The ferret may acquire an orthopneic position while breathing (**Fig. 32**). After evaluation of heart rate, rhythm, murmurs, pulse, capillary refill time, and thoracic percussion for fluid presence, radiographs should be obtained. Assessment of the vertebral heart scale (VHS) is a rapid, but limited technique that may assist the nonexpert radiologist in evaluating the cardiac silhouette (right lateral VHS reference interval: 5.2–5.5 vertebrae; **Fig. 33**).[61] Thoracic ultrasonography and ECG are typically needed to make a definitive diagnosis.

Depending on the cause of CHF, different emergency treatments should be planned:

- Oxygen, provided both via flow-by (4–6 L/min) and in an oxygen cage, should be administered to hypoxic ferrets.

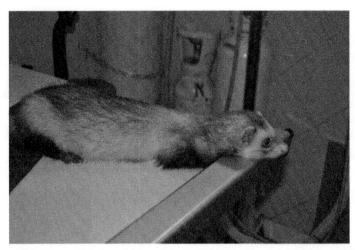

Fig. 32. Orthopneic position in a ferret with CHF. This position is also observed in healthy ferrets and should not be considered diagnostic.

- Suspected pulmonary edema is empirically treated with an initial IM administration of furosemide at 4 mg/kg, followed by recheck radiographs at 3 to 5 hours, and decreased to 2 or 1 mg/kg, once or twice a day (**Fig. 34**).
- In ferrets presenting with significant pleural effusion (**Fig. 35**), thoracentesis should be performed immediately for diagnostic and therapeutic purposes (**Fig. 36**; Video 5). Effusion of cardiac origin should be differentiated from chylothorax and pyothorax (eg, *Pseudomonas luteola* and *Nocardia* sp infection).[62,63] Chylous effusion may have a "milky" appearance (**Fig. 37**) or may be transparent;

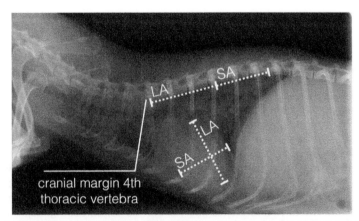

Fig. 33. Radiographic measurement of the VHS in a cardiopathic ferret (6 vertebrae, reference interval: 5.2–5.5). The long axis (LA) is the length of the heart from ventral border of bifurcation of the mainstem bronchi to the apex. The short axis (SA) is the maximal width of the heart perpendicular to the long axis. The 2 measurements are placed on the cranial margin of the 4th thoracic vertebra, and the number of vertebrae are counted to the nearest 0.25 vertebra.

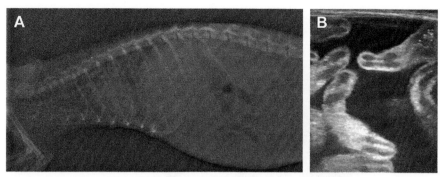

Fig. 34. Diagnostic imaging findings in a ferret with biventricular heart failure. Radiograph showing alveolar pattern (consistent with lung edema) and ascites (*A*). Abdominal ultrasound confirms ascites (*B*).

therefore, visual assessment may not be diagnostic.[64] A high effusion:serum triglyceride ratio (2–10:1) is suggestive of chylothorax.[65] In dubious cases, the presence of chylomicrons in the lipoprotein electrophoresis from the effusion is diagnostic.[64] Lymphangiography permits evaluation of the thoracic duct (see **Fig. 37**).

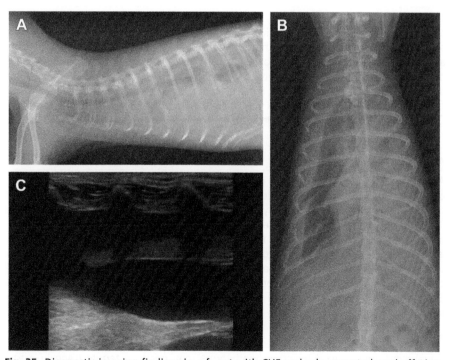

Fig. 35. Diagnostic imaging findings in a ferret with CHF and subsequent pleural effusion. Lateral (*A*) and ventrodorsal radiographs (*B*). Notice the silhouette sign and pleural fissures. Ultrasonography assists in estimation of the quantity of fluid (*C*). (*Courtesy of* Nicola Di Girolamo, Rome, Italy.)

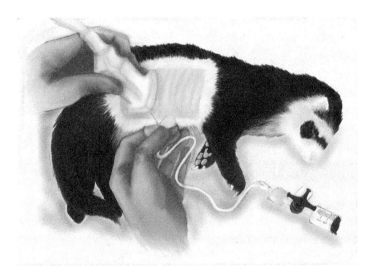

Fig. 36. Ultrasound-assisted thoracentesis is an emergency procedure that may be performed under slight sedation in the case of pleural effusion or pneumothorax. (*Courtesy of* Virginia Bua, Rome, Italy.)

Valvular Regurgitation and Cardiomyopathies

Valve incompetence is the most common cause of cardiac disease in ferrets.[60] Dilated, hypertrophic, and restrictive cardiomyopathies are less common, but often associated with CHF.[60] In the author's experience, the use of an electronic stethoscope may simplify auscultation of ferrets and usually permits the identification of murmurs (**Fig. 38**A). Valvular disorders are diagnosed by Doppler echocardiography and should be treated as in other small animals. Empirically, the author uses pimobendan (0.25–0.5 mg/kg, twice a day) and benazepril (0.5 mg/kg, once a day).[66] Chronic diuretic use of furosemide, at the lowest dose to control signs of CHF, is needed.

Atrioventricular Block

Atrioventricular block is common in ferrets, and third-degree atrioventricular block often results in CHF.[60] In most ferrets, ECG may be performed without need of chemical restraint. The ferret may be maintained in a vertical, "hanging" position (**Fig. 38**B),[67] or manually restrained in the lateral position. Administration of commercial malt paste may simplify restraint of uncooperative individuals. The ECG is interpreted as in other domestic animals (**Fig. 39**), and values of healthy individuals are detailed elsewhere.[67] Treatment options include medical therapy with sympathicomimetic medications (isoproterenol, metaproterenol) or cardiac pacing. Both epicardial and intracardial pacing have been successfully performed in ferrets.[68,69]

Filariosis

Caval syndrome caused by adult heartworms may occur in ferrets living in areas endemic of the disease. Accuracy of SNAP ELISA (enzyme-linked immunosorbent assay) -based antigen tests is unclear in ferrets, and it is suspected those tests may give false negative results. Diagnosis is based on evidence of adult worms in the heart

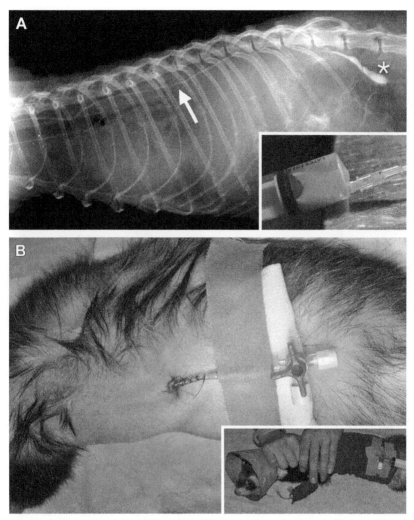

Fig. 37. Chylothorax should be differentiated from cardiogenic pleural effusion. (*A*) Lymphangiogram of the thoracic duct (*arrow*) in a ferret. Under ultrasonographic guidance, 60 mgl/kg of iohexol contrast medium was injected in the mesenteric lymph nodes. Notice the cisterna chyli (*asterisk*). Inset: typical aspect of chylous. However, transparent chylous effusion is not uncommon. (*B*) Thoracic drainage may be placed in cases of severe, recurring chylous effusion. (*Courtesy of* Nicola Di Girolamo, Rome, Italy.)

and cranial vena cava by ultrasonography. In a ferret, heartworms had been transvenously extracted.[70]

- The jugular vein is dissected; a basket endoscopic retrieval device is inserted into the vein and advanced into the cranial vena cava with fluoroscopic guidance, and heartworms are extracted.

Medical adulticide therapy using melarsomine in ferrets causes anaphylaxis in approximately half of the cases.[71] Prednisone at a dosage of 2 mg/kg may be used to mitigate clinical symptoms. Preventative medication is mandatory in endemic areas.

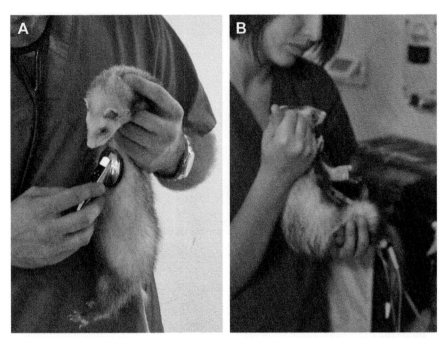

Fig. 38. Auscultation (*A*) and ECG (*B*) may be easier to perform in a vertical position in uncooperative ferrets.

Congenital Disorders

Congenital heart disorders are increasingly being diagnosed in ferrets (**Fig. 40**). Currently, ventricular septal defect, atrial septal defect, and tetralogy of Fallot are described in ferrets.[66,72,73] Often the ferrets are asymptomatic until adulthood,

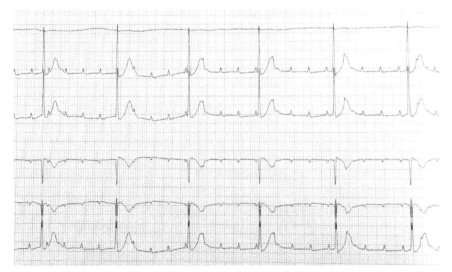

Fig. 39. ECG in a ferret with a third-degree ventricular block. Notice in lead II the dissociation of P waves and QRS complexes. The ventricular escape rhythm in ferrets is around 60 to 70 bpm.

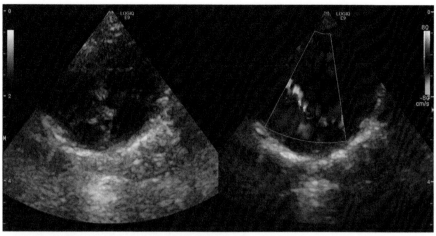

Fig. 40. Echocardiographic appearance of a ventricular septal defect in an asymptomatic ferret. A murmur was audible on auscultation. (*Courtesy of* Annalisa Nicoletti, DMV, Rome, Italy.)

when, as a consequence of severe heart remodeling, they develop CHF.[66,73] Treatment is symptomatic, because surgical correction of congenital heart disorders in ferrets has never been reported.

Hypertension and Aortic Aneurysms

Systemic hypertension may be associated with CHF and renal disease, and blood pressure should be closely monitored in ferrets with cardiac disorders (**Fig. 41**, Video 6).[74] The practitioner needs to be aware that noninvasive blood pressure measurement (with manual sphygmomanometer and Doppler probe) underestimates blood pressure in ferrets.[75] However, it remains an affordable technique

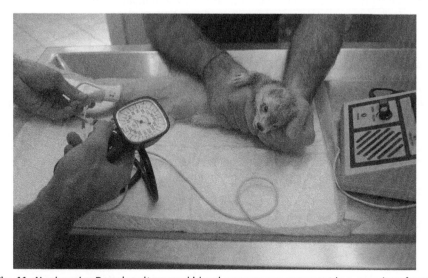

Fig. 41. Noninvasive Doppler ultrasound blood pressure measurement in a conscious ferret. (*Courtesy of* Nicola Di Girolamo, Rome, Italy.)

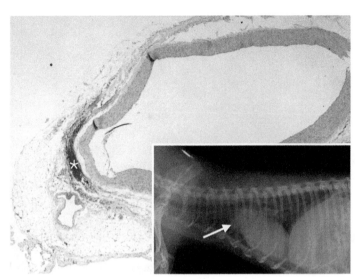

Fig. 42. Dissecting aneurysm of the aorta in a ferret with severe systemic hypertension. Notice thickening of the tunica media and presence of erythrocytes in the vascular wall (*asterisk*). Inset: lateral radiograph of the ferret showing an area of increased opacity cranial to the heart consistent with the aorta (*arrow*). (*Courtesy of* Laura Bongiovanni, Teramo, Italy; and [*inset*] Nicola Di Girolamo, Rome, Italy.)

for blood pressure monitoring. As a rule of thumb, 30 mm Hg may be added after Doppler measurement (based on published data, mean difference: −28 mm Hg, 95% confidence interval approximately 4 to 60 mm Hg).[75] Systemic hypertension in ferrets may be secondary to causes similar to other domestic carnivores, including aldosterone-secreting adrenal tumors.[76] In cases of hyperaldosteronism, administration of spironolactone and amlodipine mitigates the hypertension.[74] Uncontrolled hypertension may result in dissecting aortic aneurism and sudden death (**Fig. 42**).

TRAUMA

Given the curious nature of ferrets, they tend to escape their enclosures and suffer accidents, including falling from windows or balconies, electrocution, washing machine–related injuries, and so on. Fractures in ferrets should be managed in a similar fashion as in other small animals. Spinal and pelvic fractures occasionally occur as a consequence of falling, and standard orthopedic treatment should be considered.[77] In general, standard diagnostic and therapeutic principles developed in small animal emergency medicine should be used in case of trauma.[78]

ACKNOWLEDGMENTS

Dr Tommaso Collarile is kindly acknowledged for suggestions, images, and assistance for some of the cases described in this article. Dr Annalisa Nicoletti, Dr Ulrich Zeyen, and Dr Paolo Fonti are kindly acknowledged for assistance regarding diagnostic imaging interpretation.

SUPPLEMENTARY DATA

Supplementary data related to this article can be found online at http://dx.doi.org/10.1016/j.cvex.2016.01.006.

REFERENCES

1. Beal MW. Approach to the acute abdomen. Vet Clin North Am Small Anim Pract 2005;35:375–96.
2. Donnelly TM. Neurological diseases of ferrets. In: Proceedings of the Annual Conference of the Association of Exotic Mammal Veterinarians. Seattle (WA): 2011. p. 75–82.
3. Brauer C, Jambroszyk M, Tipold A. Metabolic and toxic causes of canine seizure disorders: a retrospective study of 96 cases. Vet J 2011;187:272–5.
4. Caplan ER, Peterson ME, Mullen HS, et al. Diagnosis and treatment of insulin-secreting pancreatic islet cell tumors in ferrets: 57 cases (1986-1994). J Am Vet Med Assoc 1996;209:1741–5.
5. Ehrhart N, Withrow SJ, Ehrhart EJ, et al. Pancreatic beta cell tumor in ferrets: 20 cases (1986–1994). J Am Vet Med Assoc 1996;209:1737–40.
6. Weiss CA, Williams BH, Scott MV. Insulinoma in the ferret: clinical findings and treatment comparison of 66 cases. J Am Anim Hosp Assoc 1998;34:471–5.
7. Syme HM, Scott-Moncrieff JC. Chronic hypoglycaemia in a hunting dog due to secondary hypoadrenocorticism. J Small Anim Pract 1998;39:348–51.
8. Lee EJ, Moore WE, Fryer HC, et al. Haematological and serum chemistry profiles of ferrets (Mustela putorius furo). Lab Anim 1982;16:133–7.
9. Summa NM, Eshar D, Lee-Chow B, et al. Comparison of a human portable glucometer and an automated chemistry analyzer for measurement of blood glucose concentration in pet ferrets (Mustela putorius furo). Can Vet J 2014;55:865–9.
10. Petritz OA, Antinoff N, Chen S, et al. Evaluation of portable blood glucose meters for measurement of blood glucose concentration in ferrets (Mustela putorius furo). J Am Vet Med Assoc 2013;242:350–4.
11. Bennett KR, Gaunt MC, Parker DL. Constant rate infusion of glucagon as an emergency treatment for hypoglycemia in a domestic ferret (Mustela putorius furo). J Am Vet Med Assoc 2015;246:451–4.
12. de Matos RE, Connolly MJ, Starkey SR, et al. Suspected primary hypoparathyroidism in a domestic ferret (Mustela putorius furo). J Am Vet Med Assoc 2014; 245:419–24.
13. Martinez C, Sabater M, Giner J, et al. Spontaneous primary hypoparathyroidism in a ferret (Mustela putorius furo). J Exot Pet Med 2015;24:333–9.
14. Wilson GH, Greene CE, Greenacre CB. Suspected pseudohypoparathyroidism in a domestic ferret. J Am Vet Med Assoc 2003;222:1093–6.
15. Lainson R. The demonstration of Toxoplasma in animals, with particular reference to members of the Mustelidae. Trans R Soc Trop Med Hyg 1957;51:111–8.
16. Garner MM, Ramsell K, Morera N, et al. Clinicopathologic features of a systemic coronavirus-associated disease resembling feline infectious peritonitis in the domestic ferret (Mustela putorius). Vet Pathol 2008;45:236–46.
17. van Zeeland Y, Schoemaker N, Passon-Vastenburg M, et al. Vestibular syndrome due to a choroid plexus papilloma in a ferret. J Am Anim Hosp Assoc 2009;45:97–101.
18. Rozengurt N, Stewart D, Sanchez S. Diagnostic exercise: ataxia and incoordination in ferrets. Lab Anim Sci 1995;45:432–4.

19. Malka S, Hawkins MG, Zabolotzky SM, et al. Immune-mediated pure red cell aplasia in a domestic ferret. J Am Vet Med Assoc 2010;237:695–700.

20. Kociba G, Caputo CA. Aplastic anemia associated with estrus in pet ferrets. J Am Vet Med Assoc 1981;178:1293–4.

21. Sherrill A, Gorham JR. Bone marrow hypoplasia associated with estrus in ferrets. Lab Anim Sci 1985;35:280–6.

22. Rosenthal KL, Peterson ME, Quesenberry KE, et al. Hyperadrenocorticism associated with adrenocortical tumor or nodular hyperplasia of the adrenal gland in ferrets: 50 cases (1987-1991). J Am Vet Med Assoc 1993;203:271–5.

23. de Wit M, Schoemaker NJ, van der Hage MH, et al. Signs of estrus in an ovariectomized ferret. Tijdschr Diergeneeskd 2001;126:526–8 [in Dutch].

24. Martínez A, Martinez J, Burballa A, et al. Spontaneous thecoma in a spayed pet ferret (Mustela putorius furo) with alopecia and swollen vulva. J Exot Pet Med 2011;20:308–12.

25. Ryland LM. Remission of estrus-associated anemia following ovariohysterectomy and multiple blood transfusions in a ferret. J Am Vet Med Assoc 1982;181:820–2.

26. Fox GJ, Bell JA. Diseases of the genitourinary system. In: Fox JG, Marini RP, editors. Biology and diseases of the ferrets. 3rd edition. Oxford (United Kingdom: Wiley Blackwell; 2014. p. 335–62.

27. Manning DD, Bell JA. Lack of detectable blood groups in domestic ferrets: implications for transfusion. J Am Vet Med Assoc 1990;197:84–6.

28. Lichtenberger M. Transfusion medicine in exotic pets. Clin Tech Small Anim Pract 2004;19:88–95.

29. Pignon C, Donnelly TM, Todeschini C, et al. Assessment of a blood preservation protocol for use in ferrets before transfusion. Vet Rec 2014;174:277.

30. Shoemaker NJ, Schuurmans M, Moorman H, et al. Correlation between age at neutering and age at onset of hyperadrenocorticism in ferrets. J Am Vet Med Assoc 2000;216:195–7.

31. Mead RA, Joseph MM, Neirinckx S. Optimal dose of human chorionic gonadotropin for inducing ovulation in the ferret. Zoo Biol 1988;7:263–7.

32. Goericke-Pesch S, Wehrend A. The use of a slow release GnRH-agonist implant in female ferrets in season for oestrus suppression. Schweiz Arch Tierheilkd 2012;154:487–91.

33. Lennox AM, Wagner R. Comparison of 4.7-mg deslorelin implants and surgery for the treatment of adrenocortical disease in ferrets. J Exot Pet Med 2012;21:332–5.

34. Kuijten AM, Schoemaker NJ, Voorhout G. Ultrasonographic visualization of the adrenal glands of healthy ferrets and ferrets with hyperadrenocorticism. J Am Anim Hosp Assoc 2007;43:78–84.

35. Dunayer E. Toxicology of ferrets. Vet Clin North Am Exot Anim Pract 2008;11:301–14.

36. Fox JG, Zeman DH, Mortimer JD. Copper toxicosis in sibling ferrets. J Am Vet Med Assoc 1994;205:1154–6.

37. DeClementi C. Prevention and treatment of poisoning. In: Gupta RC, editor. Veterinary toxicology: basic and clinical principles. New York: Elsevier; 2007. p. 1139–58.

38. Richardson JA, Balabuszko RA. Ibuprofen ingestion in ferrets: 43 cases. January 1995–March 2000. J Vet Emerg Crit Care 2001;11:53–9.

39. Means C. Rodenticides and avicides: anticoagulant rodenticides. In: Plumlee KH, editor. Clinical veterinary toxicology. St Louis (MO): Mosby; 2004. p. 444–6.

40. Benson KG, Paul-Murphy J, Hart AP, et al. Coagulation values in normal ferrets (Mustela putorius furo) using selected methods and reagents. Vet Clin Pathol 2008;37:286–8.

41. Mullen HS, Scavelli TD, Quesenberry KE, et al. Gastrointestinal foreign body in ferrets: 25 cases (1986–1990). J Am Anim Hosp Assoc 1989;28:13–9.

42. Geyer NE, Reichle JK. What is your diagnosis? Gastric dilatation-volvulus (GDV) with secondary peritoneal effusion and splenic congestion or torsion. J Am Vet Med Assoc 2012;241:45–7.

43. Hauptman K, Jekl V, Knotek Z. Extrahepatic biliary tract obstruction in two ferrets (Mustela putorius furo). J Small Anim Pract 2011;52:371–5.

44. Huynh M, Guillaumot P, Hernandez J, et al. Gall bladder rupture associated with cholecystitis in a domestic ferret (Mustela putorius). J Small Anim Pract 2014;55: 479–82.

45. Quesenberry KE, Orcutt C. Basic approach to veterinary care. In: Quesenberry KE, Carpenter JW, editors. Ferrets, rabbits and rodents: clinical medicine and surgery. 3rd edition. St Louis (MO): Saunders Elsevier; 2012. p. 174–82.

46. Ferguson DC. Idiopathic hypersplenism in a ferret. J Am Vet Med Assoc 1985; 186:693–5.

47. Martorell J, Vrabelova D, Reberte L, et al. Diagnosis of an abdominal splenosis in a case of ambulatory paraparesis of the hind limbs in a ferret (Mustela putorius furo). J Exot Pet Med 2011;20:227–31.

48. Lu D, Lamb CR, Patterson-Kane JC, et al. Treatment of a prolapsed lumbar intervertebral disc in a ferret. J Small Anim Pract 2004;45:501–3.

49. Srugo I, Chai O, Yaakov D, et al. Successful medical management of lumbar intervertebral disc prolapse in a ferret. J Small Anim Pract 2010;51:447–50.

50. Couturier J, Huynh M, Boussarie D, et al. Autoimmune myasthenia gravis in a ferret. J Am Vet Med Assoc 2009;235:1462–6.

51. Ramsell KD, Garner MM. Disseminated idiopathic myofasciitis in ferrets. Vet Clin North Am Exot Anim Pract 2010;13:561–75.

52. Draper WE, Schubert TA, Clemmons RM, et al. Low-level laser therapy reduces time to ambulation in dogs after hemilaminectomy: a preliminary study. J Small Anim Pract 2012;53:465–9.

53. Pollock CG. Disorders of the urinary and reproductive systems. In: Quesenberry KE, Carpenter JW, editors. Ferrets, rabbits and rodents: clinical medicine and surgery. 3rd edition. St Louis (MO): Saunders Elsevier; 2012. p. 46–61.

54. Martorell J, Vilalta L, Dominguez E, et al. Hydronephrosis secondary to congenital bilateral ureteral stenosis in a ferret (Mustela putorius furo). In: Proceedings of the Annual Conference of the Association of Exotic Mammal Veterinarians. Orlando (FL): 2014.

55. Di Girolamo N, Carnimeo A, Nicoletti A, et al. Retrocaval ureter in a ferret. J Small Anim Pract 2015;56:355.

56. Nolte DM, Carberry CA, Gannon KM, et al. Temporary tube cystostomy as a treatment for urinary obstruction secondary to adrenal disease in four ferrets. J Am Anim Hosp Assoc 2002;38:527–32.

57. Phair KA, Carpenter JW, Schermerhorn T, et al. Diabetic ketoacidosis with concurrent pancreatitis, pancreatic β islet cell tumor, and adrenal disease in an obese ferret (Mustela putorius furo). J Am Assoc Lab Anim Sci 2011;50:531–5.

58. Hess L. Insulin glargine treatment of a ferret with diabetes mellitus. J Am Vet Med Assoc 2012;241:1490–4.

59. Hume DZ, Drobatz KJ, Hess RS. Outcome of dogs with diabetic ketoacidosis: 127 dogs (1993-2003). J Vet Intern Med 2006;20:547–55.

60. Malakoff RL, Laste NJ, Orcutt CJ. Echocardiographic and electrocardiographic findings in client-owned ferrets: 95 cases (1994-2009). J Am Vet Med Assoc 2012;241:1484–9.

61. Stepien RL, Benson KG, Forrest LJ. Radiographic measurement of cardiac size in normal ferrets. Vet Radiol Ultrasound 1999;40:606–10.

62. Martínez J, Martorell J, Abarca M, et al. Pyogranulomatous pleuropneumonia and mediastinitis in ferrets (Mustela putorius furo) associated with Pseudomonas luteola infection. J Comp Pathol 2012;146:4–10.

63. Schoemaker N, Valtolina C, van Zeeland Y. Successful treatment of a suspected Nocardia-related pyothorax in two ferrets. In: Proceedings of the Annual Conference of the Association of Exotic Mammal Veterinarians. San Antonio (TX): 2015. p. 365.

64. Staats BA, Ellefson RD, Budahn LL, et al. The lipoprotein profile of chylous and nonchylous pleural effusions. Mayo Clin Proc 1980;55:700–4.

65. Center SA. Fluid accumulation disorders. In: Willard MD, Tvedtend H, editors. Small animal clinical diagnosis by laboratory methods. 5th edition. St Louis (MO): Elsevier; 2012. p. 226–59.

66. Di Girolamo N, Critelli M, Zeyen U, et al. Ventricular septal defect in a ferret (Mustela putorius furo). J Small Anim Pract 2012;53:549–53.

67. Dudás-Györki Z, Szabó Z, Manczur F, et al. Echocardiographic and electrocardiographic examination of clinically healthy, conscious ferrets. J Small Anim Pract 2011;52:18–25.

68. Sanchez-Migallon Guzman D, Mayer J, Melidone R, et al. Pacemaker implantation in a ferret (Mustela putorius furo) with third-degree atrioventricular block. Vet Clin North Am Exot Anim Pract 2006;9:677–87.

69. Schoemaker NJ, van Zeeland YRA. Ferret cardiology. In: Proceedings of the Annual Conference of the Association of Exotic Mammal Veterinarians. Oakland (CA): 2011. p. 12–8.

70. Bradbury C, Saunders AB, Heatley JJ, et al. Transvenous heartworm extraction in a ferret with caval syndrome. J Am Anim Hosp Assoc 2010;46:31–5.

71. Antinoff N. Clinical observations in ferrets with naturally occurring heartworm disease and preliminary evaluation of treatment with ivermectin with and without melarsomine. Proc Recent Advances in Heartworm Disease: Symposium, Batavia, IL; 2001. p. 45–7.

72. Williams JG, Graham JE, Laste NJ, et al. Tetralogy of Fallot in a young ferret (Mustela putorius furo). J Exot Pet Med 2011;20:232–6.

73. van Schaik-Gerritsen KM, Schoemaker NJ, Kik MJ, et al. Atrial septal defect in a ferret (Mustela putorius furo). J Exot Pet Med 2013;2013(22):70–5.

74. Di Girolamo N, Zeyen U, Fecteau K, et al. High-grade aortic insufficiency secondary to hypertension in a ferret with elevated serum aldosterone. In: Proceedings of the Annual Conference of the Association of Exotic Mammal Veterinarians. Indianapolis (IN): 2013.

75. Olin JM, Smith TJ, Talcott MR. Evaluation of noninvasive monitoring techniques in domestic ferrets (Mustela putorius furo). Am J Vet Res 1997;58:1065–9.

76. Desmarchelier M, Lair S, Dunn M, et al. Primary hyperaldosteronism in a domestic ferret with an adrenocortical adenoma. J Am Vet Med Assoc 2008;233:1297–301.

77. Pignon C, Krumeich N, Vallefuoco R, et al. Orthopedic pelvic fracture repair in a ferret (Mustela putorius furo). In: Proceedings of the Annual Conference of the Association of Exotic Mammal Veterinarians. Indianapolis (IN): 2013.

78. Kaelble MK. Multi-systemic trauma in a ferret. J Vet Emerg Crit Care 2000;10:13–8.

Common Emergencies in Small Rodents, Hedgehogs, and Sugar Gliders

Alicia McLaughlin, DVM*, Anneliese Strunk, DVM, DABVP (Avian)

KEYWORDS

- Rodents • Hedgehogs • Sugar gliders • Emergency • Critical care

KEY POINTS

- Small exotic mammals are prone to a variety of health problems, and require specialized husbandry care to remain healthy.
- Small exotic mammals often present to emergency hospitals in critical condition. Veterinarians should pursue diagnostic workups and initiate supportive care to maximize chances of survival.
- This article provides an overview of common emergencies in small rodents, hedgehogs, and sugar gliders.

INTRODUCTION

Small exotic mammal pets such as rats, mice, hamsters, gerbils, degus, hedgehogs, and sugar gliders are becoming more popular. Many people obtain exotic pets without appropriately researching their husbandry needs. As a result, these animals often suffer from preventable diseases. Veterinary clinicians must know what is "normal" for each species and be familiar with appropriate handling and restraint techniques to examine these patients safely, accurately identify and interpret abnormal examination findings and inappropriate husbandry situations, and provide standard of care. Emergency clinicians should familiarize themselves with the veterinary literature before adding small exotic mammals to their case load (**Box 1**).[1–18]

Patient Evaluation Overview

Small rodents

Small rodents that are commonly kept as pets include rats (*Rattus norvegicus*), mice (*Mus musculus*), gerbils (*Meriones unguiculatus*), Syrian/golden hamsters (*Mesocricetus auratus*), Siberian/dwarf hamsters (*Phodopus sungorus*), Chinese hamsters

The authors have nothing to disclose.
Center for Bird and Exotic Animal Medicine, 11401 NE 195th Street, Bothell, WA 98011, USA
* Corresponding author.
E-mail address: drmclaughlin@theexoticvet.com

Box 1
Handwashing before handling small exotics

Veterinarians should always wash their hands before and after handling small exotic mammals. This ensures that hands do not smell like a predator species, minimizing stress and risk of bites from the patient, and reduces the risk of the veterinarian contracting a zoonotic disease.

(*Cricetus griseus*), and degus (*Octodon* sp.). All of these species, except for Degus, have 4 continuously growing incisor teeth, and cheek teeth that do not grow after eruption. Degus are hystricomorphs, similar to guinea pigs and chinchillas, and all of their teeth grow continuously. Normal physiologic parameters for these species are listed in **Table 1**, and appropriate phlebotomy, catheterization, and injection sites are listed in **Table 2**.

Because many of these animals are used in laboratory research, a significant body of literature exists documenting their health problems (natural or induced).[19] The reader is encouraged to reference laboratory animal literature when researching handling/diagnostic techniques, diseases, and treatment options for small rodents (**Fig. 1**).

Hedgehogs

African Pygmy Hedgehogs (hedgehogs; *Atelerix albiventris*), are nocturnal insectivores native to central Africa. Their dorsum is covered with smooth spines, which serve as their defense mechanism; hedgehogs who feel threatened will curl up tightly into a ball. Restraint can be challenging in this species. Some individuals may be scruffed (**Fig. 2**), and will unroll in a shallow pan of water, but they often require sedation or general anesthesia for complete examination. Normal physiologic parameters for hedgehogs are listed in **Table 3**, and appropriate phlebotomy, catheterization, and injection sites are listed in **Table 4**.

Sugar gliders

Sugar gliders (*Petaurus breviceps*) are nocturnal marsupials native to New Guinea and Australia. They are arboreal and social, sharing their nests with small groups of adults and young. They have a gliding membrane (patagium) extending between their front feet to their distal hind limbs, and can use this membrane to glide through the air.

Table 1
Normal physiologic parameters of small rodents

Species	Life Span (y)	Average Weight (g)	Rectal Temperature	Heart Rate (bpm)	Respiratory Rate (bpm)
Rats	2–3.5	Males: 270–500 Females: 225–325	100.4°F (38°C)	310–500	70–150
Mice	1–2.5	Males: 20–40 Females: 20–60	99.5°F (37.5°C)	420–700	100–250
Gerbils	2–3	Males: 46–131 Females: 50–55	99.3–102.2°F (37.4–39°C)	260–600	85–160
Hamsters	1.5–2	Males: 87–130 Females: 95–130	97.2–99.5°F (36.2–37.5°C)	300–470	40–110
Degus	7–10	176–315	98.2–99.7°F (36.8–37.6°C)	Not published	Not published

Data from Refs.[1,9]

Table 2
Phlebotomy, IV/IO catheterization, and injection sites for small rodents[1,2,9,15,16,19]

Reported Phlebotomy Sites[a]	IV Catheterization Sites[a]	IO Catheterization Sites[a]	Injection Sites
Cranial vena cava	Cephalic vein	Proximal tibia, through tibial crest	IM: quadriceps, gluteal, biceps, triceps
Jugular vein			
Femoral vein	Lateral saphenous vein		SQ: intrascapular, dorsum, flank
Lateral saphenous vein		Proximal femur, through trochanteric fossa	IV: cephalic, lateral saphenous, lateral tail vein
Cephalic vein			
Ventral coccygeal vein	Lateral tail vein		
Lateral tail vein			

Abbreviations: IM, intramuscular; IO, intraosseous; IV, intravenous; SQ, subcutaneous.
[a] General anesthesia is required for almost all venipuncture and any attempts at catheterization.

Some clinically important anatomical features are highlighted in **Box 2** and **Figs. 3–5**. Care should be taken when handling to avoid bites. Anesthesia may be required for complete examination. Normal physiologic parameters for sugar gliders are listed in **Table 5**, and appropriate phlebotomy, catheterization, and injection sites are shown in **Table 6**.

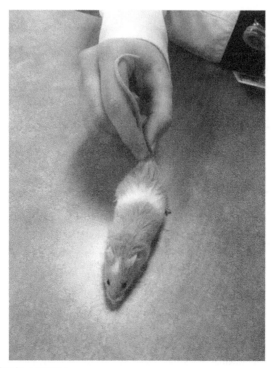

Fig. 1. Tail restraint in a mouse.

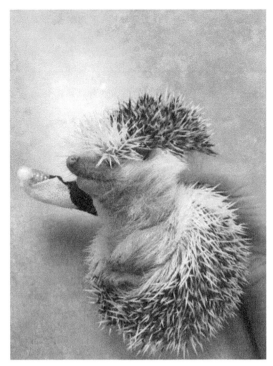

Fig. 2. Scruffing restraint in a hedgehog.

Table 3
Normal physiologic parameters of African pygmy hedgehogs

Life Span	Average Weight	Rectal Temperature	Heart Rate	Respiratory Rate
4–7 y	Males: 400–600 g Females: 400–500 g	95.7–98.6°F (36.1–37.2°C)	180–280 bpm	25–50 bpm

Adapted from Ivey E, Carpenter J. African Hedgehogs. In: Quesenberry K, Carpenter J, editors. Ferrets, rabbits, and rodents: clinical medicine and surgery. 3rd edition. St Louis (MO): Elsevier; 2012.

Table 4
Phlebotomy, IV/IO catheterization, and injection sites for African pygmy hedgehogs[10,14,17]

Reported Phlebotomy Sites[a]	IV Catheterization Sites[a]	IO Catheterization Sites[a]	Injection Sites
Cranial vena cava Jugular vein Femoral vein Lateral saphenous Cephalic	Cephalic	Proximal tibia, through tibial crest Proximal femur, through trochanteric fossa	IM: triceps, quadriceps, gluteal SQ: flank, junction of furred and spined skin midbody

Abbreviations: IM, intramuscular; IO, intraosseous; IV, intravenous; SQ, subcutaneous.
[a] General anesthesia is required for venipuncture and any attempts at catheterization.

Box 2
Clinically important sugar glider anatomy/physiology differences

Marsupial anatomy and physiology varies significantly from that of domestic species

- The "cloaca" is a common terminal opening for the rectum, urinary tract, and genital tract.

- Intact males have a pendulous scrotal sac suspended by a thin stalk cranial to the penis. Their penis is bifurcated (forked). Males also have scent glands on the forehead, chest, and cloaca (paracloacal glands), which may be mistaken for areas of alopecia. Females have a pouch on their ventral abdomen that contains scent glands; the pouch can be used to differentiate them from a neutered male on examination.

- Sugar gliders have slow metabolisms (two-thirds of that of placental mammals). They have a lower overall body temperature and do not regulate their body temperature well; as a result, they are more susceptible to temperature fluctuations compared with other mammals.

- The first digits of the hind feet do not have a toenail, and the second and third digits of the hind feet are syndactylous, functioning as a single digit that aids in grooming.

Data from Johnson-Delaney C. Marsupials. In: Meredith A, Johnson-Delaney C, editors. BSAVA manual of exotic pets. Gloucester: British Small Animal Veterinary Association; 2010. p. 103–26.

EMERGENCY MEDICINE

Small exotic mammals usually hide symptoms of illness until they are too weak to do otherwise. Many patients presenting to an emergency hospital are suffering from chronic illness, although their owners may complain of an acute presentation, and may be affected by more than one disease process. It is important for the veterinarian to look beyond the presenting complaint and evaluate for husbandry problems as well to identify hidden issues. Malnutrition and improper housing environment are common contributing factors to disease.

The importance of appropriate diagnostic workup and prompt medical attention in these patients cannot be overemphasized. Many emergency clinicians who do not specialize in exotic animals resort to minimalistic treatment approaches out of a combination of unfamiliarity with the species and fear of causing harm. In some cases, this is effective (ie, it is usually not wrong to place an animal who is in respiratory distress in

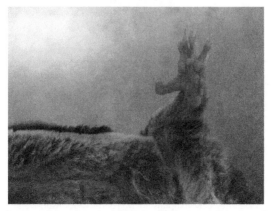

Fig. 3. Hind foot of sugar glider, showing digit 1 with no toenail and syndactylous grooming toe (fused digit 2–3).

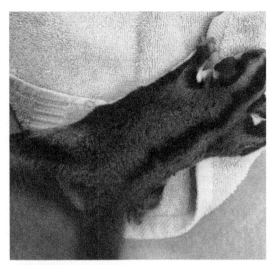

Fig. 4. Patagium of a sugar glider.

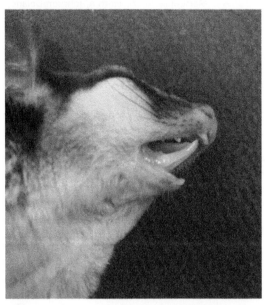

Fig. 5. Normal mandibular incisors in a sedated sugar glider; these are significantly longer than the maxillary incisors.

Table 5 Normal physiologic parameters of sugar gliders				
Life Span	**Average Weight**	**Temperature**	**Heart Rate**	**Respiratory Rate**
12–14 y in captivity	Males: 115–160 g Females: 95–135 g	Average cloacal temperature 89.6°F (32°C); rectal temperature 97.3°F (36.3°C)	200–300 bpm	16–40 bpm

Adapted from Johnson-Delaney C. Marsupials. In: Meredith A, Johnson-Delaney C, editors. BSAVA manual of exotic pets. Gloucester (United Kingdom): British Small Animal Veterinary Association; 2010. p. 104; with permission.

Table 6
Phlebotomy, IV/IO catheterization, and injection sites for sugar gliders[3,11,13]

Reported Phlebotomy Sites[a]	IV Catheterization Sites[a]	IO Catheterization Sites[a]	Injection Sites
Cranial vena cava[a]	Cephalic	Proximal tibia, through tibial crest	IM: quadriceps, gluteal, biceps, triceps
Jugular vein[a]	Lateral saphenous		
Cephalic			
Lateral saphenous		Proximal femur, through trochanteric fossa	SQ: intrascapular, flank
Femoral			
Ventral coccygeal vein			IV: cephalic, lateral tail, pouch vein
Lateral tail vein			
Medial tibial artery			

Abbreviations: IM, intramuscular; IO, intraosseous; IV, intravenous; SQ, subcutaneous.

[a] General anesthesia is required for jugular and cranial vena cava approaches to venipuncture as well as for any attempts at catheterization. It should be considered for other venipuncture locations in all but the most docile of sugar gliders.

oxygen; subcutaneous fluids and prompt administration of antibiotics can be life-saving). However, in other cases, delaying more aggressive supportive care techniques can result in death of the patient. Emergency clinicians should develop a toolkit for these species in order to be able to provide appropriate care (**Box 3, Fig. 6**).

Triage

Emergency veterinarians may be asked to triage cases over the phone. As a general rule, if an owner of one of these small mammal patients is calling to ask if their pet should be seen on emergency, it probably should, because illness is rarely recognized

Box 3
Small exotic mammal emergency toolkit

- A clear, flat-bottomed, plastic container with a lockable lid and air holes drilled in the sides, to safely contain the patient when obtaining a weight
- Gram scale – this is absolutely imperative to appropriately dose these animals with medications
- Ophthalmoscope and light source
- Otoscope with smallest available cone
- Large otoscope cone, modified for use as a laryngoscope (see also **Fig. 7** for an example of a rat-sized 3D printed laryngoscope)
- Nonrebreathing anesthesia system with 0.25 to 0.5 L bag
- Several different sizes of anesthesia masks that can either be used as an induction chamber for small patients or to provide oxygen support via facemask (see **Fig. 6**)
- 26-G intravenous catheters
- Spinal catheters for use in intraosseous catheter placement
- 4-0 and 5-0 suture
- Bandaging materials that have been cut into more narrow widths to fit smaller patients
- Appropriately sized surgical tools

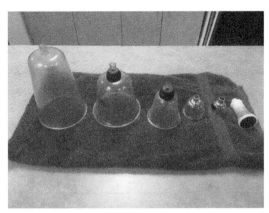

Fig. 6. Anesthetic masks used for small exotic mammals.

in early stages. Triage of small exotic mammal emergencies otherwise follows similar principles to triage of canine/feline emergencies.

Cardiopulmonary Cerebral Resuscitation

The entire medical team must be trained and prepared for administration of cardiopulmonary cerebral resuscitation (CPCR) in exotic species to maximize the chances of patient survival. CPCR guidelines for dogs and cats can be used in small exotic mammals, with some exceptions. **Table 7** provides dosages of common emergency drugs in these species.

Respiratory support

Intubate the patient if possible. A size 1.0 to 2.0 uncuffed tube is suitable for many of the species seen; alternatively, a red rubber tube, tomcat catheter, or 22-G to 18-G intravenous (IV) catheter can be used.[20] Because many rodents are obligate or dependent nasal breathers, with recessed larynxes, large tongues, small oral cavities, and small larynx/tracheas, tracheal intubation is very difficult, although it can be performed endoscopically.[21] An otoscope tube may be modified as a laryngoscope for some of these patients, particularly rats; alternatively, a 3-dimensional printer can be used to create your own laryngoscope (**Fig. 7**).[22] Hedgehogs and sugar gliders can be intubated relatively easily with a small laryngoscope.

If the larynx cannot be visualized, a needle can be used to puncture the tracheal lumen, and a wire stylet can be retrograded into the oral cavity and used to thread an endotracheal tube into the trachea.[23] Tracheotomies can also be performed, but should be reserved as a last resort owing to the risk of long-term complications.[24]

A nonrebreathing system should be used with a 0.25- or 0.5-L bag to provide intermittent positive pressure ventilation with oxygen at a rate of 20 to 30 breaths per minute. If airway access cannot be established, and a tracheotomy is not possible or desirable, a well-fitting mask can be used to attempt intermittent positive pressure ventilation in rodents as they are obligate nasal breathers.[25]

Cardiovascular support

Direct auscultation or palpation of the heart allows evaluation for cardiac arrest, arrhythmias, or other abnormalities. Electrocardiographic leads can be connected quickly to rapidly declining patients to diagnose arrhythmias. Treatment for arrhythmias should be initiated as in other species. If the patient is in cardiac arrest, the

Table 7
Emergency drug dosages for small rodents, hedgehogs, and sugar gliders

Emergency Drugs	Small Rodent Dose	Hedgehog Dose	Sugar Glider Dose
Epinephrine	0.003 mg/kg IV, IM	0.003 mg/kg IV, IM	0.003 mg/kg IV, IM
Atropine	0.05–0.4 mg/kg IV, IM	0.05–0.2 mg/kg IV, IM, SQ	0.01–0.04 mg/kg IV, IM, SQ
Glycopyrrolate	0.01–0.02 mg/kg IV, IM	0.01–0.02 mg/kg IV, IM, SQ	0.01–0.02 mg/kg IV, IM, SQ
Doxapram	5–10 mg/kg IV, IM, SQ	2–10 mg/kg IV, IM, SQ	2 mg/kg IV, IM, SQ
Lidocaine	1–2 mg/kg IV Rabbit dose for treatment of ventricular tachycardia	Dose unpublished, extrapolate from other species	Dose unpublished, extrapolate from other species
Calcium gluconate	100 mg/kg slow IV, IM	100–150 mg/kg slow IV, IM	100 mg/kg slow IV, IM, SQ
Dexamethasone	0.5–5 mg/kg SQ, IM, IV (use with caution)	1–4 mg/kg SQ, IM, IV (use with caution)	0.1–2 mg/kg SQ, IM, IV (use with caution)
Diazepam	1–2 mg/kg IV, IM prn for seizures	0.5–2 mg/kg IV, IM prn for seizures	1–2 mg/kg IV, IM prn for seizures
Midazolam	1–2 mg/kg IV/IM For seizures or sedation Better IM absorption than diazepam	0.25–0.5 mg/kg IV/IM For seizures or sedation Better IM absorption than diazepam	0.25–0.5 mg/kg IV/IM For seizures or sedation Better IM absorption than diazepam
Furosemide	1–10 mg/kg IV, IM, SQ, PO q 4–12 hours prn	2.5–5 mg/kg IV, IM, SQ, PO q8h prn	1–5 mg/kg IV, IM, SQ, PO q6-12h prn

Abbreviations: IM, intramuscular; IO, intraosseous; IV, intravenous; prn, as needed; SQ, subcutaneous.
Data from Carpenter J. Exotic animal formulary. 4th edition. St Louis (MO): Elsevier Saunders; 2013.

clinician should use his or her thumb and index/third finger to apply chest compressions directly over the heart (using the "cardiac pump") at as close to the normal heart rate as possible.[26]

Catheterization
Intravenous catheter placement can be very challenging in small exotic patients. The authors have good success in placing 26-G IV catheters in hedgehogs, sugar gliders, and rats (**Tables 2**, **4**, **6**). For hedgehogs and sugar gliders, the best site for IV catheterization is the cephalic vein (**Figs. 9** and **10**). In rats, the cephalic, lateral saphenous, and superficial lateral tail veins are easiest to use.

For smaller rodent patients or patients in severe hypovolemic shock, IV catheterization may not be possible. Intraosseous catheterization is an excellent alternative in these patients.[27,28] The most common intraosseous catheter sites in small exotic mammals are either the proximal tibia or proximal femur (**Figs. 8** and **9**).

Fluid therapy should always be part of the CPCR strategy. Volume overload is easy to induce in small exotics. Shock doses of fluids should only be used in cases of severe blood loss/ongoing losses (see Brian Roberts: Basic Shock Physiology and Critical Care, in this issue).

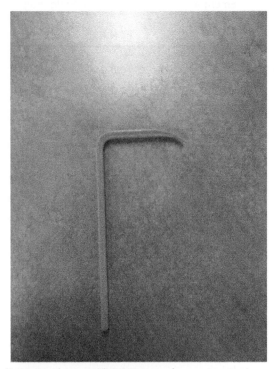

Fig. 7. Custom 3-dimensional printed laryngoscope for use in rats.

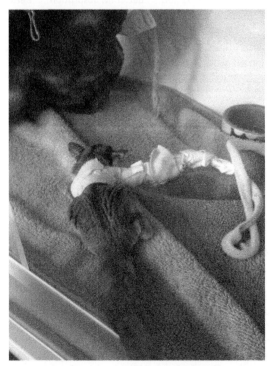

Fig. 8. This sugar glider was attempting to remove its catheter and chew on its intravenous (IV) line. An Elastikon (Johnson & Johnson Consumer Products Company, Skillman, NJ) vest and IV line cover helped it to receive the fluid therapy that it needed.

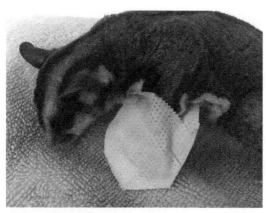

Fig. 9. "Tape sandwich" bandage (Zonas porous tape, Johnson & Johnson Consumer Products Company, Skillman, NJ) over feet to prevent catheter removal in a sugar glider.

Reviews of principles of CPCR in exotic animals have been published, and readers are encouraged to consult these papers for more information.[26,29]

Critical Care Assessment and Treatment

The physical examination may have to be performed gradually depending on the patient's stability.[30] If signs of stress are noted, including changes in respiratory rate or depth, changes to attitude or behavior, and so on, the patient should be set down immediately and allowed to rest. Sedation should be considered for some patients to minimize stress, depending on the degree of illness present, and is usually necessary for hedgehog examinations. Treatment for respiratory distress and trauma should be initiated immediately, if present, by providing the patient with oxygen support and achieving hemostasis.

Hypothermia is considered a seriously life-threatening situation. In a recent study, rabbits that were hypothermic on admission were 3 times more likely to die than rabbits without hypothermia.[31] Temperature should be determined during the initial triage process. Hypothermic patients should be provided with heat support immediately and monitored intensively both during and after the rewarming process. Heat support should also include the administration of warmed fluids (**Box 4, Fig. 10**).

Fluid support

Many small exotic mammal patients present in early decompensatory hypovolemic shock, showing symptoms of hypothermia, bradycardia, normal to decreased blood

---

Box 4
Temperature regulation issues of small exotic mammals

- Cold shock can lead to a stuporous state similar to hibernation in hedgehogs.
- Sugar gliders are prone to both hypothermia and hyperthermia owing to their low metabolism.
- Small patients have a high body surface area and are more prone to heat loss.
- Temperature monitoring should be continued after normothermia has been initially achieved.

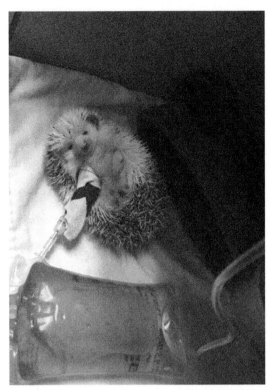

Fig. 10. Warm saline bag laid over intravenous line of critical patient to serve as a fluid warmer (food coloring used to differentiate saline bags used for warming from bags of fluids used for fluid therapy).

pressure, pale mucous membranes, prolonged capillary refill time, and mental depression.[29] Aggressive fluid therapy and supportive care are necessary to save these patients. An excellent review of the use of fluids in exotic species was published in 2004, and should be referenced for further information (**Box 5**).[32]

Fluid rates should be calculated as in dogs and cats. Reported maintenance rates for small exotic mammals range from 40 to 150 mL/kg per day, depending on species; gerbils are at the lowest end of the dose range owing to their desert adaptations, whereas mice are at the highest end of the dose range.[33] The dehydration percentage can be calculated based on clinical examination findings using the same parameters as in dogs and cats. Fluid rates should be adjusted as needed based on the patient's response to treatment and packed cell volume changes. Syringe pumps are usually necessary to administer the appropriate fluid rates owing to patient size. In very small patients, or in cases where clinicians do not have access to a syringe pump, hourly fluid boluses can be administered slowly IV.

The need for a whole blood transfusion should be assessed based on degree of clinical signs, continued or severe acute blood loss, character of anemia, and presence of clotting disorders.[34] If a transfusion is indicated, a step-by-step description of the process is available elsewhere.[35]

Treatment with synthetic colloids such as hydroxyethyl starch compounds (Hespan, B. Braun Medical Inc, Bethlehem, PA) is controversial at this time, because

---

Box 5
Recommendations for fluid route of administration

- Oral fluids can be given if the patient is stable and <5% dehydrated.

- Subcutaneous fluids should ideally only be used when venous or interosseous access cannot be obtained, and/or when the patient is <5% dehydrated.
  - Caveat: In clinical practice, patients who are more than 5% dehydrated have received subcutaneous fluids and seemed to benefit from them. In severely debilitated and hypovolemic patients, a small (1/4–1/2 maintenance) bolus of subcutaneous fluids may be administered on intake, which may help to facilitate intravenous catheter placement after assessment and discussion with the owner.

- Patients who are >5% dehydrated should receive intravenous or intraosseous fluid replacement to maximize their chances of survival.

---

several studies in humans have shown there is an increased risk of renal compromise and coagulopathy, and a correlation with poor treatment outcome.[36–38] Although there is currently no evidence to confirm a similar risk correlation in exotic animals, these fluids should be used as a last resort until further studies have been performed.[39]

Pain medication

Small exotic mammals that are suffering from painful conditions should be provided with analgesic support as soon as possible, because pain can lead to increased morbidity and mortality.[40] Symptoms of pain include lethargy, depressed mentation, reclusive or aggressive behavior, a hunched body posture, piloerection, poor grooming, chewing, licking, or overgrooming the site where pain is occurring, and vocalization.[30] Some small mammals with obviously painful conditions may not demonstrate any of these signs owing to their instinct to hide signs of illness, but should be treated with analgesics regardless. In critical patients, the dose of pain medication used should be reduced to decrease the risk of side effects. Clinicians should refer to Carpenter's Exotic Animal Formulary, 4th edition, for suggested doses of analgesics.[41]

Diagnostic Testing

Testing should be prioritized to minimize stress to the patient. Clinicians should consider collecting diagnostic samples over the course of several hours to give the patient periods of rest and to reduce the length of time that the patient has to be restrained at any one time. Alternatively, diagnostic samples may be collected after sedating or anesthetizing the patient for a short time period. It is absolutely imperative to have everything necessary for the procedure(s) ready in advance so that the animal can be restrained for the shortest time possible.

Anesthesia of small exotic mammals may be necessary for sample collection, catheter placement, or other treatment procedures, and can be performed using the same chemical restraint techniques used in dogs and cats. A variety of anesthesia protocols are published for small exotic mammal patients.[41,42] Isoflurane or sevoflurane gas is often used for very short procedures. A benzodiazepine combined with an opioid can alternatively be used to reduce anxiety, sedate the patient, and provide pain control. Because many of these emergency patients are extremely debilitated, the lowest effective doses of anesthetic/sedation agents should be used, a multimodal protocol should be selected whenever possible, and the patient should be monitored intensively throughout (**Box 6**).[43] For more information regarding anesthesia see Sandra Allweiler: How to Improve Anesthesia and Analgesia in Small Mammals, in this issue.

Most tests that can be performed in other species can be performed in these animals, although there are some limitations owing to patient size.[44] Complete blood count and serum chemistry should be considered part of the minimum database in most of these emergency patients, and can be collected from all but the smallest patients. It is always important to calculate the amount of blood that is safe to draw in these smaller patients. It is generally considered safe to draw approximately 1% of the body weight of a healthy small exotic mammal (approximately 7%–10% of total blood volume). However, no more than 0.5% of the body weight should be collected for sampling in a sick small exotic mammal.[45]

Potential locations for phlebotomy in these species are listed in **Tables 2**, **4**, and **6**. It can be very challenging to collect large volumes of blood from peripheral blood vessels owing to their tendency to collapse. Rubber bands can be used as tourniquets, and the site can be warmed to improve vasodilation and maximize volume obtained.[46]

In the authors' experience, drawing blood in these species from the cranial vena cava under isoflurane anesthesia allows rapid collection of adequate blood volumes for the purpose of diagnostic testing with minimum stress to the patient (**Fig. 11**). Risks of this technique include hemorrhage into the thoracic cavity and/or pericardial sac and cardiac puncture; however, these risks are minimized with a good understanding of anatomy, general anesthesia at the time of the blood draw, and use of a 25-G needle or smaller.[45]

Urine can be collected via ultrasound-guided cystocentesis, palpation-guided cystocentesis (if the clinician has a good familiarity with species anatomy and/or does not have access to ultrasound), and free catch samples (which may be collected in a sterile container with gentle bladder expression or via a catch tray within the cage). Catheterization in these species may be difficult or impossible owing to the small size of their urethras.

Radiographs are extremely helpful for screening patients for a variety of illnesses. In debilitated patients, radiographs may be taken without sedation. However, for healthier, aggressive, stressed patients, and most hedgehogs, sedation is often necessary for diagnostic image collection. Tape can be used to keep the radiographer's hands out of the radiographic beam. The spines of hedgehogs should be lifted away from the body and taped to the x-ray plate on lateral views to minimize interference with the radiographic image (**Fig. 12**). Orthogonal views should always be

---

Box 6
Anesthetic monitoring tools

Anesthetic monitoring tools that can be used in exotic patients

- Direct auscultation
- Visual observation of respiratory excursions (shallowing of excursions is often the first sign of an anesthetic complication)
- Electrocardiogram
- Body temperature
- CO_2 output (if intubated)
- Pulse oximetry
- Indirect blood pressure (not always accurate in these patients owing to small size)
- Doppler assessment of pulse/heartbeat

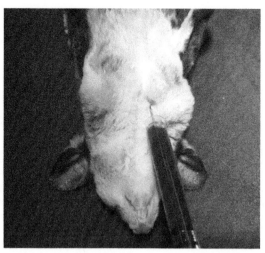

Fig. 11. Drawing blood from the cranial vena cava in an anesthetized sugar glider using an 0.5-mL insulin syringe.

obtained. There are a variety of references available to obtain normal images for comparison.[47–49]

Abdominal ultrasonography is somewhat limited by size of the patient. However, most ultrasound machines present in veterinary practices can still be used to identify urinary bladders and obvious abnormalities such as abdominal fluid, pleural effusion, pericardial effusion, and masses. Advanced diagnostic imaging (CT, MRI, etc) may be extremely helpful in diagnosing/staging certain disease processes, although availability varies.[44]

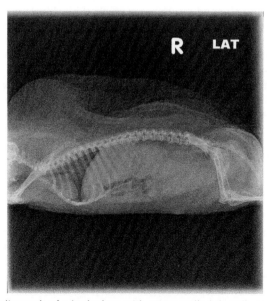

Fig. 12. Lateral radiograph of a hedgehog with spines pulled dorsally to minimize artifact.

If an infectious disease is suspected, bacterial and (if indicated) fungal cultures should be performed. Microbial resistance to antibiotics is becoming very common, and obtaining a culture at the outset of treatment could be the difference between life and death. Traumatic wounds should always be cultured.

COMMON PRESENTING COMPLAINTS ON EMERGENCY

The reader is encouraged to consult other reviews of emergencies in small exotic mammals for additional information/perspectives in these cases.[20,25,30,43,45,50,51]

Anorexia and Lethargy

Decreased appetite and energy levels are one of the most common reasons for small exotic mammal patients to arrive at the emergency hospital. These symptoms are seen with almost every presenting health problem. Because small exotic mammals hide symptoms of illness for as long as possible, an animal that is showing signs of anorexia and lethargy is probably seriously ill. The history and physical examination may help to determine the systems involved. In the absence of physical findings, a minimum database of bloodwork and radiographs should be performed. Supportive care should be initiated until a definitive diagnosis can be identified.

Trauma

Traumatic injuries are common. In general, the stabilization methods used in dogs and cats can be extrapolated to small exotic mammals (**Box 7**). Animal bites are arguably the most common traumatic injury seen in small exotic mammals. Wounds may come from a cage mate, from other household animals, or from wild animals if the patient was housed outdoors (**Fig. 13**). Severity of injuries may vary from mild to life threatening, depending on the animal involved. Many patients will present in shock owing to pain and blood loss.

Blunt trauma, fractures, and/or spinal injuries may be seen associated with falling or being dropped, being stepped on, or being crushed by objects such as furniture or damage from things within the cage wheels, and so on. Tooth damage and/or ocular proptosis are common sequelae. Fractures may be seen secondary to nutritional secondary hyperparathyroidism in sugar gliders; in these cases, the animal will usually be showing concurrent symptoms of hypocalcemic tetany.

Electric shock may occur in patients that have access to electrical wires. Symptoms may include difficulty breathing, loss of appetite (owing to burn wounds on the tongue, lips, gums, and palate), muscle spasms or seizure activity, and secondary infections owing to burn wounds. Burn damage will not be able to be fully assessed for up to several days after the injury.

If the tip of the tail is grabbed or caught in gerbils and some rats, the skin in this area can slough, resulting in necrosis of the underlying tendons and bone known as "fur/skin slip."

Respiratory Distress

Any small exotic mammal patient exhibiting dyspnea should be provided with oxygen support immediately, after checking the airway for possible obstruction and removing any obstructions that are present. Oxygen support is usually best provided via oxygen cages or chambers to minimize handling and patient stress, although severely debilitated patients may allow facemask oxygen delivery. Consider sedation with butorphanol with or without midazolam to reduce anxiety and improve inspiratory depth.

Box 7
Diagnostic workup and treatment of trauma patients

Diagnosis

- Diagnostic imaging (radiographs and ultrasound, as indicated) to assess for fractures, pulmonary contusions/edema, and internal hemorrhage. If a spinal injury is suspected, advanced imaging (CT, MRI, etc) should be considered.

- All wounds should be cultured.

- Bloodwork may be beneficial to look for concurrent disease processes, but may be unwise depending on patient size and amount of blood already lost.

- In electric shock victims, blood gas monitoring and electrocardiogram should be performed to assess respiratory and cardiac function. Diuretics may be necessary if pulmonary edema is present.

Treatment

- Aggressive fluid, antibiotic, and analgesic support is critical. Oxygen/respiratory support may be necessary, especially with electric shock patients.

- Any bleeding should be addressed with direct pressure to the source. Depending on the type of wound, a variety of methods above and beyond direct pressure may be required to achieve hemostasis, including:
  - Silver nitrate/styptic powder[52];
  - Ligation of compromised blood vessel;
  - Cautery of compromised blood vessel;
  - Anesthesia to drop blood pressure and allow clot formation; and
  - Topical epinephrine to induce vasoconstriction.

- Wounds necessitating surgical closure should be covered with a sterile dressing until the patient is stable enough for anesthesia and wound repair. Open wound management should be considered, at least initially, because abscesses are common sequelae to premature closure. Wounds should be thoroughly flushed with sterile saline before closure.

- Both hedgehogs and sugar gliders are prone to self-mutilation and should be prevented from accessing their wounds. Hedgehogs may ingest topical medications by "anointing" with them.[53]

- Surgical repair should be performed as in other species. When possible, intradermal sutures should be used in the final closure layer to minimize the risk of postoperative dehiscence owing to self-trauma.

- In cases of fur/skin slip, the tail should be amputated several vertebrae proximal to the site of skin sloughing. This procedure can be performed as in a dog or cat.

- Fractures may be stabilized surgically or splinted depending on the location/severity of the fracture, age of patient, and concurrent disease. The same principles of fracture management for dogs and cats apply to exotic mammals.
  - Some small mammal patients are intolerant of both splinting and surgical management. If the fracture is closed, 4 to 6 weeks of cage rest may be an acceptable method of treating these patients. However, there may be complications associated with healing, and amputation of a fractured limb may need to be considered as an alternative, depending on the case.

- Spinal injuries cannot currently be treated with surgery in these small patients. Antiinflammatory analgesics, muscle relaxants, and 4 to 6 weeks of cage rest may result in return to partial or full function, depending on severity of the injury. In other patients, the damage will be permanent. Quality of life should be monitored closely.

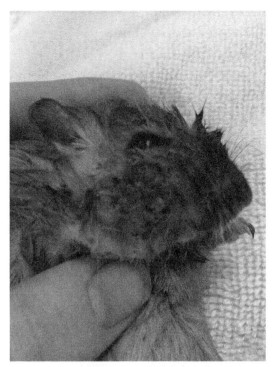

Fig. 13. Cage mate trauma in a gerbil.

Although bacterial pneumonia is a very common cause of respiratory distress in small exotic mammals, there are a wide variety of noninfectious disease processes that can also cause respiratory distress, including choking, cardiac disease, and neoplasia, in addition to atypical infectious diseases (**Table 8**). The emergency practitioner must systematically rule out these other diseases with a thorough diagnostic workup. Radiographs are perhaps the most valuable initial diagnostic test to perform, because the presence of infectious disease is not always reflected in complete blood count results. Additional imaging, including chest ultrasonography and a computed tomography scan, may be necessary to confirm the diagnosis.

Respiratory infections in rodents are often caused by a complex multifactorial syndrome involving multiple bacterial and viral pathogens.[1,12] *Mycoplasma pulmonis* is endemic to most pet rodent populations, and causes disease when concurrent infection is present or when ammonia levels are high in the environment. Common infectious organisms in rats and mice include *Streptococcus pneumoniae*, cilia-associated respiratory bacillus, and Sendai virus. Other rodents may develop disease from *Pasteurella*, *Klebsiella*, *Bordetella*, and *Staphylococcus* species.[12] Hedgehogs can develop pneumonia associated with *Pasteurella*, *Bordetella*, and *Corynebacterium* species, and there is a report of a hedgehog with disseminated histoplasmosis.[54] In addition to antibiotic therapy, the use of nebulization, bronchodilators, and other supportive treatments should be considered (**Fig. 14**, **Table 9**).

Cardiovascular disease is extremely common in small exotic mammals (see **Table 10**). Clinical signs of cardiovascular disease may include dyspnea or open mouth breathing, cyanotic mucous membranes, sternal recumbency, neck extension,

Table 8
Cause and recommended diagnostic testing/treatment for respiratory distress

Cause of Respiratory Distress	Diagnostics/Treatment
Choking	Thorough oral examination using an otoscope or endoscope; endoscopic assisted removal of foreign body to clear the airway (may be removed via the oral cavity using instrumentation or pushed into esophagus if it is a food bolus).
Bacterial pneumonia	Radiographs, CBC, tracheal wash/culture, antibiotics, supportive care (see **Table 9**)
Fungal pneumonia	Radiographs, CBC, tracheal wash/cytology/culture, fungal PCR, CT scan, antifungals
Viral pneumonia	Radiographs, CBC, PCR tests for individual viral diseases
Cardiac disease	Radiographs, echocardiogram, ECG, blood pressure measurement, CBC, chemistry (to assess kidney function), Diuretics, ACE inhibitors, other cardiac supportive medications as indicated
Neoplasia	Radiographs, CT, ultrasound guided FNA/cytology, biopsy, treatment depends upon type/stage of tumor but may include chemotherapy or radiation

Abbreviations: ACE, angiotensin-converting enzyme; CBC, complete blood count; CT, computed tomography; ECG, electrocardiograph; FNA, fine needle aspiration; PCR, polymerase chain reaction.

distended jugular veins, severe lethargy, and abnormal or absent respiratory and/or cardiac sounds.[51] There may be a history of "seizures" (syncopal episodes). Exophthalmia has been reported as being indicative of underlying cardiac disease owing to severe venous congestion[57]; another potential rule out for exophthalmia is a cranial mediastinal mass.

Neoplasia, as in other species, is more common in older patients, but can also be seen in juveniles. Symptoms for neoplasia can be very similar to that of an infectious pneumonia. Treatment options depend on the type of tumor identified and the stage at which it was diagnosed.

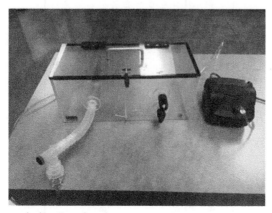

Fig. 14. Mouse in a nebulization chamber.

Table 9
Alternatives to oral antibiotic therapy for treatment of infectious pneumonia in small exotic mammals

Nebulization	Bronchodilators	Antiinflammatory Drugs	Mucolytics	Sildenafil
Antibiotics that can be nebulized include aminoglycosides, fluoroquinolones, tetracyclines, and cephalosporins.[41] Both amphotericin B and terbinifine can be nebulized in cases of fungal pneumonia.[41]	Aminophylline, theophylline, and albuterol can be nebulized or administered orally. (Use dog/cat doses for albuterol[55]; published doses exist for aminophylline and theophylline)	Steroids may be considered in severe cases of respiratory distress.[41] Their use must be carefully evaluated in light of possible side effects such as immunosuppression. Route of administration may be oral, injectable, or nebulized.	N-Acetylcysteine can be used as a mucolytic.[41] The injectable form can be nebulized. May cause respiratory tract irritation; should be used after a bronchodilator.	Sildenafil (5 mg/kg orally once daily) may help manage pulmonary hypertension in rats with chronic infectious respiratory disease.[56]

Table 10		
Causes of cardiovascular disease in small mammals, hedgehogs, and sugar gliders		
Small Mammals	**Hedgehogs**	**Sugar Gliders**
Cardiomyopathy	Cardiomyopathy (incidence	Cardiomyopathy
Atrial thrombosis	approached 40% in one	Myonecrosis
Dystrophic/metastatic	report)[58]	(both associated with
mineralization, calcifying	○ Dilated cardiomyopathy	malnutrition)
vasculopathy	○ Multifocal degeneration and	
Coronary arteriosclerosis	mineralization of cardiac	
Endocardial hyperplasia	myofibers	
Endocardiosis	○ Vascular thrombosis	
Endocarditis/myocarditis		
Toxicity		
Amyloidosis		
Vitamin deficiency/excess		
Septicemia		
Rhabdomyomatosis		
Ventricular septal defect		
Hyperadrenocorticism		
cardiovascular disease		
complex		
Focal myocardial degeneration		
Pericardial effusion/cardiac		
tamponade		
Dilated cardiomyopathy		
Arteriosclerosis		
Aortic rupture		

Heatley J. Cardiovascular anatomy, physiology, and disease of rodents and small exotic mammals. Vet Clin Exot Anim 2009;12:99–113.

Neurologic Disorders

Causes of neurologic disorders include trauma, toxin exposure (such as heavy metal toxicosis), bacterial, viral, fungal, or parasitic infections, tumors, and metabolic abnormalities (see **Box 8**). There are several case reports of intervertebral disc disease in hedgehogs, including one case with concurrent herpes simplex infection.[59,60]

Box 8
Diagnostic workup and treatment of neurologic disorders

Diagnosis

- Radiographs/CT/MRI

- Complete blood count/chemistry/ionized calcium

- Urinalysis

- Fecal analysis to check for signs of parasites

- Toxin screens

Treatment

- Seizures should be managed as in other species

- Provide fluid/nutritional support and nonsteroidal antiinflammatory drugs until the cause of neurologic symptoms can be identified and treated.

A variety of tumors have been noted to affect the central nervous system in small exotic mammals, including pituitary tumors in rats[61] and both astrocytoma and spinal osteosarcoma in hedgehogs.[62–64] There is also a report of a peripheral nerve sheath tumor in a hedgehog.[65] Symptoms may include change in behavior, dull or depressed mentation, head tilt, seizures, and self-mutilation, among others. Computed tomography (CT) or MRI is usually necessary to definitively diagnose a central nervous system tumor, although a strong index of suspicion may be created based on the physical examination findings. The prognosis for these tumors is generally poor. In rats with pituitary tumors, cabergoline at 0.6 mg/kg q72 hours has been used to decrease expression of symptoms and improve quality of life.[41,66]

Head tilts can be caused by central or peripheral vestibular disease. Potential causes for head tilts include otitis media/interna, pituitary tumors in rats, *M pulmonis* infections in rats, and stroke, among others. Cases of suspected strokes are relatively common in older rats.

Wobbly hedgehog syndrome is a disease of unknown etiology, although a genetic component is suspected, that results in a vacuolization of the white matter of the brain and spinal cord, and associated neurogenic muscle atrophy. The symptoms typically progress from mild ataxia to complete paralysis over a variable time period. It usually manifests in hedgehogs under the age of 2 years, although it can occur at any age. There are currently no premortem diagnostic tests available.[67]

The most common cause for seizures and tremors in sugar gliders is hypocalcemia related to nutritional secondary hyperparathyroidism caused by inappropriate husbandry. However, the clinician must be careful to rule out other disease processes in these animals as well.

Sugar gliders and hedgehogs are prone to self-mutilation owing to pain; sugar gliders may also self-mutilate owing to behavioral problems arising from isolation housing.[50] It is very important to use appropriate intraoperative and postoperative pain management protocols in this species to minimize the risk of self-trauma.

Ophthalmic Disorders

Proptosis

Traumatic exophthalmia is very common in hedgehogs owing to their shallow orbital rim.[68] Other potential causes for proptosis include retrobulbar abscessation, potentially related to dental disease, and retrobulbar tumor formation.[69] Hedgehogs suffering from wobbly hedgehog syndrome seem to be especially prone to unilateral exophthalmos, with 1 report listing an incidence rate of 28% of confirmed wobbly hedgehog syndrome cases.[67]

Proptosis can occur iatrogenically in hamsters from being scruffed. If the proptosis is noticed immediately, gentle manipulation may suffice to replace the globe within the orbit (**Box 9**).[70]

Chromodacryorrhea (porphyrin discharge)

Rodents secrete an irritating substance known as porphyrin from the Harderian glands during periods of stress or respiratory illness. The substance is reddish brown and will commonly stain the fur around the eyes, nose, and inside of the front legs (where the patient is grooming). Pet owners who are unfamiliar with this phenomenon may suspect that their pet is bleeding. A Wood's lamp can be used to confirm the diagnosis, as porphyrin fluoresces.[73] Although this symptom is not pathogenic in and of itself, the clinician should seek to identify the underlying reason for the porphyrin discharge.

Box 9
Diagnostic workup and treatment of proptosis

Diagnosis

- A thorough medical history and detailed examination of the dentition and skull may be sufficient to identify the underlying cause.

- Fluorescein stain should be used to evaluate for corneal ulceration if the eye is not going to be enucleated.

- Radiographs (both dental and skull), with or without CT scan, should be performed to rule out a retrobulbar abnormality.

Treatment

- Depending on how quickly the problem is identified, in some cases replacement of globe within the socket followed by a temporary tarsorrhaphy can be curative, or at least lead to a phthisical eye. Butterfly catheter tubing may be used to create stents for tarsorrhaphy sutures. The tarsorrhaphy procedure is otherwise performed as in other species. The tarsorrhaphy sutures should be removed 1 week postoperative and the globe should be examined; if it seems to be healing well, the sutures should be replaced for another week, then removed permanently.[71]

- In many cases, enucleation is necessary. Many small exotic mammals have an orbital sinus that can bleed profusely if it is damaged. A thorough understanding of the ocular anatomy is necessary for this procedure, and Gelfoam or a similar hemostasis product should be available at the time of surgery in case of hemorrhage.[72]

Miscellaneous

Corneal ulcers, eye infections, and other ocular disorders in small exotic mammals are generally managed as in other species. Degus are prone to diabetes when fed a diet high in sugar, and may develop cataracts as a result.[74] Degus with cataracts should be presumed diabetic until proven otherwise.

Gastrointestinal Disorders

Dental disorders

Rodents that do not have appropriate items to gnaw on are prone to incisor overgrowth/malocclusion. Some rodents will chew on metal cage bars, which can result in tooth fractures. Traumatic injuries to the teeth and/or jaws (which are common in cases where the animal is dropped) can also lead to incisor malocclusion. In severe cases, the incisors can grow into the gingiva, hard palate, sinuses, and other anatomic structures, resulting in severe pain and abscessation. Degus can also suffer from overgrowth of the cheek teeth with similar results. Common symptoms include drooling, inappetence, and weight loss.

Hedgehogs and sugar gliders are both prone to oral osteomyelitis, gingivitis, and calculus related to dental disease. Hedgehogs with dental disease will often develop a profound gingival hyperplasia associated with this condition. Hedgehogs are also extremely prone to oral neoplasias, primarily squamous cell carcinoma.[75] These tumors are often found surrounding the dental arcades or tucked up between the maxillary arcades ventral to the hard palate. They are usually very locally invasive, but rarely metastasize. The most common symptoms for dental disease and/or oral tumors are decreased appetite, change in food preference, and weight loss (**Box 10**).

Diarrhea and vomiting

Diarrhea in small exotic mammals is always considered an emergency. These animals can become critically ill and dehydrated within hours of initial symptom presentation.

Box 10
Diagnostic workup and treatment of oral/dental disease

Diagnosis

- Incisor malocclusion can easily be diagnosed on physical examination. If wounds are present, they should be cultured.

- If dental disease is suspected, dental radiographs should be performed to assess for subgingival disease.

- In hedgehogs with either gingival hyperplasia or oral masses, biopsies should always be collected before confirming the diagnosis. Benign processes may be confused with malignant tumors otherwise.

Treatment

- Rodents with incisor malocclusion should be treated for any existing wounds. Their incisors should be trimmed regularly with a high-speed dental drill or cutting disk on a high-speed Dremel tool (toenail trimmers should never be used owing to the risk of causing longitudinal dental fractures below the gingival margin). Alternatively, the incisors can be surgically removed to prevent ongoing overgrowth. Rodents can prehend food well without incisors, although hard food items will need to be broken into small pieces or moistened before feeding.

- Overgrown cheek teeth in degus should be trimmed/managed similarly to rabbits, guinea pigs, and chinchillas.

- Both traumatic fractures of the teeth/jaw, and dental disease of hedgehogs and sugar gliders, should be managed as in a dog or cat.

- Surgical removal of hedgehog oral tumors can be attempted, but it may be difficult to remove the entire tumor, and there is a high rate of reoccurrence. If treatment is attempted, follow-up with chemotherapy, radiation, or cryotherapy under the guidance of a veterinary oncologist should be considered.

Adapted from Heatley J. Cardiovascular anatomy, physiology, and disease of rodents and small exotic mammals. Vet Clin Exot Anim 2009;12:99–113.

Causes of diarrhea include infections (bacterial, viral, fungal, or parasitic), gastrointestinal dysbiosis owing to rapid changes in diet, metabolic disorders, and toxins, among others. Dysbiosis can also be induced iatrogenically by administration of certain antibiotics (see Pharmacologic Species Contraindications under Treatments) to herbivorous rodents such as hamsters and degus. Prolapse of the gastrointestinal tract may be seen associated with severe diarrhea, especially if the animal is also hypocalcemic.

Diarrhea is one of the most common emergency presenting complaints for hamsters. Known to lay people as "wet tail," there are actually many different recorded causes for this symptom. A survey of hamsters from a commercial breeding facility had the following potential pathogens identified in their gastrointestinal tracts: *C piliforme* (Tyzzer's disease), *C difficile* toxins, *Campylobacter* spp., cestodiasis (*Hymenolepis nana*), protozoal infections (Giardia, Entamoeba, *Spironucleus muris*, Trichomonas), *Torulopsis/Candida* yeast, and *Helicobacter*-type spiral organisms.[76] In young hamsters (<10 weeks of age), *Lawsonia intracellularis* infections are reported to be the most common cause of diarrhea; this organism induces proliferative ileitis and a high mortality rate. Other causes for diarrhea in hamsters include *Salmonella*, *Y pseudotuberculosis*, *C perfringens*, and *E coli* infections (**Box 11**).[76,77]

Vomiting may be seen in hedgehogs and sugar gliders, but is not possible in rodents owing to esophageal anatomy.

Box 11
Diagnostic workup and treatment of diarrhea/vomiting

Diagnosis

- Full fecal analysis, including fecal direct/wet mount, fecal float, fecal gram stain cytology, and culture should always be performed in these patients. In many cases, the cause for diarrhea can be identified based on fecal analysis alone.

- Diagnostic imaging (radiographs/ultrasound) is helpful to rule out intussusception, foreign body, obstruction, and/or neoplasia

- Complete blood count/chemistry should be performed to assess for signs of systemic illness (infection and/or organ dysfunction) and degree of dehydration

- Patients should be screened for any suspected toxin exposure.

Treatment

- The most important treatment for diarrhea and/or vomiting in small exotic mammals is fluid support to prevent life-threatening dehydration.

- The underlying cause of illness should be addressed while correcting fluid deficits.

- Cholestyramine may help to bind bacterial enterotoxins. Treating primary or secondary bacterial infections is very important. A good combination therapy to consider is enrofloxacin/metronidazole. If *Lawsonia intracellularis* is suspected, chloramphenicol should be included in the treatment protocol.

- Probiotics and high-fiber liquid critical care diets should also be provided.

- Metoclopramide seems to be an effective antinausea medication in these species.

Urogenital Emergencies

Female hedgehogs very commonly develop reproductive tract tumors, and rats are also prone to reproductive neoplasia (**Fig. 15**).[78–80] If urogenital bleeding is seen, it is very important to perform diagnostic imaging (radiographs, ultrasound imaging) to search for a tumor, in addition to urinalysis. The urine sample should ideally be taken via ultrasound-guided cystocentesis to avoid inadvertently aspirating a fluid-filled uterus, which can be mistaken for a bladder on palpation. Bladder stones, bladder

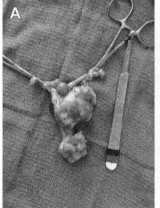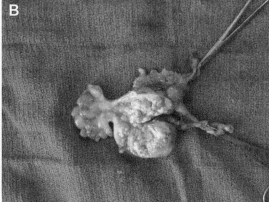

Fig. 15. (*A, B*) Uterine tumor with a necrotic center in a rat.

infections, prostatic disease, and cystic ovaries can also lead to hematuria or stranguria (**Box 12**).

Dystocia is rarely seen in rodents and hedgehogs, but the authors have seen several cases. If it occurs, it is usually secondary to poor calcium supplementation within the diet during pregnancy or fetal malposition or fetal death. It is possible that the animal may be pregnant without the owner being aware, because many exotic pet owners are not able to identify the sex of their pet(s). Dystocia in sugar gliders is not reported because of the marsupial reproductive process.

Hypocalcemic sugar gliders are prone to penile prolapses, and animals experiencing dystocias and/or hypocalcemia related to pregnancy may prolapse their uterus. Pouch infections have been reported in female sugar gliders.[11] Pyometra and mucometra have been reported in small rodents.[1]

Skin Disease

Small exotic mammals may present to the emergency hospital for masses that "just appeared." These masses may be bleeding, either secondary to self-trauma from the patient, or owing to sheer size of the mass and resulting environmental damage. In many cases, the mass will have been present for extended time periods because the owner does not frequently examine the pet. However, in some cases, such as abscesses and certain types of aggressive tumors, masses can seem to develop practically overnight (see **Box 13**).

Abscesses in these species are often secondary to bite wounds or dental disease. Small exotic mammal pus is usually caseous and does not drain well. Abscesses should be surgically addressed (**Fig. 16**).

Tumors are extremely common in both small rodents and hedgehogs, and may be either benign or malignant. Mammary tumors are the most frequently seen tumors in rats. The tumors are estrogen mediated, and spaying female rats at 3 months or less of age significantly decreases their risk of formation.[81] Tumors can arise over most of the body, and can become nearly as large as the rat itself. It is common for these masses to become traumatized from dragging on the ground or self-inflicted wounds. The tumors are usually benign in rats; however, in hedgehogs, mammary tumors are usually malignant and may metastasize.[79,82] Scent gland tumors may be found in gerbils and

---

Box 12
Diagnostic workup and treatment for urogenital disorders

Diagnosis

- An animal suspected of a urogenital disorder should, at bare minimum, undergo radiographs, an ultrasound of the urogenital tract, complete blood count/chemistry with or without ionized calcium (if a sugar glider or pregnant animal), and urinalysis.
- If a tumor is removed, it should be submitted for histopathology.
- If an infection is suspected, a culture should be submitted.

Treatment

- Varies depending on the underlying disease.
- Bleeding uterine tumors and pyometras should be surgically addressed as soon as possible.
- Dystocias can be managed medically or surgically depending on presentation.
- Prolapses should be reduced, and the underlying cause corrected.
- Infections should be treated based on culture results.

Box 13
Diagnostic workup and treatment of skin disorders

Diagnosis

- A fine needle aspirate/cytology of skin masses is sometimes diagnostic, but an excisional biopsy may be necessary to confirm the diagnosis. Radiographs and serum chemistry should be recommended as a way to screen for metastasis if malignant tumors are suspected. A complete blood count can serve as a staging tool for response to abscess treatment.

- If dermatitis is present, a thorough diagnostic workup includes skin scrape/cytology (gram stain and oil mount), dermatophyte culture, bacterial culture, and skin biopsy.

- In severe cases of pododermatitis, radiographs of the affected feet should be performed to check for osteomyelitis.

Treatment

- In most cases, surgical removal of masses is indicated. Abscesses may be marsupialized in some cases, but require extensive follow-up care by the owner.

- If possible, rats with mammary masses should be spayed at time of mass removal or soon thereafter.

- Treatment for dermatitis depends on the underlying cause. Pododermatitis cases can often be managed with bandaging, topical and systemic antibiotics/antiinflammatory drugs, and removal of environmental precursors.

- If a constriction lesion is present, remove the constricting object. This may require sedation and magnifying loupes to find fibers or contracted tissue related to swelling and pain. Wounds should be cultured, and radiographs should be performed if osteomyelitis is suspected. Wounds should be kept covered with a nonadherent bandage until healed. Amputation of the affected tissues is necessary if necrosis is present.

---

hamsters. These tumors usually are found on ventral midline, commonly become abscessed, and are often malignant.[83]

Dermatitis may present as a primary or secondary disease condition in emergency cases. Pododermatitis is common in animals housed on wire flooring, and can also be seen in animals with unclean bedding and/or inappropriately small enclosures, animals with abnormal weight bearing due to lameness, obese animals, and animals with toenails that are severely overgrown. It can be severe enough to result in osteomyelitis and require amputation of the affected limb. All of these animals are prone to ringworm (usually *Trichophyton* spp.), bacterial dermatitis, and a variety of parasitic diseases (fleas, mites, etc).[84] Cutaneous lymphoma is another important rule-out in cases of diffuse alopecia and/or crusting of the skin.[85,86]

Constriction lesion skin wounds may be seen in small exotic mammals with rope or towel substrates. Fibers can wrap around the extremities, cutting off blood supply and resulting in necrosis if not addressed promptly. Young rats housed in low humidity environments are also predisposed to annular constrictive lesions of the tail base, known as "ring tail".[2]

Toxin Exposure

Small exotic mammal toxicity presentations in emergency practice include a variety of plant toxins (often caused by a child feeding the pet or the pet having access to houseplants), topically applied toxins (exposure to flea and tick products, antiseptic solutions, etc), lead-based paint, and accidental access to human medications. Ironically, many pet rodents suffer from rodenticide toxicity when they are allowed to roam the house unsupervised.[87] Toxicities can also arise from owners choosing

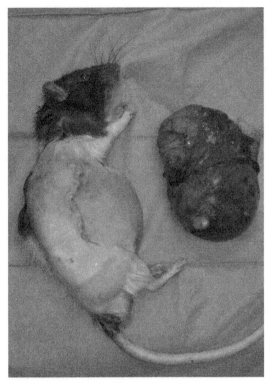

Fig. 16. Rat after surgical removal of an encapsulated abscess.

to medicate their pets without veterinary advice based on information obtained from the Internet.

Diagnosis and treatment for toxicities varies widely depending on the type of intoxicant. There are animal poison control centers that offer toxicologist consulting services, often providing detailed information regarding exotic animal intoxication cases, recommended treatments, and prognosis.[88] This is an excellent resource for the emergency clinician.

TREATMENT

Treatment of small exotic mammal patients is complicated by a general lack of peer-reviewed, evidence-based recommendations. There are a variety of formularies in other textbooks available, but the single most helpful, most applicable resource at this time is Carpenter's Exotic Animal Formulary, 4th edition, which provides dosages for many drug classes in all of the species discussed in this article.[41] The authors strongly advise that anyone considering treatment of these small exotic mammals purchase a copy of this textbook for reference.

There are a number of important pharmacological contraindications in these species (**Box 14**). The dog and cat literature should also be examined for other potential contraindications when developing treatment plans for small exotics.

Nutritional Support

Small exotic mammals can develop serious complications if food is withheld for longer than 12 to 24 hours. Although feeding these patients should a top priority, it

> **Box 14**
> **Pharmacologic species contraindications.**
>
> Hamsters and degus should not receive the following antibiotics orally:
> - Penicillins
> - Cephalosporins (particularly first generation)
> - Lincosamides
> - Macrolides
>
> These medications can induce clostridial enterotoxicity in strictly herbivorous rodents.
>
> *Note:* This rule does not apply to rats, mice, gerbils, hedgehogs, or sugar gliders.
>
> Streptomycin and procaine (Novocain) should not be used in mice.
>
> Nitrofurantoin (Macrobid) should not be used in rats.
>
> Dihydrostreptomycin (Vibriomycin) and streptomycin should not be used in gerbils.
>
> Tylosin (Tylan) should be avoided/only used with extreme caution in hamsters.
>
> *Data from* Lennox A, Bauck L. Small rodents: basic anatomy, physiology, husbandry, and clinical techniques. In: Quesenberry K, Carpenter J, editors. Ferrets, rabbits, and rodents: clinical medicine and surgery. 3rd edition. St Louis (MO): Elsevier; 2012. p. 339–53; and Carpenter J. Exotic animal formulary. 4th edition. St Louis (MO): Elsevier Saunders; 2013.

should not be initiated until the following abnormalities have been addressed: fluid deficit, electrolyte abnormalities, acid–base abnormalities, and body temperature abnormalities.[89] Once these issues have been corrected and pain is under control, most small exotic mammal patients will start eating on their own. It is important to offer a diet that the patient is familiar with, because some of these animals will develop strong dietary preferences and will not eat an unfamiliar food item, especially when ill.

If the patient does not want to eat on its own, careful syringe feeding of a liquid diet such as Oxbow Critical Care or Emeraid Critical Care (Oxbow Animal Health, Murdock, NE; Emeraid LLC, Cornell, IL) can be performed. In general, small exotic mammals should receive 5% to 20% of their body weight in grams in milliliters of food per day, split into multiple feedings; smaller patients require a higher volume of food relative to body weight. Dyspneic patients should be fed with caution, because feeding can lead to choking. Placement of feeding tubes (esophagostomy, gastrostomy, etc) may be considered in persistently anorexic patients.[90]

Surgical treatment options

Surgical intervention may be necessary in some cases (**Box 15**). The most common reason to consider emergency surgery in a small exotic patient is to address internal or external hemorrhage. The general principles of surgery and aseptic technique in exotic mammal species are the same as for other species.

Because it is beyond the scope of this paper to cover all of the possible surgical procedures that may be considered in these species, the reader is encouraged to refer to exotic mammal literature if surgery is being considered for a particular problem.[13,14,91–93]

Treatment complications

Small rodents, hedgehogs, and sugar gliders may be difficult to medicate at home. It is important to teach owners how to appropriately restrain and medicate patients before discharge. Because many of these animals' medications must be compounded owing

---

Box 15
Surgical considerations

- Patients should ideally never be taken to surgery until they have been adequately stabilized. The exception is cases of uncontrolled hemorrhage.

- Intraoperative and postoperative monitoring and supportive care is crucial to a positive outcome. It is important to note that a decrease in ventilatory depth is often one of the first signs of anesthetic complications.

- Anatomy of these species does vary, and should be taken into account when preparing for and performing surgery.

- Please note that in many rodent species, the GI tract is extensive and should be handled with the utmost care to prevent trauma.

---

to their small size, consider tailoring the flavoring of the compounded medication to the individual patient's taste to improve acceptance.

Small rodents and sugar gliders are extremely prone to self-traumatic dehiscence of surgical incisions. Ways to reduce the risk of dehiscence include closing with an intradermal pattern, providing excellent preoperative, intraoperative, and postoperative multimodal analgesia, and in some cases, applying an Elizabethan collar or bandage (body wrap) to prevent the patient from accessing the surgery site. It is important to monitor appetite, drinking, and eliminations to make sure that patients are functioning well with a collar or bandage.

Without correction of underlying husbandry problems, many animals will fail to respond to treatment. Detailed and compassionate communication with the owner, with both verbal and written discharge instructions, will maximize the chance of positive outcomes.

Humane euthanasia of small exotic mammals

Unless a catheter is already present, the authors do not recommend catheter placement before euthanasia to minimize patient stress. Euthanasia should consist of

Table 11
Euthanasia agents and dosages

Euthanasia Agents	Small Exotic Mammal Dose
Butorphanol/dexmedetomidine/tiletamine/ zolazepam (Telazol) combination; "TTDex" (Reconstitute Telazol powder with 2.5 mL Butorphanol and 2.5 mL dexmedetomidine)	0.1–0.2 mL intramuscularly provides deep surgical plane anesthesia for all species discussed. Excellent premedication due to low volume of injection. Variable pain on initial injection. Administering injection SQ in small rodents decreases discomfort.
Ketamine/midazolam/butorphanol	10–20 mg/kg ketamine, 2 mg/kg midazolam, and 1–2 mg/kg butorphanol will typically provide surgical plane anesthesia.
Ketamine/xylazine (Anased)	Ketamine 10–20 mg/kg for all species; xylazine 1–5 mg/kg for hedgehogs/sugar gliders, 5–10 mg/kg for small rodents.
Sodium pentobarbital (Euthasol) – for use once patient is unconscious	0.1–0.5 mL intravenous, intracardiac, or intrahepatic

Data from Carpenter J. Exotic animal formulary. 4th edition. St Louis (MO): Elsevier Saunders; 2013; and Ko J, Berman A. Anesthesia in shelter medicine. Top Companion Anim Med 2010;25(2):92–7.

premedication with either isoflurane gas or an overdose of an intramuscular sedative injection followed by injection of sodium pentobarbital or similar agent (**Table 11**).

SUMMARY

There is still a paucity of peer-reviewed, evidence-based clinical information available for the veterinary practitioner. Further research is needed to establish the best treatment recommendations when dealing with various illnesses and efficacy of treatments.

REFERENCES

1. Sayers I, Smith S. Mice, rats, hamsters, and gerbils. In: Meredith A, Johnson-Delaney C, editors. BSAVA manual of exotic pets. 5th edition. Gloucester (United Kingdom): British Small Animal Veterinary Association; 2010. p. 1–27.
2. Lennox A, Bauck L. Small rodents: basic anatomy, physiology, husbandry, and clinical techniques. In: Quesenberry K, Carpenter J, editors. Ferrets, rabbits, and rodents: clinical medicine and surgery. 3rd edition. St Louis (MO): Elsevier; 2012. p. 339–53.
3. Carboni D, Tully T. Marsupials. In: Mitchell M, Tully T, editors. Manual of exotic pet practice. St Louis (MO): Saunders, Elsevier; 2009. p. 299–325.
4. Brown C, Donnelly T. Rodent husbandry and care. Vet Clin North Am Exot Anim Pract 2004;7(2):201–25, v.
5. Simone-Freilicher E, Hoefer H. Hedgehog care and husbandry. Vet Clin North Am Exot Anim Pract 2004;7(2):257–67, v.
6. Dierenfeld E. Feeding behavior and nutrition of the African pygmy hedgehog (Atelerix albiventris). Vet Clin North America Exot Anim Pract 2009;12(2):335–7.
7. Booth R. Sugar gliders. Seminars in Avian and Exotic Pet Medicine 2003;12(4): 228–31.
8. Dierenfeld E. Feeding behavior and nutrition of the sugar glider (Petaurus breviceps). Vet Clin North Am Exot Anim Pract 2009;12:209–15.
9. Johnson-Delaney C. Guinea pigs, chinchillas, degus, and duprasi. In: Meredith A, Johnson-Delaney C, editors. BSVMA manual of exotic pets. 5th edition. Gloucester (United Kingdom): British Small Animal Veterinary Association; 2010. p. 28–62.
10. Johnson D. African pygmy hedgehogs. In: Meredith A, Johnson-Delaney C, editors. BSAVA manual of exotic pets. 5th edition. Gloucester (United Kingdom): British Small Animal Veterinary Association; 2010. p. 139–47.
11. Johnson-Delaney C. Marsupials. In: Meredith A, Johnson-Delaney C, editors. BSVMA manual of exotic pets. Gloucester (United Kingdom): British Small Animal Veterinary Association; 2010. p. 103–26.
12. Brown C, Donnelly T. Disease problems of small rodents. In: Quesenberry K, Carpenter J, editors. Ferrets, rabbits, and rodents: clinical medicine and surgery. 3rd edition. St Louis (MO): Elsevier; 2012. p. 354–72.
13. Ness R, Johnson-Delaney C. Other small mammals: sugar gliders. In: Quesenberry K, Carpenter J, editors. Ferrets, rabbits, and rodents: clinical medicine and surgery. 3rd edition. St Louis (MO): Elsevier; 2012. p. 393–410.
14. Ivey E, Carpenter J. African hedgehogs. In: Quesenberry K, Carpenter J, editors. Ferrets, rabbits, and rodents: clinical medicine and surgery. 3rd edition. St Louis (MO): Elsevier; 2012. p. 411–27.
15. Tully T. Mice and Rats. In: Mitchell M, Tully T, editors. Manual of exotic pet practice. St Louis (MO): Saunders Elsevier; 2009. p. 326–44.

16. Heatley J, Harris M. Hamsters and gerbils. In: Mitchell M, Tully T, editors. Manual of exotic pet practice. St Louis (MO): Saunders, Elsevier; 2009. p. 406–32.

17. Heatley J. Hedgehogs. In: Mitchell M, Tully T, editors. Manual of exotic pet practice. St Louis (MO): Saunders, Elsevier; 2009. p. 433–55.

18. Lightfoot T. Clinical examination of chinchillas, hedgehogs, prairie dogs, and sugar gliders. Vet Clin North Am Exot Anim Pract 1999;2(2):447–69.

19. Anderson L, Otto G, Pritchett-Corning K, et al. Laboratory animal medicine. 3rd edition. American College of Laboratory Animal Medicine Series. Oxford (UK): Elsevier; 2014.

20. Antinoff N. Small mammal critical care. Vet Clin North Am Exot Anim Pract 1998; 1(1):153–75.

21. Johnson D. Endoscopic intubation of exotic companion mammals. Vet Clin North Am Exot Anim Pract 2010;13:273–89.

22. Vongerichten A, Aristovich K, Sato dos Santos G, et al. Design for a 3-dimensional printed laryngoscope blade for the intubation of rats. Laboratory Animals 2014;43(4):140–2.

23. Corleta O, Habazettl H, Kreimeier U, et al. Modified retrograde orotracheal intubation technique for airway access in rabbits. Eur Surg Res 1992;24(2):129–32.

24. Lennox A, Capello V. Tracheal intubation in exotic companion mammals. J Exotic Pet Med 2008;17(3):221–7.

25. Lichtenberger M, Lennox A. Critical care of the exotic companion mammal (with a focus on herbivorous species): the first twenty-four hours. J Exotic Pet Med 2012; 21:284–92.

26. Costello M. Principles of cardiopulmonary cerebral resuscitation in special species. Seminars in Avian and Exotic Pet Medicine 2004;13(2):132–41.

27. Lennox A. Intraosseous catheterization of exotic animals. J Exotic Pet Med 2008; 17(4):300–6.

28. Tein T, Hafeez W. Intraosseous access. EMedicine Journal 2008;1. Available at: http://www.emedicine.com/proc/topic80431.htm. Accessed November 1, 2015.

29. Lichtenberger M. Shock and cardiopulmonary-cerebral resuscitation in small mammals and birds. Vet Clin North Am Exot Anim Pract 2007;10:275–91.

30. Johnson D. Emergency presentations of the exotic small mammalian herbivore trauma patient. J Exotic Pet Med 2012;21:300–15.

31. Di Girolamo N, Toth G, Selleri P. At-admission hypothermia and mortality in hospitalized pet rabbits: why measurement of rectal temperature is critical. Proc Assoc. Exotic Mammal Conf 2014.

32. Lichtenberger M. Principles of shock and fluid therapy in special species. Seminars in Avian and Exotic Pet Medicine 2004;13(3):142–53.

33. Orcutt C. Fluid therapy in small mammals. NAVC Conf. Proc 2005.

34. Lichtenberger M. Transfusion medicine in exotic pets. Clin Tech Small Anim Pract 2004;19(2):88–95.

35. Raymundo V. Small mammals: blood transfusion. In: Mayer J, Donnelly T, editors. Clinical veterinary advisor: birds and exotic pets. St. Louis (MO): Elsevier Saunders; 2013. p. 551–2.

36. Hand W, Whiteley J, Epperson T, et al. Hydroxyethyl starch and acute kidney injury in orthotopic liver transplantation: a single-center retrospective review. Anesth Analg 2015;120(3):619–26.

37. Kancir A, Johansen J, Ekeloef N, et al. The effect of 6% hydroxyethyl starch 130/ 0.4 on renal function, arterial blood pressure, and vasoactive hormones during radical prostatectomy: a randomized controlled trial. Anesth Analg 2015;120(3): 608–18.

38. Perner A, Haase N, Guttormsen A, et al. Hydroxyethyl starch 130/0.42 versus Ringer's acetate in severe sepsis. N Engl J Med 2012;367(2):124–34.
39. Cazzolli D, Prittie J. The crystalloid-colloid debate: Consequences of resuscitation fluid selection in veterinary critical care. Journal of Veterinary Emergency and Critical Care 2015;25(1):6–19.
40. Barter L. Rabbit analgesia. Vet Clin North Am Exot Anim Pract 2011;14(1):93–104.
41. Carpenter J. Exotic animal formulary. 4th edition. St Louis (MO): Elsevier Saunders; 2013.
42. Longley L. Anaesthesia of Exotic Pets. St. Louis (MO): Saunders Elsevier; 2008.
43. Lennox A. Critical rodents and other small exotic mammal emergencies. NAVC Conf. Proc 2008.
44. Evans E, Souza M. Advanced diagnostic approaches and current management of internal disorders of select species (rodents, sugar gliders, hedgehogs). Vet Clin North Am Exot Anim Pract 2010;13:453–69.
45. Hawkins M, Graham J. Emergency and critical care of rodents. Vet Clin North Am Exot Anim Pract 2007;10:501–31.
46. Dyer S, Cervasio E. An overview of restraint and blood collection techniques in exotic pet practice. Vet Clin Exot Anim 2008;11:423–43.
47. Capello V, Lennox A. Clinical radiology of exotic companion mammals. Ames (IA): Wiley-Blackwell; 2013.
48. Krautwald-Junghanns M, Pees M, Reese S, et al. Diagnostic imaging of exotic pets: birds, small mammals, reptiles. Hannover (Germany): Schlutersche; 2010.
49. Silverman S, Tell L. Radiology of rodents, rabbits, and ferrets: an atlas of normal anatomy and positioning. St Louis (MO): Elsevier; 2005.
50. Lennox A. Emergency and critical care procedure in sugar gliders (Petaurus breviceps), African hedgehogs (Atelerix albiventris), and prairie dogs (Cynomys spp.). Vet Clin North Am Exot Anim Pract 2007;10:533–55.
51. Schnellbacher R, Olson E, Mayer J. Emergency presentations associated with cardiovascular disease in exotic herbivores. J Exotic Pet Med 2012;21(4):316–27.
52. Howe N, Cherpelis B. Obtaining rapid and effective hemostasis: Part I: Update and review of topical hemostatic agents. J Am Acad Dermatol 2013;69(5):659.e1–17.
53. Hernandez-Divers S. Principles of wound management of small mammals: hedgehogs, prairie dogs, and sugar gliders. Vet Clin North Am Exot Anim Pract 2004;7:1–18.
54. Snider T, Joyner P, Clinkenbeard K. Disseminated histoplasmosis in an African pygmy hedgehog. J Am Vet Med Assoc 2008;232(1):74–6.
55. Plumb D. Plumb's veterinary drug handbook. 8th edition. Ames (IA): Wiley-Blackwell; 2015.
56. Knafo S. Sildenafil citrate as a pulmonary protectant in chronic murine mycoplasma pulmonis infection. Proc Assoc. Exot. Mam. Vet. Conf 2014.
57. Reusch B. Investigation and management of cardiovascular disease in rabbits. In Practice 2005;27:418–25.
58. Raymond J, Garner M. Cardiomyopathy in captive African hedgehogs (Atelerix albiventris). J Vet Diagn Invest 2000;12:468–72.
59. Raymond J, Aguilar R, Dunker R, et al. Intervertebral disc disease in African hedgehogs (Atelerix albiventris): four cases. J Exotic Pet Med 2009;18(3):220–3.
60. Allison N, Chang T, Steele K, et al. Fatal herpes simplex infection in a pygmy African hedgehog (Atelerix albiventris). J Comp Pathol 2002;126(1):76–81.

61. Thompson S, Huseby R, Fox M, et al. Spontaneous tumors in the Sprague-Dawley rat. J Natl Cancer Inst 1961;27(5):1037–57.

62. Nakata M, Miwa Y, Itou T, et al. Astrocytoma in an African hedgehog (Atelerix albiventris) suspected wobbly hedgehog syndrome. J Vet Med Sci 2011;73(10): 1333–5.

63. Gibson C, Parry N, Jakowski R, et al. Anaplastic astrocytoma in the spinal cord of an African pygmy hedgehog (Atelerix albiventris). Vet Pathol 2008;45(6):934–6.

64. Rhody J, Schiller C. Spinal osteosarcoma in a hedgehog with pedal self-mutilation. Vet Clin North Am Exot Anim Pract 2006;9(3):625–31.

65. Martin K, Johnston M. Forelimb amputation for treatment of a peripheral nerve sheath tumor in an African pygmy hedgehog. J Am Vet Med Assoc 2006; 229(5):706–10.

66. Eguchi K, Kawamoto K, Uozumi T, et al. In vivo effect of cabergoline, a dopamine agonist, on estrogen-induced rat pituitary tumors. Endocr J 1995;42(2):153–61.

67. Graesser D, Spraker T, Dressen P, et al. Wobbly hedgehog syndrome in African pygmy hedgehogs (Atelerix spp.). J Exotic Pet Med 2006;15(1):59–65.

68. Wheler C, Grahn B, Pocknell A. Unilateral proptosis and orbital cellulitis in eight African hedgehogs (Atelerix albiventris). J Zoo Wildl Med 2001;32(2):236–41.

69. Fukuzawa R, Fukuzawa K, Abe H, et al. Acinic cell carcinoma in an African pygmy hedgehog (Atelerix albiventris). Vet Clin Pathol 2004;33(1):39–42.

70. Keller D. Small mammals: hamsters: ocular disorders. In: Mans C, Mayer J, Donnelly T, editors. Clinical veterinary advisor: birds and exotic pets. St Louis (MO): Elsevier Saunders; 2013. p. 293–5.

71. Miller P. Ocular Emergencies. Slatter's fundamentals of veterinary ophthalmology. Philadelphia: Saunders; 2013. p. 437–44.

72. Holmberg B. Ophthalmology of Exotic Pets. Slatter's fundamentals of veterinary ophthalmology. Philadelphia: Saunders; 2013. p. 445–61.

73. Beaumont S. Ocular disorders of pet mice and rats. Vet Clin North Am Exot Anim Pract 2002;5:311–24.

74. Lee T. Octodon degus: a diurnal, social, and long-lived rodent. ILAR J 2004; 45(1):14–24.

75. Raymond J, White M. Necropsy and histopathological findings in 14 African hedgehogs (Atelerix albiventris): a retrospective study. J Zoo Wildl Med 1999; 30(2):273–7.

76. Barron H, Richey L, Hernandez-Divers S, et al. Etiology, pathology, and control of enterocolitis in a group of hamsters. Proc Assoc. Avian Vet Conf 2007.

77. Frisk C, Wagner J. Hamster enteritis: a review. Lab Anim 1977;11:79–85.

78. Done L, Deem S, Fiorello C. Surgical and medical management of a uterine spindle cell tumor in an African hedgehog (Atelerix albiventris). J Zoo Wildl Med 2007; 38(4):601–3.

79. Wellehan J, Southorn E, Smith D, et al. Surgical removal of a mammary adenocarcinoma and a granulosa cell tumor in an African pygmy hedgehog. Can Vet J 2003;44(3):235–7.

80. Mikaelian I, Reavill D, Practice A. Spontaneous proliferative lesions and tumors of the uterus of captive African hedgehogs (Atelerix albiventris). J Zoo Wildl Med 2004;35(2):216–20.

81. Hotchkiss C. Effect of surgical removal of subcutaneous tumors on survival of rats. J Am Vet Med Assoc 1995;206(10):1575–9.

82. Raymond J, Garner M. Spontaneous tumors in captive African hedgehogs (Atelerix albiventris): a retrospective study. J Comp Pathol 2001;124:128–33.

83. Jackson T, Heath L, Hulin M, et al. Squamous cell carcinoma of the midventral abdominal pad in three gerbils. J Am Vet Med Assoc 1996;209(4):789–91.

84. Ellis C, Mori M. Skin diseases of rodents and small exotic mammals. Vet Clin North Am Exot Anim Pract 2001;4(2):493–542.

85. Chung T, Kim H, Choi U. Multicentric epitheliotropic T-cell lymphoma in an African hedgehog (Atelerix albiventris). Vet Clin Pathol 2014;43(4):601–4.

86. Spugnini E, Pagotto A, Zazzera F, et al. Cutaneous T-cell lymphoma in an African hedgehog (Atelerix albiventris). In Vivo 2008;22(1):43–5.

87. Lichtenberger M, Richardson J. Emergency care and managing toxicoses in the exotic animal patient. Vet Clin North Am Exot Anim Pract 2008;11:211–28.

88. ASPCA Animal Poison Control Center. 2015. Avaialable at: http://www.aspcapro. org/poison. Accessed November 1, 2015.

89. Remillard R. Nutritional support in critical care patients. Vet Clin North Am Small Anim Pract 2002;32(5):1145–64.

90. Whittington J. Esophagostomy feeding tube use and placement in exotic pets. J Exotic Pet Med 2013;22(2):178–91.

91. Capello V, Lennox A. Gross and surgical anatomy of the reproductive tract of selected exotic pet mammals. Proc Assoc. Avian Vet Conf 2006;19–28.

92. Johnson D. Exotic companion mammal surgeries that you need to know. Western Veterinary Conference Proc 2013.

93. Bennet R. Small rodents: soft tissue surgery. In: Quesenberry K, Carpenter J, editors. Ferrets, rabbits, and rodents: clinical medicine and surgery. 3rd edition. St Louis: Elsevier; 2012. p. 373–91.

Critical Care of Pet Birds

Jeffrey Rowe Jenkins, BS, DVM, DABVP (Avian Practice)

KEYWORDS

- Avian • Critical care • Triage • Trauma • Shock • Fluid therapy

KEY POINTS

- Success with the critical bird patient is founded on preparation and planning.
- Triage begins with first client contact.
- Assessment of the critical patient must coincide with the initiation of care.
- The intensive care environment requires heat and oxygen in a manner that conserves the patient's energy.
- Fluids are best administered at body temperature via an intraosseous route.

Prepare: to put in proper condition or readiness (dictionary.com); to make ready beforehand for some purpose, or, to put in a proper state of mind (merriam-webster.com).

Plan: to arrange a method or scheme beforehand for any work, enterprise, or proceeding (dictionary.com); to devise or project the realization or achievement of (merriam-webster.com).

The successful treatment of the critical avian emergency is predicated on the preparation and planning of doctors, supportive staff, and the avian hospital as well as knowledge of the facility. Preparation leads to an ability to foresee those activities and routines that will be necessary to affect the desired results. Preparation requires a thorough education that includes understanding the basics of basics of avian anatomy, physiology, and pathophysiology of birds, the study of avian behavior, knowledge of avian species and their differences, pharmacology, and the mechanics of avian therapeutics. Last, knowledge of avian disease is needed/necessary. Likewise, the hospital or emergency facility requires preparation by the accumulation of obtaining necessary equipment, supplies, pharmaceuticals, and personnel.

Planning to a great extent involves a path or protocol that is expected to lead to a successful conclusion. These plans start from initial client contact, patient intake, the signing of informed consent and financial estimates, and protocols for the care of patients with specific signs or complaints.

The author has nothing to disclose.
Avian & Exotic Animal Hospital, Inc, San Diego, CA, USA
E-mail address: drexotic@aol.com

Vet Clin Exot Anim 19 (2016) 501–512
http://dx.doi.org/10.1016/j.cvex.2016.01.014
1094-9194/16/$ – see front matter © 2016 Elsevier Inc. All rights reserved.
vetexotic.theclinics.com

Planning assumes that one can control the various elements required to bring to pass their goals. Preparing, on the other hand, focuses on the ultimate goal. Planning is often less flexible, indicating a process and timeframe. Preparation allows flexibility to adapt to the changing situations. Having both in place will greatly aid in the successful treatment of the critical patient.

The purpose of this article is to aid in that preparation and planning with the goal of a smooth progression of events from initial contact, through patient stabilization and eventual release.

TRIAGE

Triage: sorting of and allocation of treatment to patients and especially battle and disaster victims according to a system of priorities designed to maximize the number of survivors; the sorting of patients (as in an emergency room) according to the urgency of their need for care (merriam-webster.com).

The triage of the critical avian patient begins long before the arrival of the patient. An understanding, and preparation, by both doctors and staff of the urgency associated with signs of disease and trauma is necessary. Some signs, such as bleeding or significant trauma, are obvious, whereas others, such as hypothermia, dehydration, and anemia, are not as apparent. It is therefore of great importance to assess the indicators of these parameters. The rapid metabolism of the avian patient acts as a multiplier and makes many situations that may not be immediately life threatening more critical. In some rare cases, the avian patient responds better than the more familiar mammal patient. Your triage preparation should include a plan or protocol of how the flow of information from client, to staff, to doctor, and back to the client, is executed and how patients are processed once presented at the hospital.[1]

PHONE CONTACT

Effective initial contact improves communication and speeds response in critical cases. Information should be gathered that allows hospital staff and equipment to be ready at the time the patient arrives. Hospital staff that answer phones and make appointments must be trained and allowed to make judgments as to what is an emergency situation needing immediate attention and effectively communicate that information to the client and to doctors and staff. Information must be gathered including the nature of the emergency, and the client and patient information. If time permits, a brief history of events leading to the emergency and history of prior health problems may be helpful. This information should be made available to doctors and nursing staff immediately so that preparations for the patient's arrival can be made.

It should be made certain that the client knows the address of and the directions to the hospital. The client should call back or stay on the line for turn-by-turn directions if they are not familiar with where they are going or if the location is difficult to find.

PRESENTATION

The physical evaluation aspect of triage begins at presentation and is often the responsibility of reception and nursing staff and most often involves inspection of the patient as presented. If the bird is in a cage or transport carrier, visual inspection may be possible. If the bird is held or restrained by the client, it should be transferred to a clear container where it may be observed. Alert, eupneic, perching birds may be placed in an examination room awaiting further evaluation by a veterinarian. Birds with more significant signs of distress, including fluffed feathers and hunched posture (sick bird signs), dyspnea, weakness (unable to perch and/or recumbent), or that are notably cyanotic or pallid, are moved to a supportive environment immediately. Heat, oxygen, and physical support in the form of foam or towel bolsters that can be used as perches are included. Patients that are bleeding, experiencing seizures, or have open fractures require immediate intervention by doctor and staff.

INFORMED CONSENT/EMERGENCY CARE RELEASE AND ESTIMATE

The owner's signature should be secured on a document of informed consent and authorization to treat before providing any services. The key points of informed consent include information on medical and surgical alternatives (including the need for restraint, sedation, or anesthesia), an explanation of the planned procedure, and explanation of the anticipated outcome, discussion of serious complications (including death), the type and extent of additional services that will be needed, and an estimate of fees and how payment must be made. Obviously, much of this material will not be available at presentation of the critical patient. This material should be included once it becomes available. Alternatively, an Emergency Care Release and Estimate should be signed authorizing initial emergency evaluation and lifesaving treatment.[1] This document should cover those items above and make clear that there are risks in treatment and that there is no guarantee of outcome with treatment.

HISTORY

Anamnesis: a recalling; preliminary case history of a medical or psychiatric patient (merriam-webster.com).

History may be collected by staff or by the veterinarian and should include signalment, any events leading up to the emergency, a description of symptoms noted by the owner and their duration, treatments performed by the owner or other veterinarian, a brief history of the bird's origin, cage or aviary habitat, diet, and exposure to other birds (including boarding or grooming). Specific questions should be asked regarding mental awareness, strength, problems walking/perching/flying, and eating and appetite. The presence of polyuria, polydipsia, the change of color of droppings, regurgitation, bleeding, and loss of coordination or seizures should be noted.

PHYSICAL EXAMINATION

Examination: the act of looking at something closely and carefully; the act of examining something; close and careful study of someone or something to find signs of illness or injury.

The bird should be visually observed before restraint when possible. A plan of action should be formed based on this initial observation, and necessary equipment and supplies gathered. The strategy should allow for completion of the examination, collection of laboratory and/or physiologic data, along with initial treatment at one time to minimize the duration, and hence, minimize the stress of restraint. With some critical patients, it may be necessary to allow periods of rest along with supplemental oxygen between stressful or painful restraint and treatments.

Once restrained, physical examination should include an assessment of overall condition (body score), mental attitude, state of hydration, color of mucous membranes, brief palpation of body and limbs, auscultation of heart, lungs, air sacs, and airways, and examination of integument for signs of bruising, hemorrhage, or trauma in the physical examination. Special attention should be given to eyes and adnexal tissue. Head trauma commonly results in damage to the eye. A neurologic examination should be performed, including assessment of cranial nerve function, on birds with head trauma as well as birds with other neurologic abnormalities.

Placement of an abdominal air sac tube is a priority in patients that are markedly dyspneic due to respiratory obstruction. Isoflurane or sevoflurane anesthesia is preferred to protracted restraint in some critically ill birds. If these patients are stable with oxygen supplementation, addressing hypotension and hypothermia should have priority.

CLINICAL TESTING

Data: factual information (as measurements or statistics) used as a basis for reasoning, discussion, or calculation; information output by a sensing device or organ that includes both useful and irrelevant or redundant information and must be processed to be meaningful (merriam-webster.com).

The laboratory data that should be collected will vary with the bird and the presenting condition. It is recommended that you collect a minimum of a blood smear, hematocrit or packed cell volume, and measurement of total solids be collected.[1]

RADIOLOGY

Radiology: the science of radioactive substances and high-energy radiations: a branch of medicine concerned with the use of radiant energy (as X-rays or ultrasound) in the diagnosis and treatment of disease (merriam-webster.com).

Radiology is a powerful tool in avian medicine, the scope of which is beyond that of this article. There are cases, however, whereby a radiograph is necessary for the evaluation of a critical patient. Ingested foreign material, especially heavy metals, may be ruled out with a quick radiograph.[1] In some cases, the anesthesia and/or restraint necessary for proper positioning may not be possible. In these cases, less than perfect positioning may provide an answer. More suitable studies can be performed once the patient is stabilized.

SPECIAL DIAGNOSTIC PROCEDURES

Protocol: a detailed plan of a scientific or medical experiment, treatment, or procedure (merriam-webster.com).

Several other special diagnostic procedures may be appropriate in assessing the critical patient. Measurement of body temperature (seldom measured in the clinically normal patient), heart rate, and blood flow using an ultrasonic Doppler blood flow detector (Doppler; Parks Medical Electronics, Inc, Aloha, OR, USA),[1] electrocardiogram, blood gas, ultrasound, transillumination, and other procedures might be included in this group. Again, it is important to be mindful of the stress of restraint and manipulation early in the treatment of the critical patient.

PATIENT SUPPORT

Support: to maintain in condition, action, or existence (merriam-webster.com).

FLUID SUPPORT

Circulation: the movement of blood through the vessels of the body that is induced by the pumping action of the heart and serves to distribute nutrients and oxygen to and remove waste products from all parts of the body (merriam-webster.com).

Shock: a state of profound depression of the vital processes of the body that is characterized by pallor, rapid but weak pulse, rapid and shallow respiration, reduced total blood volume, and low blood pressure and that is caused usually by severe especially crushing injuries, hemorrhage, burns, or major surgery (merriam-webster.com).

The benefits of fluid therapy for the critical patient have long been recognized. Restoration of blood volume and normalization of cardiac output and tissue oxygenation all depend on the return of normal fluid volume.

FLUID PHYSIOLOGY

There has been a repeated discussion in avian medical literature, including by the author of this article, about shock and the physiologic processes associated with it in mammals and birds.[1,4,5] The conclusion of this discussion is that shock is ultimately a state resulting in inadequate distribution of systemic blood flow, and hence, oxygen and nutrients, to tissues. It is best classified in the avian patient functionally as hypovolemic, cardiogenic, or vasogenic. Hypovolemic shock, due directly from hemorrhage or indirectly from fluid losses secondary to vomiting, diarrhea, or polyuria, is the most common. Dehydration and electrolyte imbalance often accompany this form of shock. Cardiogenic shock is the result of impaired cardiac function and decreased output. Cardiac failure resulting from pulmonary hypertension is the most common cause seen in the author's practice, but arrhythmia, pericardial effusion or mass, and cardiomyopathy may also result in decreased cardiac function. Vasogenic shock is most often associated with sepsis, endotoxemia, and toxicosis and is seen in the terminal stages of overwhelming infectious disease.[4]

Regardless of the cause, shock results in inadequate circulation of blood and tissue perfusion. Correcting blood volume and improving tissue oxygenation are therapeutic priorities. Electrolyte, pH, and other imbalances will be corrected if adequate perfusion to vital organs is corrected and maintained.

ROUTE

Oral fluids, most often in the form of oral alimentation, are adequate for the patient who is not in shock or significantly dehydrated or the debilitated bird is at risk of regurgitation. This route is safe and economical in many cases. It is often inadequate for the critical patient, however. Subcutaneous fluids are the mainstay for maintenance of fluids in avian medicine. They are similarly safe, economical, and less likely to cause complications than IO or intravenous (IV) routes.

Both IO and IV routes are preferred in critically ill patients. IO catheters may be placed quickly, are easy to maintain, and are stable and reliable. IV catheters may be used for initial fluid therapy, but do not have the stability of an IO catheter. IV catheter placement involves somewhat prolonged restraint, which has to be taken into account for the stressed patient or the patient in shock. Fluids may be given in a large bolus IO unlike the IV route. The tibiotarsus and ulna may be used for catheter placement. The jugular and cutaneous ulnar veins are the most common sites for indwelling catheter placement. The medial metatarsal vein may be used in large species.

Placement of the IO catheter begins with proper site preparation, similar to epithelial preparation for an IV catheter. A 22-gauge, 1.5-inch spinal needle is the catheter of choice in most psittacine cases, although any size needle may be used, provided that a stylet is inserted into the needle before placement of the IO catheter into the medullary cavity of the bone. When the IO catheter is placed in the distal ulna, the distal wing tip is flexed and the needle is inserted at a 45° to 60° angle; this angle is reduced once the catheter enters the cortex. When using the proximal tibiotarsal bone, the stifle is flexed and the needle is advanced through the insertion of the patellar tendon at the cnemial crest. The needle should be advanced to the hub; the stylet should be removed, and the catheter should be flushed with heparinized saline.[2]

CHOICE OF FLUIDS

Crystalloids, aqueous solutions of mineral salts or other water-soluble molecules, are the fluid of choice for avian patients in critical decompensation and dehydrated conditions. Crystalloids are highly effective at replacing fluids within the interstitial compartments, expanding circulating fluid volume, and enhancing diuresis, which facilitates elimination of toxic byproducts. Crystalloid fluids rapidly leave the circulation and equilibrate in the interstitial fluid compartment. Only 25% of isotonic fluids, such as lactated Ringer's solution (LRS) or 0.9% NaCl solution, remain in the vascular compartment 30 minutes after administration.

Many critical patients are in a state of acidosis. LRS is the fluid of choice for these patients. Lactate is metabolized to bicarbonate by the liver. In severe states of persistent acidosis, LRS should be supplemented with bicarbonate. A dose of 1 mEq/kg of sodium bicarbonate may be given every 15 to 30 minutes to a maximum of 4 mEq/kg. Hyperkalemia may result from severe tissue trauma or extreme catabolic state such as prolonged starvation. The amount of potassium in LRS is not enough to endanger these patients; however, the addition of calcium gluconate at 5 mg/kg as a cardioprotectant and glucose, which facilitates the movement of potassium as cross-cell membranes, is advisable. Hypokalemia may result from regurgitation or aggressive fluid therapy, requiring potassium supplementation. Potassium chloride may be added to LRS at a dose of 0.1 to 0.3 mEq/kg to a maximum of 11 mEq/kg per day. Infusion of a large volume of crystalloid fluids reduces colloidal osmotic pressure and predisposes to pulmonary and peripheral edema and impaired peripheral tissue oxygen exchange.[1,4]

Birds that are hypovolemic from blood loss may benefit from treatment with hypertonic (7.5%) saline or colloidal fluids. Hypertonic saline is recommended for cases of acute blood loss, endotoxemia, or hypotension. When it is given at 5 ml/kg, it can result in a rapid improvement in cardiac function. Cardiac contractility and output increase from the expanded vascular volume and the direct inotropic effect on the heart. These effects are transient however, lasting only 2 to 3 hours in the dog and 15 to 20 minutes in the cat. The effect may be even shorter in birds. The use of colloids (6% Dextran 70) to the solution prolongs the effects. In cases of hydropericardium, pulmonary edema, or increased intracranial pressure without hemorrhage, hypertonic saline may be useful.

Synthetic colloids (hetastarch and dextrans) have a similar effect as hypertonic saline but with a longer half-life (24 hours in mammals). A dose of 10 to 20 mL/kg is safely used at the author's hospital.

Fluids should be warmed before administration, and bolus fluids can be given with relative safety IO or IV over a 3- to 5-minute period. Once the fluid deficit is replaced and the bird is eating and drinking normally for 1 to 2 days, the maintenance hydration therapy can be discontinued (**Fig. 1**).

SUPPORTIVE ENVIRONMENT/INTENSIVE CARE ENVIRONMENT

Patient support includes the enclosure, thermal support, and oxygen support.

THERMAL SUPPORT

The goal of the intensive care environment (ICE) is to provide support for metabolic needs while minimizing energy expenditure so that the patient may focus on returning

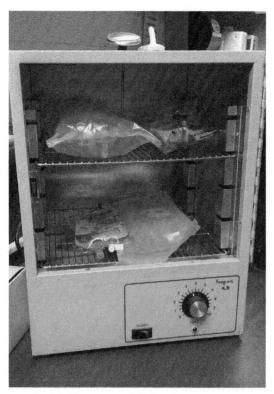

Fig. 1. Fluids incubator. Fluids for subcutaneous, IV, or IO treatments are kept at 101.0 F (38.0 C).

to physiologic normality. A healthy bird's energy needs, reflected in its basic metabolic rate, is greater than that of a mammal and is greater in passerine birds than in some non-passerine birds. It is also greater in a bird laying eggs, fighting an infection, or healing from an injury. When an animal is no longer able to meet its energy needs, there is a critical point of decompensation, which is the cause of physiologic crisis. Correcting this energy imbalance, then supporting the healing patient, is one of the most important goals of critical care.[1]

The ICE is the most important tool to correct the energy balance of the avian patient. It should maintain a temperature that will keep the patient at or just above its thermoneutral zone (TNZ). The TNZ is the temperature range wherein an animal's rate of heat production is in equilibrium with the rate of loss to the environment (Mosby's Medical Dictionary, 9th edition. 2009, Elsevier). An animal's TNZ is related to its metabolic rate, or how much energy is being produced or consumed to provide ongoing physiologic functions. In adult humans, TNZ is typically reported to be 64°–72°F (18°–22°C). In the author's hospital, critical avian patients are kept at 90°–95°F (32°–35°C).

Birds are best heated by conduction from a heated surface, and radiation from an infrared heat source, such as a heat lamp or infrared heat panel. Convection (moving, heated air), at least from commercially available forced air units, did not perform well and was far too expensive in the author's high volume of bird, reptile, and small mammal practice. In addition, they were difficult and expensive to clean, sterilize, and maintain and dimensionally not engineered for the sick bird (tall versus long).

OXYGEN SUPPORT

Oxygen is widely used in avian critical care, yet there is surprisingly little evidence guiding its use. Titrating oxygen levels and monitoring the patient to maintain a normal level of tissue oxygenation are not practical in most patients. As a consequence, a significant portion of critically ill patients are subjected to hyperoxia. That said, the use of oxygen supplementation clearly improves prognosis of the avian patient and is commonly used. However, the risks and the negative consequence of hyperoxia may be as great as those of hypoxia.[3] The ICE therefore must be oxygen safe. Any electrical connections must be outside the oxygenated chamber to eliminate the risk of oxygen fires or explosions.

INTENSIVE CARE ENVIRONMENTS

The author used several products over the years to create this ICE, from bird cages to baby incubators and radiant heat baby warmers, to custom-made water-jacketed "avian brooders." The author currently uses clear plastic food storage boxes (Camwear Boxes and Camwear Flat Lids; Cambro USA, Huntington Beach, CA, USA) kept on shelves heated with flexible heat tape (Flexwatt Heat Tape; Calorique, West Wareham, MA, USA). The temperature is controlled using feedback thermostats (DBS-1000 Advanced Temperature Control System; Helix Controls Systems, Inc, Vista, CA, USA) and monitored using thermometers within the environment. These storage boxes allow for good utilization of space and allow many patients to be observed by nursing staff in a small area. They are inexpensive, unbreakable, and easily cleaned and sterilized. The boxes nest when stacked so storage of unused units takes only the space of a single box (**Fig. 2**).

COMFORT

The author recommends lining the floor of the ICE with 16×20 Huck surgical towels. They are inexpensive, easily cleaned, and easily sterilized. Occasionally, he uses underpads (Chux; Dynarex Disposable Underpad; Dyranex, Orangeburg, NY, USA). These liners are highly absorbent and are used in human medicine for incontinence and obstetrics. Newspaper is slippery, and bulk bedding material is messy and

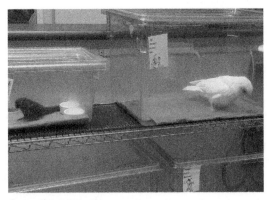

Fig. 2. ICE used in the author's practice.

expensive and insulates the patient from the heat source. Rolled towels or foam bumpers are used to support weak, uncoordinated, or recumbent patients.

FLAT SURFACES VERSUS PERCHES

The author does not recommend using perches or perching surfaces in critical bird environments. He has found that compromised patients do better kept on a flat surface. A bird on the flat surface burns less energy, is more likely to eat and drink, and is less likely to fall or be injured.

NUTRITIONAL SUPPORT

Nutrition: the act or process of affording nutriment or nourishment (merriam-webster. com).

Nutritional support is required for the successful treatment of the critical avian patient. Providing energy and avoiding energy loss are the primary concerns initially, but more complete nutrition is necessary for the patient to thrive. Parenteral alimentation has been investigated and had limited use but requires an intraosseous (IO) catheter or vascular access devise and is significantly more stressful and costly to perform. Enteral nutrition is much more practical and is the common route used in avian practice. It is important to provide nutritional support early in the treatment of the critical patient, but the patient must be at a point where it can process and absorb the material it is being fed. The strength of the patient, its ability to remain upright and support its head, its state of hydration (see above) must be evaluated prior to initiating tube feeding, or other forms of enteral nutrition.

In the past, hand feeding formula designed for hand feeding avian neonates was used and is still a reasonable choice. The author's hospital uses Nutri-Start's Baby Bird Formula (Lafeber Co, Cornell, IL, USA). Commercial enteral nutritional formulas made for humans have been recommended and used successfully. They are typically liquid, and care must be used that they are more easily aspirated by weak birds. Products designed for the avian patient are currently used in the author's hospital: Roudybush Formula AA Acute Care (Roudybush, Inc, Woodland, CA, USA) and Emeraid Omnivore (LafeberVet, Cornell, IL, USA).

ORAL GAVAGE

Oral gavage is one of the most dangerous procedures performed with an avian patient. Crop burns and perforation of the cervical esophagus are all too common injuries that occur when care is not taken. Staff should be trained and supervised when performing this skill until well experienced. The manufacturer's directions should be followed to produce a gruel consistency. Formula should be fed at body temperature (101°–105°F, 38°–40°C). A thermometer should be used to assess this temperature. An appropriate sized syringe is filled with formula and the largest diameter feeding needle is attached that may be passed into the patient's beak, reducing the chance of perforation of the esophagus. Both steel and plastic (Instech Laboratories, Inc, Plymouth Meeting, PA, USA) needles are available. The patient should be restrained in a towel with the thumb of the left hand placed under the right mandible. The right hand is used to pass the tube from the bird's left to right from the commissure of the beak toward the right side of the oral pharynx. No force should be required. The tube passing should be palpated into and down the esophagus under your left thumb. The tube is then slid into the crop. It is wise to have another person palpate that the tube is in the correct location before injecting formula into the crop. The crop is filled to capacity (**Table 1**). Overfilling may result in regurgitation with risk of aspiration. Feeding should

Table 1	
Approximate adult crop/tube feeding volumes of common species	
Budgerigars	1–2 mL
Lovebirds	2–3 mL
Cockatiels	3–6 mL
Conures	4–12 mL
Amazons	15–35 mL
Cockatoos	20–40 mL
Macaws	35–60 mL

be the last treatment done at that handling, and the bird should be set down immediately after. Further handling after feeding may result in regurgitation.

Circulation: the movement of blood through the vessels of the body that is induced by the pumping action of the heart and serves to distribute nutrients and oxygen to and remove waste products from all parts of the body (merriam-webster.com).

Shock: a state of profound depression of the vital processes of the body that is characterized by pallor, rapid but weak pulse, rapid and shallow respiration, reduced total blood volume, and low blood pressure and that is caused usually by severe especially crushing injuries, hemorrhage, burns, or major surgery (merriam-webster.com).

CARDIOPULMONARY RESUSCITATION

Resuscitation: to bring (someone who is unconscious, not breathing, or close to death) back to a conscious or active state again (merriam-webster.com).

Avian patients are commonly presented at or near death, and with cessation of effective circulating blood flow and ventilation, cardiopulmonary arrest (CPA) ensues. As with mammal patients, signs of CPA in birds include loss of consciousness, collapse, lack of a palpable pulse, no auscultable heartbeat, pale or cyanotic mucous membranes, lack of effective respirations, and lack of measurable blood pressure. Cardiopulmonary resuscitation (CPR) typically refers to re-establishing blood flow by performing manual cardiac and thoracic compressions and manual ventilation until spontaneous circulation and ventilation occurs.

In a perfect world, the avian patient would be intubated, and thoracic compressions would cause cardiac contractions resulting in a pulse that would be palpable or detectable with Doppler. Unfortunately, that is not the case. A bird's heart is surrounded by highly compressible air sacs, and sternal compressions do not typically result in circulation.

It is a fact that successful resuscitation is not common for the avian patient, but success is possible. The physiologic chemical changes associated with respiration and parenteral fluid administration may be what stimulates some patient's hearts to beat, or, it may be that thoracic compressions stimulate the heart just enough to initiate a beat. **Box 1** is a flowchart for avian CPR.

MEDICAL THERAPY

Chemotherapy: the use of chemical agents in the treatment or control of disease or mental disorder (merriam-webster.com).

Antibiotic Choices

In critically ill patients, the source of infection may not be apparent at the time of admission to the intensive care unit (ICU). In such patients, IV empirical antibiotics

---

Box 1
Flow chart for avian cardiopulmonary resuscitation

1. Assess patient thoroughly
   a. Carefully observe for breathing, examine oral cavity for obstruction
   b. Auscult for sounds of respiration and heartbeat
   c. Breathing and heart beating, go to step 5
   d. Not breathing/no heartbeat, go to step 2

2. Intubate
   a. Open the mouth and sweep out any debris using a cotton swab
   b. Use appropriate size noncuffed tube
   c. Attach oxygen source when possible

3. Begin positive pressure respiration
   a. Apply forceful intermittent positive pressure ventilations at 3- to 5-second intervals with 100% oxygen
   b. Allow full expiration between breaths
   c. Breathing and heart beating, go to step 5
   d. Not breathing/no heartbeat, go to step 4

4. Begin thoracic compressions
   a. Use 2 to 3 fingers on keel and make sharp firm compressions every 1 to 2 seconds
      i. This action likely does not cause meaningful cardiac compressions but may improve respirations or just move the heart around enough that it stimulates a beat.

5. Place IO catheter
   a. Proximal tibiotarsus is preferable site

6. Give rapid bolus of crystalloid fluids followed by more fluids (crystalloid or colloidal)
   a. 2 mL/100 g body weight (20%) over 30 to 60 seconds
   b. Follow additional 2 mL over next several minutes
   c. Breathing and heart beating, go to step 10
   d. Not breathing/no heartbeat, go to step 7

7. Give atropine 0.2 mg/kg IO
   a. Breathing and heart beating, go to step
   b. Not breathing/no heartbeat, go to step 8

8. Give sodium bicarbonate 4 mEq/kg IO
   a. Breathing and heart beating, go to step 9
   b. Not breathing/no heartbeat, go to step 10

9. Give epinephrine by intracardiac injection at 0.10 mg/kg
   a. Breathing and heart beating, go to step 9
   b. Repeat steps: not breathing/no heartbeat
   c. Repeat at 0.20 mg/kg, then 0.50 mg/kg if no response, repeat steps 3 to 9

10. Start fluids/begin monitoring/get diagnostics
    a. LRS with 5% dextrose, and bicarbonate at 5 to 10/mL per hour using syringe/IV
    b. Monitor heart and respiratory rate/monitor blood pressure if possible

---

must be started as early as possible within the first hour of recognition of severe sepsis and septic shock. Each hour of delay can and will decrease the chances of prognosis for survival of the patient. Antibiotics chosen for the critical patient before confirmation of a specific agent should be broad spectrum and bactericidal. The author's antibiotics of choice include piperacillin-tazobactam, cefotaxime, and amikacin.

PAIN MANAGEMENT

The prevention and alleviation of pain are important aspects of critical care. Not only the humane consideration of providing relief for pain in animal patients but also the pain itself creates its own undesirable metabolic and behavioral side effects. Any disease or injury that causes tissue inflammation and damage is likely to cause pain as part of its clinical picture. Analgesia should be included in the treatment of avian patients. Recent studies have shown the apparent role of the κ receptor in avian pain and support the use of κ-agonist opioids such as butorphanol for management of pain in birds. Butorphanol has become the most commonly recommended analgesic for avian patients and can be used as a primary analgesic in trauma cases. Butorphanol doses range 0.5 to 2.0 mg/kg depending on the situation, in most cases given at 1 to 2 mg/kg IM q 6-12 hours in the author's experience. The major disadvantage of butorphanol is the need for frequent dosing. It appears the analgesic effects of these drugs do not last longer than 4 hours, necessitating frequent redosing for analgesic coverage. Liposome encapsulated butorphanol has a much longer duration of action, and it seems that this formulation lasts longer.

Nonsteroidal anti-inflammatory drugs (NSAIDs), primarily meloxicam, have proven to be effective in avian patients as well. Birds seem to be fairly NSAID tolerant, although it would be ideal to have documented normal uric acid and aspartate aminotransferase/bile acids before administering NSAIDs. In the author's hospital, they typically do not use NSAIDs in birds that are hypoperfused or dehydrated. In parrots, they dose meloxicam at 0.5 mg/kg intramuscularly frequently and continue this dose orally twice daily for as long as is necessary.[6,7]

CONTINUED CARE

The transition from critical ICU patient to more stable hospital patient occurs when the patient has reached a state of physiologic homeostasis under treatment. At this point, more significant diagnostic testing may be performed, and treatment of specific disease processes and/or trauma may begin.

REFERENCES

1. Jenkins JR. Avian critical care and emergency medicine. In: Altman RB, Clubb SL, Dorrestein GM, editors. Avian medicine and surgery. Philadelphia: WB Saunders Co; 1997. p. 839–63.
2. Jenkins JR. Hospital techniques and supportive care. In: Altman RB, Clubb SL, Dorrestein GM, editors. Avian medicine and surgery. Philadelphia: WB Saunders Co; 1997. p. 232–52.
3. Hope J, Kilgannon J, Jones A, et al. Relationship between supranormal oxygen tension and outcome after resuscitation from cardiac arrest. Circulation 2011; 123(23):2717–22.
4. Hernandez M, Aguilar RF. Steroids and fluid therapy for treatment of shock in the critical avian patient. In: Fudge AM, Jenkins JR, editors. Seminars in avian and exotic pet medicine: critical care. Philidelphia: WB Saunders Co; 1994. p. 190–9.
5. Lichtenberger M. Principles of shock and fluid therapy in special species. In: Fudge A, Jenkins ERS, editors. Seminars in avian and exotic pet medicine: emergency medicine, vol. 13. Philidelphia: WB Saunders Co; 2004. p. 142–53, 3.
6. Machin K. Avian pain: physiology and evaluation. Compend Contin Educ Pract Vet 2005;27(2):98–109.
7. Hawkins MG, Paul-Murphy J. Avian analgesia. Vet Clin North Am Exot Anim Pract 2011;14(1):61–80.

Common Emergencies in Pet Birds

Jane D. Stout, VMD

KEYWORDS

- Emergency • Bird • Dyspnea • Regurgitation • Dystocia • Seizure • Trauma • Toxin

KEY POINTS

- Regardless of the emergency presentation of a pet bird, initiation of supportive care to stabilize the patient is the clinician's primary goal.
- Additional therapeutics and diagnostics should only be attempted once the patient is stable and may be better implemented by an avian veterinarian.
- The duration and severity of the avian patient's disease and the clinician's initiation of appropriate therapy often determines clinical outcome.

INTRODUCTION

Treating avian emergencies can be a challenging task. Pet birds often mask signs of illness until they are critically ill. Also, during regular and illness examinations, metabolic stress resulting from prolonged restraint, diagnostics, and treatment may result in further decompensation of the avian patient. Likewise, a bird's small stature and high metabolic rate may cause additional stress related to hypothermia, dehydration, and blood loss, all of which are experienced more acutely than in cats or dogs. Accordingly, quick identification of the patient's affliction and initiation of appropriate supportive care are essential. This article discusses common avian emergency presentations, diagnostics, and initial treatment options that clinicians may implement in the emergency room.

EMERGENCIES THAT PRESENT WITH RESPIRATORY SIGNS

Birds commonly present with respiratory clinical signs. These patients can be categorized as critical and may decompensate quickly. Accordingly, rapid and minimal handling is often required. Luckily, a thorough history, observation of the bird before handling, and a brief examination can often assist the clinician in identifying the region of respiratory disease (**Tables 1** and **2**).[1]

The author has nothing to disclose.
Avian & Exotic Animal Hospital, 1276 Morena Boulevard, San Diego, CA 92110, USA
E-mail address: jane.stout@gmail.com

Vet Clin Exot Anim 19 (2016) 513–541
http://dx.doi.org/10.1016/j.cvex.2016.01.002
1094-9194/16/$ – see front matter © 2016 Elsevier Inc. All rights reserved.

Table 1
History, clinical signs, and common etiologies of respiratory disease categorized by location within the respiratory tract

	History	Clinical Signs	Differential Diagnoses
Upper Airway (nares and sinus)	• Poor diet • Exposure to new bird • Exposure to a mild respiratory irritant • Sneezing, yawning, head shaking, or beak rubbing behavior • History of ocular or nasal discharge	• Inflamed nares ± discharge • Nasal foreign body • Ocular discharge • Conjunctivitis • Blunted choanal papillae ± choanal discharge or abscesses • Swollen periorbital sinuses • Possible nasal stridor • May have increased RR but usually no increase in RE or respiratory distress • If there is bilateral occlusion of the nares there may be open mouth breathing	• Bacterial infection (consider gram-negative spp., *Chlamidophial psittaci,* and *Mycoplasma* spp.) • Fungal infection (consider *Aspergillus* spp.) • Papillomas • Nutritional deficiencies (hypovitaminosis A) • Respiratory irritants • Allergies • Nasal foreign bodies • Neoplasia
Lower airway (glottis, trachea, syrinx)	• History of recent surgery or anesthetic procedure with intubation • Acute onset of labored breathing while eating • Acute respiratory distress • History of a voice change	• Inspiratory stridor • Canaries with tracheal mites have a respiratory click • Increased RR/RE • Respiratory distress with neck extended and open mouth breathing in cases of complete tracheal obstruction • Physical examination may otherwise be normal	• Parasitic infection (Trichomonas, tracheal mites) • Viral (Amazon tracheitis, papilloma) • Granuloma (*Aspergillus,* bacterial, hypovitaminosis A) • Foreign body obstruction • Compressive extraluminal mass (Goiter in budgerigars, neoplasia) • Tracheal fibrinous seal secondary to endotracheal tube compression • Neoplasia
Lower airway (bronchi, lungs, air sacs)	• Exposure to respiratory irritant or toxin • Macaw housed with a cockatoo or African gray parrot • A history of lethargy, decreased appetite, and weight loss • May have a history of vomiting • Exercise intolerance	• Poor body condition • Tail bob or increased RR/RE • Open mouth breathing • Expiratory wheeze • Cough	• Exposure to respiratory irritants or toxin • Pulmonary hypersensitivity of blue and gold macaws • Aspiration pneumonia • Infectious pneumonia (bacterial or fungal) • Air sacculitis (bacterial or fungal) • Air sac rupture

Abbreviations: RE, respiratory effort; RR, respiratory rate.
Data from Refs.[2–5]

Table 2			
History, clinical signs, and common etiologies of extrarespiratory disease resulting in dyspnea			
	History	**Clinical Signs**	**Differential Diagnoses**
Coelomic cavity disease	• A history of lethargy and decreased appetite • Wide-based stance or seems off balance • Exercise intolerance	• Poor body condition • Distended coelom • Palpable egg or mass • Ascites	• Ascites (liver failure, peritonitis (egg yolk vs other), protein losing nephropathy, neoplasia) • Obesity • Cardiovascular failure • Coelomic mass (neoplasia, egg) • Organomegaly • Anemia

Data from Refs.[2,3,5]

Physical Examination

The physical examination of a bird that presents with signs of respiratory disease should begin with examination of the bird at rest in its carrier or in a hospital oxygenated incubator. The patient's general demeanor, respiratory rate and effort, and any audible respiratory sounds should all be noted and described. Restraint for physical examination should be minimized and the clinician should focus on auscultation and palpation of the coelomic cavity. Detection of ascites, organomegaly, or any coelomic masses indicate potential extrarespiratory cause for the observed dyspnea (see **Table 2**).[2–4,6] The examination may require staging depending on the patient's stability. The avian respiratory anatomy differs greatly from that of mammals.[7] Important clinical variations are listed in **Table 3**.

Treatment and Diagnostics of Common Respiratory Emergencies

Rhinitis/sinusitis

Birds that present with rhinitis or sinusitis are often fairly stable and can usually handle minimal restraint without oxygen supplementation. Common causes are listed in **Table 1**. The goal of the emergency doctor should be to clear the upper airway and implement appropriate pharmaceutical therapy if indicated.

- Nasal foreign bodies, debris, and rhinoliths may be removed with atraumatic forceps, a cotton-tipped applicator, or a curette. Larger rhinoliths should be removed under general anesthesia (**Fig. 1**).[2,3]
- Nasal flushes remove debris and mucous from the nares and often improve respiratory flow (**Fig. 2**). The clinician may perform cytology or culture and sensitivity on collected samples.[1–5] If the cytology indicates bacterial or fungal infection, or if an infectious etiology is suspected, appropriate therapies include:
  - Medicated nasal flushes
  - Intranasal antibiotics and antifungals (ophthalmic preparations may be used in the nares)
  - Systemic antibiotics and antifungals
- Birds with marked periorbital sinus swelling may benefit from a sinus aspirate (**Fig. 3**). Sinus aspirates should be performed in the anesthetized patient to avoid accidental piercing of the eye. Again, samples may be used for cytology or culture and sensitivity.[2–4]

Table 3
Unique features of the avian respiratory anatomy

	Description	Clinical Significance
Choanal slit	This is a V-shaped slit opening in the soft palate that connects the nasal cavity to the oropharynx. In many species the slit has triangular shaped papillae.	Blunting of the choanal papillae is often seen in respiratory disease. Mucoid drainage and abscessation may also be seen.
Glottis	There is no epiglottis covering the glottis in birds.	The lack of epiglottis often makes birds easier to intubate than mammals but may put them at a higher risk for aspiration.
Trachea	The avian trachea has complete cartilaginous rings.	Because the avian trachea cannot expand, the use of a cuffed endotracheal tube in a bird may result in pressure necrosis.
Syrinx	This vocal organ is found at the termination of the trachea.	A voice change may indicate disease at the level of the syrinx. This organ may also be a common site for tracheal foreign bodies to become lodged.
Diaphragm	There is no diaphragm in birds. A thin membrane called the oblique septum separates the thoracic and abdominal cavities. Birds breathe through the contraction and relaxation of intercostal and abdominal muscles, changing the intracoelomic pressure, which forces air in and out of the air sacs.	Preventing a bird from expanding its chest during restraint may lead to suffocation.
Air sacs	These are membrane—thin, saclike extensions of the lungs that expand and contract with respiration.	Compression of the air sacs by fluid, enlarged organs, or masses may result in respiratory compromise.

Data from Refs.[2,3,7]

Parasitic tracheal infections

- The tracheal mite, *Sternostoma tracheacolum*, most frequently affects the airways of canaries and finches. Clinical signs include an audible respiratory click and dyspnea. Mites may be seen by transtracheal illumination.[2–4] Ivermectin at

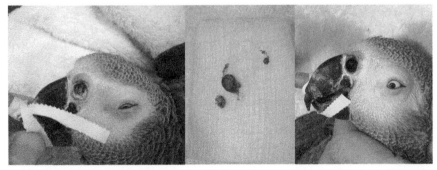

Fig. 1. The removal of a large fungal rhinolith from the nostril of an African gray parrot was performed under anesthesia.

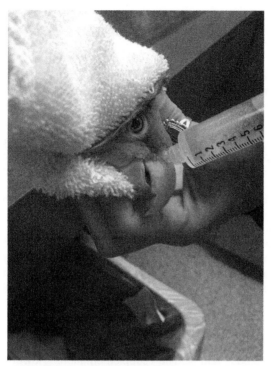

Fig. 2. Performing a nasal flush. To perform a nasal flush, the bird should be restrained head down so that the saline will flow out the nares and mouth and minimize the risk of aspiration. A 3- to 12-mL syringe filled with warm saline is applied directly to the patient's nostril. The saline is gently flushed into one nostril and then the other.

a dose of 0.2 mg/kg orally, subcutaneously, or intramuscularly may be used as treatment.[8]

- Trichomoniasis is most commonly seen in pet pigeons and doves but also has been documented in psittacines. Lesions appear as white or yellow caseous plaques of the oral cavity and may cause obstruction of airways and subsequent

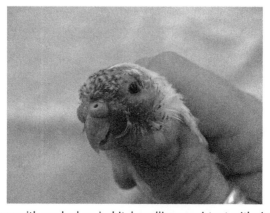

Fig. 3. A budgerigar with marked periorbital swelling consistent with sinusitis.

dyspnea. The organism may be visualized by preparing a wet mount slide of a plaque sample.[2,3] Metronidazole at a dose of 10 to 30 mg/kg orally every 12 hours treats *Trichomoniasis*.[8]

Tracheal obstruction

Birds that present with a partial or complete tracheal obstruction require immediate care. Potential causes of obstruction are listed in **Table 1**. Treatment options include:

- Birds should receive oxygen supplementation in a heated incubator.
- Administration of terbutaline at a dose of 0.01 mg/kg intramuscularly every 6 to 8 hours and butorphanol at a doses of 1 to 2 mg/kg intramuscularly every 2 to 3 hours may facilitate the patient's breathing.[5]
- Birds that do not respond to the above treatments or that have a complete obstruction require placement of an air sac cannula.[2,3,5,6,9]
- Birds with suspected tracheal obstruction require cervical and thoracic radiographs to search for a syrinx granuloma or tracheal foreign body. Extraluminal tracheal compression lesions may also be observed on radiographs.[10] Foreign bodies often require removal via suction, endoscopy, or tracheotomy. These procedures are more readily performed by a veterinarian experienced in advanced avian treatment, and the patient should be transferred to an appropriately equipped facility once stabilized.
- In the United States iodine deficiency/goiter in budgerigars has become much less common secondary to the advent of better quality over-the-counter feeds and iodine supplementation. However, extratracheal compression secondary to enlarged thyroid glands should be suspected in budgerigars with a history of voice change, dyspnea, and a poor-quality seed diet. Treatment for these patients is 1 drop of 1:10 dilution iodine and water in the patient's drinking water daily. Clinical signs often resolve within 2 days of initiating treatment.[4] Appropriate supportive care for a dyspneic patient should also be initiated.

Exposure to respiratory irritant or toxin and asthma/hypersensitivity patients

Patients with a history of toxin exposure that present in severe respiratory distress have a guarded-to-poor prognosis.[3] Oxygen supplementation in a heated incubator and minimal handling is the primary treatment for these patients. Other potential treatments include:

- Terbutaline administered at 0.01 mg/kg intramuscularly every 6 to 8 hours. Terbutaline may also be nebulized.[5]
- The use of a fast-acting steroid (dexamethasone sodium phosphate 6–8 mg/kg intravenously) has been suggested.[3]

Pneumonia and air sacculitis

- Administer oxygen supplementation in a heated incubator as needed.
- Birds with a history of aspiration should receive prophylactic broad-spectrum antibiotic therapy.[3,5]
- Consider nebulization with a bronchodilator, antibiotic, or antifungal.[2,5]
- If there is suspicion of aspergillosis, consider initiating a prophylactic systemic antifungal drug.[2–5]
- Fluid and nutritional support should be provided as needed.

- Birds with pneumonia and air sacculitis require a full diagnostic workup including blood work, imaging, and infectious disease testing. These tests are often best performed once the patient is stabilized by an experienced avian veterinarian.

Subcutaneous emphysema

Subcutaneous emphysema is secondary to damage of the air sac system. Acute air sac damage related to bodily trauma is the most common cause of subcutaneous emphysema; however, subcutaneous emphysema can also be a sequela of primary air sac disease. Treatment involves deflating the skin with a needle and syringe or by making a small incision in the skin with a scalpel. This procedure often requires repeated treatments.[2–4]

Treatment and Diagnostics of Birds with Extrarespiratory Causes of Dyspnea

Extrarespiratory causes of dyspnea are listed in **Table 2**. Treatment varies depending on the etiology. All dyspneic birds should be provided supplemental oxygen as needed. Specific initial treatments for extrarespiratory disease are discussed below.

Cardiovascular failure

Cardiac disease may be difficult to detect in birds. A heart murmur or arrhythmia, limb edema, and a bluish color of the periorbital skin may suggest primary heart disease. Signs of dyspnea may be secondary to pulmonary edema or ascites.[5,11] Emergency therapies include:

- Oxygen supplementation in a heated incubator
- Furosemide, which may be administered at 2 to 4 mg/kg intramuscularly or intravenously[5,12]
- Nitroglycerine ointment, which reduces resistance to blood flow by dilating systemic arterioles applied to the patient's back[5]

Ascites

In birds, ascites has multiple etiologies (see **Table 2**). Birds that present with ascites may decompensate drastically once restrained. An oxygen-charged heated incubator should be readied before handling these patients. Coelomocentesis may be performed with the goal of extracting only enough fluid to relieve the patient's dyspnea.[2,3,5] The procedure is demonstrated in **Fig. 4**.

EMERGENCIES THAT PRESENT WITH GASTROINTESTINAL SIGNS

Anorexia, crop stasis, vomiting, diarrhea, and abnormal droppings are common reasons for a bird presenting to the emergency room. These clinical signs may present acutely or have a chronic origin (days to weeks) and may be a manifestation of primary gastrointestinal disease, systemic illness, or toxin exposure (**Table 4**).[6,12–14]

Initial Therapeutics

Some avian patients presenting with only 1 episode of vomiting or mild diarrhea may be fairly bright and alert; however, most of the emergency room cases tend to have more severe gastrointestinal signs, and the birds often present fluffed, lethargic, and dehydrated. Initial supportive care should include:

- Heat support

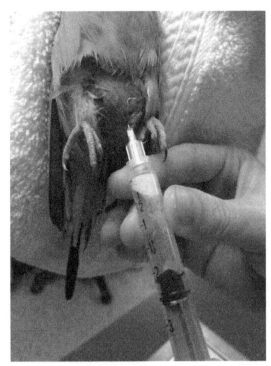

Fig. 4. Steps in performing a coelomocentesis: (1) During restraint keep the bird vertical. Because birds do not have a diaphragm, dorsal recumbency can cause respiratory distress in patients with an abdominal effusion. (2) Provide flow-by oxygen as needed. (3) If possible, perform the procedure with ultrasound guidance to reduce the risk of complication. (4) When performing a blind coelomocentesis, perform the procedure slightly cranial to the cloacal in the central third of the coelom where it is most distended. (5) A 25- to 22-gauge needle on an appropriately sized syringe or same gauge butterfly catheter can be used. (6) Remove only enough fluid to relieve the patient's dyspnea. (7) Collected fluid should be preserved for cytology or culture and sensitivity.

- Rehydration. Depending on the severity of dehydration, subcutaneous, intravenous, or intraosseous fluids may be used.
- Nutritional support. Anorexic patients should be gavage fed a commercial feeding formula.
  - Aggressive oral nutritional support is contraindicated in birds that present with vomiting or crop stasis. Initially, these patients can receive supplements of dextrose in administered fluids. Small amounts of oral Pedialyte or diluted feeding formula may also be gavaged.
- Crop gavage and massage for crop stasis patients. Small volumes of warm water or lactated ringers may be gavage fed into the crop. The crop may then be massaged to mix the hardened material with the fluid. This may allow for crop emptying. Alternatively, the mixed crop contents may be aspirated back with the gavage feeding tube. If the crop contents are not readily aspirated with the tube, the patient may need to be treated surgically with an ingluviotomy, but this procedure should be performed by an experienced avian veterinarian.[6,13]

Table 4
Differential diagnoses of common gastrointestinal signs seen in avian emergency patients

Clinical Sign	Differential Diagnoses	Clinical Sign	Differential Diagnoses
Crop stasis	• Foreign body (crop or upper GI) • Extraluminal crop compression • Crop atony secondary to overfeeding neonates • ingluvitis/enteritis (bacterial, fungal, parasitic) • Proventricular dilatation disease • Secondary to systemic disease • Neoplasia • Heavy metal toxicity	Vomiting/regurgitation	• Dietary indiscretion • Foreign body (proventriculus, ventriculus, intestinal) • Extra- or intraluminal obstruction • Enteritis (bacterial, fungal parasitic) • Proventricular dilatation disease • Secondary to systemic disease • Neoplasia • Heavy metal toxicity • Ingestion of other toxins that induce vomiting • Normal courtship display
Diarrhea	• Stress • Dietary • Enteritis • Liver disease • Pancreatitis • Toxin ingestion	Hematochezia	• Cloacal papilloma • Cloacitis or ulceration • Egg binding • Prolapse • Hemorrhagic enteritis • Lower GI neoplasia

Melena	• Ingestion of pigmented fruit (looks like melena)
	• Upper GI disease
	  ○ Enteritis
	  ○ Foreign body
	  ○ Ulcer
	  ○ Intestinal papilloma
	  ○ Neoplasia
	• Anorexia/starvation
		Undigested food	• Proventricular dilatation disease (avian bornavirus)
			• Enteritis
			  ○ Gram-negative bacteria
			  ○ Avian gastric yeast
			  ○ Candida
			  ○ Giardiasis
			• Intestinal Neoplasia

Polyuria	• Stress • Dietary • Renal disease • Enteritis • Liver disease • Pancreatitis • Sepsis	Green/yellow urates	• Liver disease
Hematuria	• Heavy metal toxicity	—	—

Abbreviation: GI, gastrointestinal.
Data from Refs.[12–14]

Possible Diagnostics

Although the emergency clinician's primary goal should be to stabilize the patient, several noninvasive diagnostics tests may provide valuable information that may further dictate the therapeutic plan.

- Cytology on crop swab or aspirate. In vomiting and crop stasis patients, evaluating crop contents for infectious agents may be beneficial. Crop contents may be sampled with a crop swab or aspirated with a gavage tube. Samples may then be smeared on a slide, stained, and evaluated microscopically.[6,12–14]

- Fecal wet mount and gram stain. Samples of a patient's feces (avoid urates) may be evaluated as a wet mount or Gram stain for evidence of parasitic, bacterial, or fungal infection (**Box 1**).[6,12–14]
- Radiographs. Radiographs may help to identify a crop foreign body or the presence of heavy metal; however, patients suffering from crop stasis are at a higher risk for aspiration. Therefore, radiographs should be performed judiciously.

As in other species presenting with signs of gastrointestinal distress, the avian patient also requires a more complete workup including a complete blood count and serum chemistry profile, infectious disease and heavy metal testing as needed, fecal culture, and advanced imaging.[6,12–14] These diagnostics are often beyond the scope of the emergency room setting and may be performed after the patient is transferred to an avian veterinarian.

Additional Initial Therapies Considered for Birds Presenting with Gastrointestinal Signs

- Initiation of antibiotic or antifungal therapy. If evidence of infection is present on crop or fecal cytology, or if there is high suspicion of enteritis, appropriate therapy should be initiated. Injectable systemic antibiotics should be selected over oral formulations for birds that present with vomiting or crop stasis. Conversely, oral antibiotics and antifungal medications that work topically may be beneficial via gavage as a localized treatment of the crop.[12,13]
- Antiparasitic therapy. Appropriate parasiticide therapy should be initiated if an organism is found on a fecal wet mount.
- Promotility medication. Promotility medications may facilitate crop emptying.[13] These medications should not be initiated until the patient is well hydrated and a foreign body or obstruction has been excluded.
- Chelation therapy. Birds suspected of experiencing heavy metal toxicity should be started on chelation therapy.[6,12–14]

Common medications used to treat gastrointestinal disease are listed in **Table 5**.

EMERGENCIES INVOLVING THE REPRODUCTIVE TRACT
Egg Binding and Dystocia

Egg binding is defined as prolonged oviposition or the failed expulsion of the egg from the oviduct. In essence, the egg has remained in the oviduct beyond normal motility

---

Box 1
Common infectious agents seen on crop cytology and fecal gram stain

- Gram-negative bacteria
- Clostridium
- Avian gastric yeast
- Budding or abundant yeast

Data from Lumeij TJ. Gastroenterology. In: Ritchie BW, Harrison GJ, Herrison LR, editors. Avian medicine: principles and application. Lake Worth (FL): Wingers Publishing Inc; 1994. p. 482–521; and Hoefer HL. Diseases of the gastrointestinal tract. In: Altman RB, Club SL, Dorrestein GM, et al, editors. Avian medicine and surgery. Philadelphia: WB Saunders; 1997. p. 419–53.

Table 5
Commonly used drugs for treatment of birds with gastrointestinal tract signs

Medication	Dose	Route	Frequency	Comments
Antibiotics				
Amoxicillin clavulanate	125 mg/kg	PO	q 8 h	Effective against clostridium.
Enrofloxacin	5–15 mg/kg	IM or PO	q 12 h	Broad-spectrum antibiotic. Oral may cause emesis. Injectable may cause muscle necrosis.
Marbofloxacin	5 mg/kg	PO	q 24 h	Less likely to cause emesis than enrofloxacin
Piperacillin/tazobactam	100 mg/kg	IM	q 6–12 h	Broad-spectrum for gram positive, gram negative (anaerobic and aerobic including pseudomonas).
Trimethoprim/sulfamethoxazole	40–50 mg/kg	PO	q 12 h	Broad-spectrum antibiotic. Also treats coccidia.
Antifungals				
Amphotericin B	100–109 mg/kg	PO	q 12 h × 10–30 d	Use injectable formulation. Treats avian gastric yeast.
Fluconazole	2–5 mg/kg	PO	q 24 h × 7–10 d	Fungistatic. Not effective against avian gastric yeast.
Ketoconazole	10–30 mg/kg	PO	q 24 h × 14 d	May cause regurgitation or liver toxicity.
Nystatin	300,000 U/kg	PO	q 12 h × 7–14 d	Not absorbed across the GI tract. Treats by direct contact.
Antiparasitics				
Fenbendazole	20–50 mg/kg	PO	q 24 h × 5 d	Treats ascarids and giardia. May be toxic in lories. If used in molting bird may cause feather destruction.
Metronidazole	10–30 mg/kg	PO	q 12 h × 10 d	Treats giardia and trichomonas.
Toltrazuril	7–10 mg/kg	PO	q 24 h × 2–3 d	Treats coccidian.
Prokinetics				
Metoclopramide	0.5 mg/kg	PO or IM	q 8–12 h	—
Cisapride	1 mg/kg	PO	q 12 h	—
Chelators				
CaEDTA	30–40 mg/kg	IM	q 12 h × 3–5 d then off 3–5 and on PRN	Ensure that patient is hydrated during use.

Abbreviations: GI, gastrointestinal; IM, intramuscularly; PO, orally; PRN, as needed.
Data from Hawkins MG, Barron HW, Speer BL, et al. Birds. In: Carpenter JW, editor. Exotic animal formulary. St Louis (MO): Elsevier Saunders; 2013. p. 184–438.

estimates for a given species. Dystocia is a more advanced form of egg binding in which the arrested egg in the distal oviduct is either obstructing the cloaca or causing prolapse through the oviductal-cloaca orifice.[15-19] Although any female bird may present with egg binding or dystocia, cockatiels and budgies are overrepresented.[20] Lovebirds, canaries, and finches are also commonly presenting species.[15,16] Common causes contributing to egg binding and dystocia are include in **Box 2**.

Clinical signs of egg binding and dystocia

Generally, birds that present with dystocia are more debilitated than those with egg binding. Clinical signs of dystocia are listed in **Box 3**. Birds with less complicated cases of egg binding may present with milder clinical signs of egg retention. In both egg binding and dystocia cases, the egg is often palpable in the caudal coelom, but some cases require radiography or ultrasonography for accurate diagnosis.[15,16]

Emergency treatment of egg binding and dystocia

For patients that present with egg binding, supportive care should be initiated, including but not limited to supplemental heat, fluids, and nutritional support. Given that malnutrition and hypocalcemia are frequent causes of egg binding, calcium supplementation at a dose of 100 mg/kg subcutaneously or orally[8] should also be started.[15-19] Often this supportive care is enough to initiate oviposition or stabilize a patient for transfer to an avian veterinarian.

Patients that are exhibiting signs of distress even after supportive care may require pharmaceutical or surgical intervention (**Table 6**).

Egg Yolk Peritonitis

Egg yolk peritonitis is inflammation of the peritoneum induced by exposure of the coelomic cavity to egg yolk material. Conditions leading to ectopic eggs and oviductal

---

Box 2
Common etiologies of egg binding and dystocia, egg yolk peritonitis, and cloacal prolapse

Egg Binding and Dystocia	Egg Yolk Peritonitis	Cloacal Prolapse
• Calcium imbalances	Ectopic egg	Female birds (prolapse of the cloaca, uterus, vagina, or distal oviduct).
• Nutritional deficiencies	• Stress	• Dystocia.
• Obesity	• Trauma	• Chronic egg laying
• Temperature changes	• Normal oviductal reverse peristalsis	• Malnutrition
• Environmental stressors		• Loss of uterine tone
• Malformed eggs	Oviductal disease	• Cloacitis or salpingitis
• Cloacal masses	• Salpingitis	• Reproductive neoplasia
• Oviductal conditions	• Oviductal impaction	Male birds (prolapse of the cloaca or phallus (waterfowl))
• Hereditary disease	• Neoplasia	• Excessive masturbation
	• Cystic hyperplasia of the oviduct	• Infection or trauma of the phallus
		Birds with a cloacal or intestinal prolapse
		• Diarrhea
		• Cloacitis/enteritis
		• Cloacaliths
		• Papillomas
		• Neoplasia

Data from Refs.[15-19]

Box 3	
Common clinical signs of dystocia and egg yolk peritonitis in birds	
Clinical Signs of Dystocia	**Clinical Signs of Egg Yolk Peritonitis**
• Generalize depression, inappetence or anorexia	• Lethargy
	• Inappetence, anorexia, and weight loss
• Abnormal posturing including hunched back, wide-based stance, and wing droop	• May have a history of recent egg laying or a cessation of egg laying
• Abdominal straining	• Wide-based stance or coelomic distention
• Dyspnea	• Ascites
• Inability to produce droppings	• Dyspnea
• Leg paresis/paralysis secondary to compression of the ischiatic nerve by the egg or hypocalcemia	
• Oviductal prolapse with the egg still contained within the reproductive tract.	
Data from Refs.[15–19]	

disease/rupture are the primary causes of egg yolk deposition into the coelomic cavity and subsequent peritonitis (see **Box 2**). Depending on the etiology, egg yolk peritonitis may be infectious or sterile.[15–19]

Clinical signs of egg yolk peritonitis

Clinical signs in birds with egg yolk peritonitis depend on the duration of the peritonitis and on whether the peritonitis is sterile or septic. Typically, birds with advanced or septic peritonitis are more debilitated and critically ill patients.[15–17] Common clinical signs of egg yolk peritonitis are included in **Box 3**.

Emergency treatment of egg yolk peritonitis

Birds that present on emergency with egg yolk peritonitis are usually those displaying more severe clinical signs, including generalized debilitation, ascites, and secondary dyspnea. Accordingly, therapeutic goals include stabilizing the patient through supportive care, providing analgesia as needed, and performing coelomocentesis to relieve the ascites induced dyspnea.[15–19]

The procedure depicting coelomocentesis is described in **Fig. 4**. Potential complications of this diagnostic and therapeutic technique include:

- Puncture of coelomic organs
- Laceration of the air sacs, subsequent leakage of fluid into the air sacs, and drowning related to a lateral approach

In birds with egg yolk peritonitis, collected fluid samples are often yellow to brown. On cytology, fat particles and yolk material may be seen. If bacteria are observed, the clinician should initiate broad-spectrum antibiotic therapy, and the fluid sample should be submitted for culture and sensitivity.[15,16,19]

Cloacal Prolapse

Cloacal prolapse most often involves the cloaca, the reproductive tract, and the gastrointestinal tract but may also encompass the ureter (**Figs. 5** and **6**). Common conditions that may result in tissue prolapse are listed in **Box 2**.

Table 6 Treatment options for dystocia cases that have not responded to initial supportive care and calcium supplementation		
	Therapeutic/Procedure Description	**Comments**
Pharmaceuticals	Prostaglandin E topical gel applied to the vent at a dose of 0.1 mL/100 g bird will cause the relaxation of the uterovaginal sphincter. It will also stimulate uterine contractions. Oxytocin at a dose of 0.5 IU/kg IM may cause uterine contractions. It may be used along with prostaglandin E for a potentiated response.	• Prostaglandin E gel is expensive and can be difficult to keep in stock. • The use of oxytocin in birds is controversial because it does not relax the uterovaginal sphincter. • The use of these pharmaceutical agents is contraindicated if the cause of dystocia is suspected to be a large or malformed egg. Radiographic evaluation of the egg before initiation of these medications is recommended.
Manual manipulation	The egg can be produced by gently massaging it from the pelvic canal. The cervix may need to be carefully expanded with hemostats before the above manipulation.	• Best performed in the anesthetized or heavily sedated patient. • Damage to the cervix, oviduct, and prolapse are potential consequences of overaggressive manipulation.
Ovocentesis	Cloacal approach: • The egg is visualized in the vagina using an otoscope cone, speculum, or ring retractor. • An 18-gauge needle is inserted via the cloaca into the egg and the egg's contents are aspirated. The egg is then collapsed. Transabdominal approach: • The egg is manipulated so that it is held adjacent to the body wall. • The needle is inserted through the abdominal wall and into the egg. The yolk contents are aspirated and the egg is collapsed.	• Best performed in the anesthetized patient. • There is a small risk of damaging the oviduct or seeding the reproductive tract or coelom with yolk material during this procedure. The collapsed egg should pass on its own in several days. The owner should be instructed that if they do not see the egg within 48 h they should recheck with their avian veterinarian.

Abbreviation: IM, intramuscularly.
Data from Refs.[9,15,16]

Clinical signs of cloacal prolapse

Cloacal prolapses are diagnosed by the obvious protrusion of tissue through the vent. Initial evaluation of the prolapse should include:

- Determining what tissue has prolapsed
- Gauging the viability of the prolapsed tissue
- Assessing whether an egg is still present in the reproductive tract if dystocia is suspected
- Evaluating the cloaca for a cloacalith, papilloma, or other abnormal tissue

Treatment of cloacal prolapses

Strategies for treating cloacal prolapses are shown in **Fig. 7**. Patients should be anesthetized before the cleaning and reduction of the prolapse. For all levels of prolapse,

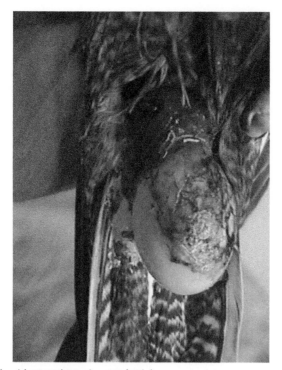

Fig. 5. Prolapsed oviduct and egg in a cockatiel.

the stability of the patient should be considered before prolapse placement, and supportive care and analgesia should be provided.[4,15–17]

EMERGENCIES OF THE NEUROLOGIC SYSTEM

Birds that present with neurologic disease may be challenging to treat and diagnose. They often require rapid initiation of critical care in the wake of little diagnostic information. Accordingly, a complete history and neurologic and physical

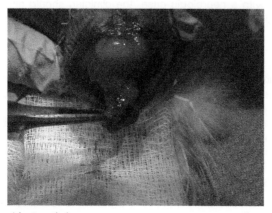

Fig. 6. Prolapsed oviduct and cloaca.

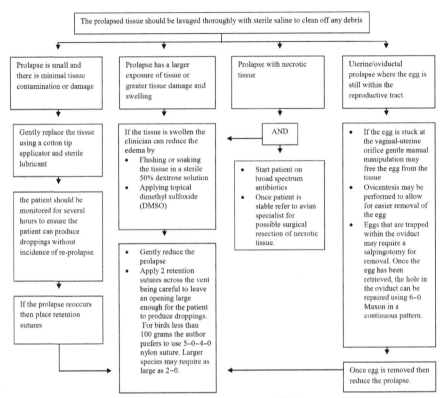

Fig. 7. Treatment of cloacal prolapses. (*Data from* Refs.[9,15-17])

examinations are invaluable when treating a bird with neurologic signs. Ideally, a complete blood count, serum blood chemistry profile, radiographs (to rule out heavy metal ingestion), infectious disease and toxin (including heavy metal) testing as needed, and even advanced imaging (MRI or CT) should be performed on birds with neurologic signs to obtain a diagnosis.[6,21-23] However, these diagnostics are often beyond the abilities of the general small-animal emergency room service. When presented with a neurologic case, the clinician should aim to stabilize and support the bird until it is transferred to a veterinarian experienced in avian medicine.

Seizures

Seizures are a common neurologic condition in birds presenting on an emergency service. Both focal and full tonic-clonic seizures may be witnessed in birds. A seizuring bird may also present fluttering on the bottom of the cage. Like mammals, birds also experience an aura phase before the seizure and a postictal phase after the seizure.[21-24] Common causes of seizures in birds are listed in **Table 7**.

The primary goal when presented with a seizuring patient is to stop the seizures. **Fig. 8** describes the common protocol for seizure management in birds. Other immediate therapeutics to consider include:

- Intravenous dextrose administration if a patient is found to have a low blood glucose level[21-24]

Table 7	
Common causes of seizures in birds	
Nutritional	• Vitamin E and selenium deficiencies • Vitamin B deficiencies • Vitamin D imbalances
Degenerative	• Hydrocephalus
Metabolic	• Hypoglycemia (neonates and raptors) • Hypocalcemia • Hepatic encephalopathy (liver failure) • Renal failure • Heat stress
Vascular/hypoxic event	• Ischemic stroke • Yolk emboli • Arteriosclerosis
Infectious	• Bacterial (chlamydiosis, granuloma, encephalitis) • Fungal (mycotoxins, aspergillosis) • Parasitic (*Sarcocystis* spp., *Baylisascaris*) • Viral (WNV, EEEV, avian bornavirus)
Trauma	• Head trauma
Toxin	• Heavy metal toxicity • Insecticides (organophosphates)
Neoplasia	• Tumor of the central nervous system
Idiopathic	• Excitatory seizures • Diagnosis of exclusion

Abbreviations: EEEV, eastern equine encephalitis virus; WNV, west nile virus.
  Data from Refs.[21–23,25,26]

- Calcium supplementation if hypocalcemia is suspected (eg, African gray parrot on a poor diet or a chronically calcium-depleted egg-laying female)[6]
- Chelation therapy if heavy metal toxicity is suspected[6,23,24]

Currently, long-term treatment of idiopathic seizures in birds involves the use of phenobarbital or potassium bromide. There are few studies or case reports evaluating the use of newer antiseizure drugs in birds and reported doses are extrapolated from cats and dogs.

Ataxia and Tremors

Clinical signs of ataxia and tremors in birds are caused by many of the same etiologies as seizures (see **Table 7**) with the additional rule out of spinal cord disease. Treatment of these patients includes:

- Supportive care (ie, heat, fluids, nutrition)
- Potential management of tremors with a benzodiazepine
- Correction of hypoglycemia, hypocalcemia, and heavy metal toxicity if suspected[6,24]

Head Trauma

Head trauma often occurs when a flighted bird flies into a window, wall, door, or ceiling fan. The author has also treated several flighted pet birds that escaped the house and were hit by a car. Initial treatment of birds that present with signs of head trauma is detailed in **Box 4**.

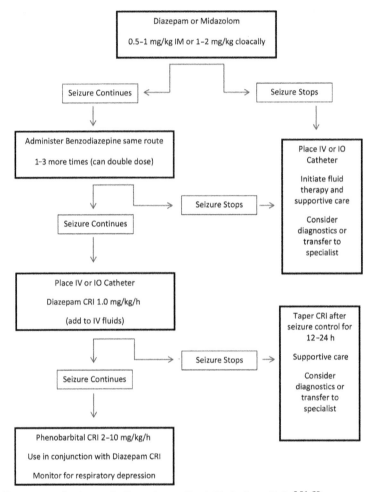

Fig. 8. Treatment of seizures in the avian patient. (*Data from* Refs.[6,21-23])

Once the head trauma patient is stabilized, the bird should be evaluated for soft tissue trauma and beak and skull fractures. The treatment of these injuries is more thoroughly discussed in the Trauma section.

Acute Onset of Leg Paresis or Paralysis

Birds may present on emergency with unilateral or bilateral paralysis or paresis, and common differential diagnoses for both are listed in **Box 5**. Initial treatment for these patients should include[24]:

- Supportive care
- Appropriate analgesia and radiographs to rule out potential fractures if trauma is suspected
- Treatment for nutritional deficiencies and suspected toxicities as described above.

Box 4
Treatment of the avian head trauma patient

- Place the bird in a dark, quiet, well-padded incubator that limits motility.

- Administer oxygen supplementation as needed.

- Placement of intravenous or intraosseus catheter and initiation of fluid support Note: aggressive fluid administration may cause an increase in intracranial pressure. Consider decreasing fluid rates by 33% to 50%.

- If brain edema is suspected or the patient does not respond appropriately to oxygen and fluid resuscitation, mannitol may be administered to lower intracranial pressure. Mannitol at a dose ranging from 0.25 to 1.0 mg/kg may be administered as a slow intravenous bolus given over 20 minutes. This dose can be repeated as needed every 4 to 6 hours with no more than 3 boluses within a 24-hour period.

- Butorphanol may be used for analgesia at a dose of 1 to 2 mg/kg intramuscularly every 4 to 6 hours.

- The use of corticosteroids in head trauma cases is controversial. In human brain trauma patients, corticosteroids may induce hyperglycemia, which has been associated with an increase in mortality. Corticosteroid administration may also cause a marked leukopenia in birds. The suggested dose for dexamethasone sodium phosphate is 2 to 6 mg/kg intramuscularly or intravenously.

- The cyclo-oxgenase inhibitor, Meloxicam, may help decrease cerebral edema and intracranial pressure when administered at a dose of 0.5 mg/kg intramuscularly every 12 hours in the hydrated patient.

- Nutritional support in the form of fluids supplemented with dextrose, gavage feeding, or free-choice feed should be provided.

Data from Refs.[6,8,22,24,27]

TRAUMA
Broken Blood Feathers

Common causes of broken blood feathers include damage to the feathers during falls or night frights and self-trauma by the bird cracking the feather sheath. There may be significant blood loss from a broken blood feather, with broken primary wing and tail feathers often resulting in the most hemorrhage.[28]

Although owners may have stopped the bleeding at home by applying flour, cornstarch, or a coagulant like styptic powder, it is still beneficial to pull the broken feather, as further trauma to the shaft may cause repeated hemorrhage. For avian patients presenting with actively bleeding feathers, immediate hemostasis and removal of the broken feather is essential (**Fig. 9**).[28]

Trauma to the Nails

Broken and avulsed toe nails are fairly common emergency presentations. These injuries may occur when a bird's nail becomes stuck in a toy, cage door, or other item. To treat broken nails:

- Trim off rough edges and cauterize with silver nitrate or styptic powder.[28,29]
- If the entire nail has been removed and the underlying bone is exposed, hemostasis may be obtained with digital pressure. The exposed tissue should then be cleaned and protected with tissue glue or a light bandage.[28,29]

Box 5	
Common causes of limb paresis/paralysis in birds	
Unilateral Paresis/Paralysis	**Bilateral Paresis/Paralysis**

Unilateral Paresis/Paralysis	Bilateral Paresis/Paralysis

• Ischiatic nerve compression
   ○ Dystocia
   ○ Ovarian/testicular enlargement/neoplasia
   ○ Renomegaly or neoplasia
   ○ Granuloma or abscess
 	
• Spinal cord disease
   ○ Ischemic vascular event
   ○ Neoplasia
   ○ Granuloma
 	
• Fractured long bone
	• Infectious
	   ○ Meningitis
	   ○ Avian bornavirus
	   ○ Newcastle disease virus
	   ○ Polyomavirus
	   ○ *Chlamidophial psittaci*
	
	• Toxicity
	   ○ Heavy metal
	   ○ Organophosphate
	
	• Nutritional
	   ○ Vitamin E or B deficiency
	   ○ Hypoglycemia
	   ○ Hypocalcemia
	
	• Metabolic
	   ○ Hepatic encephalopathy
	
	• Ischemic vascular event (brain or spinal cord)
	
	• Arteriosclerosis
	
	• Neoplasia of the central nervous system
	
	• Spinal cord disease
	   ○ Trauma
	   ○ Granuloma
	
	• Generalized weakness secondary to systemic disease

Data from Quesenberry KE, Hillyer EV. Supportive care and emergency therapy. In: Ritchie BW, Harrison GJ, Herrison LR, editors. Avian medicine: principles and application. Lake Worth (FL): Wingers Publishing Inc; 1994. p. 382–416; and Rosenthal K. Disorders of the avian nervous system. In: Altman RB, Club SL, Dorrestein GM, et al, editors. Avian medicine and surgery. Philadelphia: WB Saunders; 1997. p. 461–74.

Trauma to the Skin

Abrasions and lacerations

Keel and ventral coccygeal abrasions (**Fig. 10**) and lacerations are common in overclipped birds with a history of frequent falling or jumping from perches.[9,28] To treat these lesions:

- Wounds should be gently cleaned.
- Appropriate analgesia should be provided.
- A superficial wound may do well with a topical antibiotic, whereas deeper wounds may require systemic therapy.
- Lacerations requiring surgical intervention may be repaired in house or referred to an avian specialist.
- Avian patients may further mutilate these wounds. If there is evidence of self-mutilation, a protective collar may be needed. Care should be taken that the patient may still eat and drink while wearing the collar.[10,28]

Burns

Thermal burns occur most frequently in the avian patient when a bird flies into a boiling pot of water or hot cooking oil, stands on a hot surface, or chews an electrical cord.

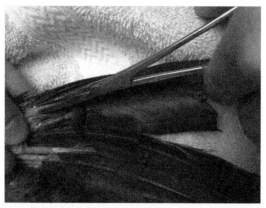

Fig. 9. Procedure for removing a blood feather: (1) Isolate the broken shaft from the surrounding feathers and apply digital pressure if the feather is still bleeding. (2) Use a pair of hemostats to grip the feather shaft at its base. With your other hand apply counter pressure at the base of the skin to prevent tearing or trauma. (3) Pull the feather ensuring that you have removed the entire shaft and apply pressure at the follicular opening to prevent continued hemorrhage.

Crop burns secondary to hot feeding formula may also be seen. Burns may range from singed feathers and mild erythema of the skin to severe, widespread lesions. Treatment should be directed toward providing analgesia and wound care.[6,28,29]

- In oil burn cases, the skin should be thoroughly rinsed with cool water to remove the oil.
- Cool water may also be used for tissue that is overheated.

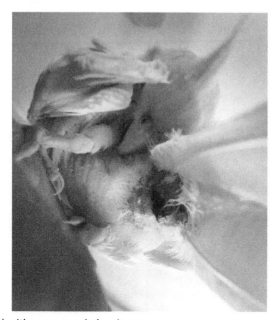

Fig. 10. Cockatiel with a coccygeal abrasion.

- Topical silver sulfadiazine cream may be applied to the burns.
- Antibiotic and antifungal therapy should be initiated in crop burn patients.
  - Crop burn patients require surgical intervention after fistula formation and should be referred to an avian specialist.

Bite wounds

Bite wounds caused by other birds most commonly are found on the cranium or on the digits and feet (**Fig. 11A**).[6,29] Bite wounds by other animals are also seen on emergency service.

- Birds kept in outdoor aviaries may be attacked by birds of prey or raccoons.
- Indoor birds may present with bite wounds caused by cats and dogs (**Fig. 11B**).

Bite wounds by mammals may range from superficial puncture wounds and bruising to large lacerations, penetration of the coelomic cavity, fractures, and traumatic limb amputations. Many of these avian patients present with signs of shock.[6] Treatment includes:

- Stabilization with supportive care, as-needed oxygen, and analgesia should be attained.
- Initiation of antibiotic therapy should target gram-negative and anaerobic bacteria.
- Superficial bite wounds to the feet may result in erythema, soft tissue swelling, and lameness. These injuries often respond to cage rest and analgesia.
- More severe wounds and fractures may require flushing, bandaging, suturing, or fracture repair. Consider transferring complicated repairs to an avian veterinarian once the patient is stable.

Trauma to the Beak

Collisions, entrapment, and bite wounds

Injuries to the beak may occur when a bird experiences a head-on collision during flight or when a bird with clipped wings falls (**Fig. 12A**). Birds may also entrap their beaks in a toy, cage, or household object (see **Fig. 12B**) or may be bitten by another animal (see **Fig. 11A**). These types of beak injuries may vary in severity from bruising, to chipped maxillary tips, to fractures and avulsions.[28,29]

- If hemorrhage is noted, hemostasis may usually be obtained by manual pressure.[28] Bleeding maxillary tip fractures can be cauterized with silver nitrate or styptic.

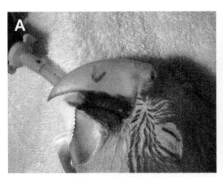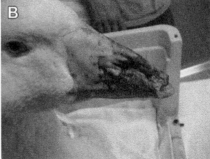

Fig. 11. (*A*) A bite wound to a green winged macaw by an avian housemate. (*B*). A bite wound to a goose by a dog.

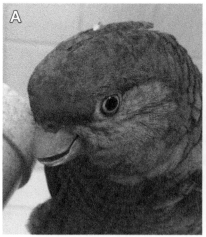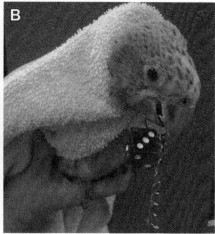

Fig. 12. (*A*) Green-cheeked Amazon parrot that lost a portion of her upper beak in a fall. (*B*) Golden conure with entrapment of the lower beak in a toy.

- Even small fractures may be painful, and the patient may need to be sedated or anesthetized for the procedure and provided with adequate analgesia.
- Small puncture wounds can be gently lavaged with sterile saline. Larger, contaminated wounds may need to be cleaned of debris and bandaged.
- More complicated beak fractures or avulsions require surgery or stabilization with acrylic.[29,30]
  ○ These procedures are preferably done by an avian specialist.
- The clinician should provide beak injury patients with soft food or gavage feeding formula.

Band Wounds and Other Constriction Injuries

Injuries secondary to leg bands are a fairly common emergency. Leg bands may be open or closed and made out of metal or plastic. Common factors leading to leg band injuries are listed in **Box 6**.

Box 6
Common etiologies of leg band injuries

- The uncinched end of an open band may become snagged on a toy, cage, or other material leading to secondary soft tissue trauma or even a fracture or dislocation of the banded leg as the bird struggles to free itself.

- Closed bands may also become caught in similar scenarios.

- Leg bands that are too small may cause constriction of the distal limb.

- Injuries that result in swelling of the foot and tarsus may be exacerbated by secondary leg band constriction.

- Birds with a history of poor nutrition may have squamous hyperplasia of the skin. This build-up of excess skin under the band may also lead to a constriction injury.

Data from Degernes LA. Trauma Medicinein. Ritchie BW, Harrison GJ, Harrison LR, editors. Avian medicine: principles and application. Lake Worth (FL): Wingers Publishing Inc.; 1994. p. 417–33; and Worell AB. Dermatological conditions affecting the beak, claws, and feet of captive avian species. Vet Clin North Am Exot Anim Pract 2013;16:777–99.

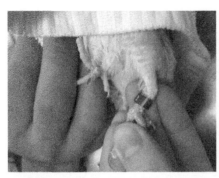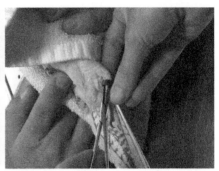

Fig. 13. Removal of an open band using hemostats.

Care should be taken when detaching leg bands, as removal can result in further soft tissue trauma or fracture of the leg.[28,29] Birds with caught leg bands may have been hanging or struggling for hours before presentation.

- Compromised patients should be allowed to rest and provided with heat support, fluids, and pain management as needed before attempting band removal.
- Depending on the extent of the band injury, the bird may need to be sedated or anesthetized for the procedure.
- Open bands may often be removed by sliding a pair of hemostats between the band and leg and opening the instrument to cause the widening of the open band gap. The leg may then be freed through this gap (**Fig. 13**).
- Closed bands will need to be cut with wire or bolt cutters of various strengths depending on the band size or material.
- Once the band is removed, the leg wounds should be treated appropriately with hemostasis, bandaging, or suturing as needed.[28,29]

Birds also often present on emergency for foreign material constriction of their digits and feet (**Fig. 14**).[29] Common materials include string material of shredded bird toys or rope perches, shredded towels, thread, and even human hair. The material may be lightly wound or causing severe constriction and pressure necrosis of the digits or feet.

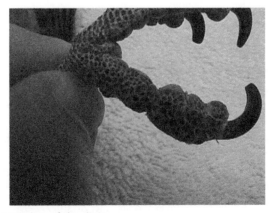

Fig. 14. String constriction of the digit.

- In more complicated entrapments, the patient may need to be sedated or anesthetized.
- For small birds or when the caught material is very fine, magnification may be helpful.
- Often, the curved end of small suture scissors can be guided under the wrapped material to cut the constriction and free the digit.
- In cases in which the material is deeply embedded in the skin, great care should be taken to make sure all foreign material is removed.

Glue Traps

Birds with unsupervised access to the household may become stuck in glue traps intended for rodent control. These patients often present in real distress from struggling to free themselves. Speedy but cautious removal of the bird from the trap and appropriate onset of supportive care are imperative for successfully treatment.

- If only a small feathered region of a bird is stuck to the glue trap, the glued feathers may be cut or gently removed while the bird is securely restrained.[6]
- When a bird is more severely entangled in a glue trap, the judicious application of a commercial mineral oil product will readily unstick feathers and limbs from the glue. Commercial automobile protectants and dish detergents may alternatively be used.[6]
- Once the bird is freed, its feathers should be cleaned of the remaining glue or applied oil residue using a commercial dish detergent and warm water (100°F–105°F). However, the unstable patient should be allowed to rest and provided with heat, fluid, and nutritional support before a bath is implemented.

Fractured Limbs

Fractures of the appendages may be secondary to flight accidents, falling, crushing accidents, or bite wounds. Pathologic fractures may also be seen. The primary goal

Table 8 Common bandages used for fracture immobilization in birds		
	Uses	**Comments**
Figure of eight bandage	Used for wing fractures, dislocations, and soft tissue injuries distal to the elbow	• Wing should be wrapped in a normal anatomic flexed position.
Wing body wrap	Used for fractures and injuries of the humerus, shoulder, and coracoid	• Combines a figure of eight bandage with a body wrap. • Ensure that the legs are not trapped in the wrap. • Ensure that the body wrap does not impede respiration.
Modified Robert Jones bandage	Used for leg fractures and injuries of the tibiotarsus, tarsometatarsus, and hock joint	• Used in birds that weigh >80 g. • A tongue depressor or half layer of thermoplastic bandage can be used for extra support.
Tape splint	Used for fractures and injuries of the digits and the leg distal to the femur	• Often used in birds that weigh <80 g • Can be used in birds that weigh up to 600 g if combined with a thermoplastic bandage

Data from Refs.[28,31]

Table 9
Common toxicologic emergencies of pet birds

	Toxin	Clinical Signs	Treatment
Heavy metal	Lead Zinc	Ataxia, seizures, weakness, vomiting, regurgitation, anemia, diarrhea or melena, hematuria or hemoglobinuia, and yellow or green urates	• Chelation therapy with CaEDTA at 30–40 mg/kg IM or IV q 12 h × 5 d • Seizure control • Supportive care
Insecticides	Organophosphates Carbamates Pyrethrins	Ataxia, tremors, seizures, Crop stasis, and diarrhea Tremors, seizures, and hyperthermia	• Seizure control • Atropine 0.01–0.1 mg/kg IM or IV • If topical exposure, wash with a commercial dish detergent and warm water (100°F–105°F) once bird is stable. • Supportive care
Anticoagulant rodenticides	First generation (warfarin) Second generation (brodifacoum and bromadiolone)	Subcutaneous hemorrhage, bleeding from the nares, and oral petechiae	• Vitamin K therapy 0.2–2.2 mg/kg IM q 8 h; once stable, IM or PO q 24 h × 14–28 d • Supportive care
Respiratory toxins	Smoke Nicotine Polytetrafluoroethylene Aerosols and air fresheners Cleaners (Ammonia and Bleach) Scented candles Hair and nail products Self-cleaning oven Burnt cooking oil	Depending on the toxin CS may vary from rhinitis and conjunctivitis to marked dyspnea. CS with PTE are severe. May also see secondary immunosuppression	• Oxygen • Bronchodilator therapy • Anxiolytic analgesic (Butorphanol) • Diuretics? • Anti-inflammatory medications • Antibiotics or antifungals if concerned with secondary infection • Supportive care
Food	Avocado	Lethargy, dyspnea, and acute death secondary to pericardial effusion and edema and congestion of the lungs and liver	• Oxygen • Gastric lavage • Activated charcoal at 1–3 g/kg • Supportive care

Abbreviations: CS, clinical signs; IM, intramuscularly; IV, intravenously; PO, orally; PTE polytetrafluoroethylene toxicity.
Data from Refs.[6,8,9,32]

of the emergency room doctor is to stabilize the patient first and the fracture second. Fractures may later be surgically repaired by an avian veterinarian.

- Unstable patients should be treated with supportive care and appropriate analgesia.
- In stable patients, radiographs should be considered.
- Fractures of stable patients should be immobilized using appropriate bandaging techniques (**Table 8**). The patient will need to be sedated or anesthetized for bandage placement.
- Antibiotic therapy should be initiated in patients with open fractures.

EXPOSURE TO TOXINS

Avian patients are most commonly exposed to potential toxins through inhalation and ingestion. Cutaneous exposure can also occur. **Table 9** lists common sources of avian toxicities that may be seen on the emergency service.

SUMMARY

Pet birds may present with a multitude of emergency conditions. Regardless of the emergency presentation, initiation of supportive care to stabilize the patient is the clinician's primary goal. Additional therapeutics and diagnostics should only be attempted once the patient is stable and may be better implemented by an avian veterinarian. The duration and severity of the avian patient's disease and the clinician's initiation of appropriate therapy often determine clinical outcome.

REFERENCES

1. Donley B, Harrison GJ, Lightfoot TL. Maximizing information from the physical exam. In: Harrison GJ, Lightfoot TL, editors. Clinical avian medicine. Palm Beach (FL): Spix Publishing Inc; 2006. p. 153–212.
2. Tully TN, Harrison GJ. Pneumonology. In: Ritchie BW, Harrison GJ, Herrison LR, editors. Avian medicine: principles and application. Lake Worth (FL): Wingers Publishing Inc; 1994. p. 556–81.
3. Voyer EV. Clinical manifestations of respiratory disorders. In: Altman RB, Club SL, Dorrestein GM, et al, editors. Avian medicine and surgery. Philadelphia: WB Saunders; 1997. p. 394–411.
4. Phalen DN. Respiratory medicine of caged birds. Vet Clin North Am Exot Anim Pract 2000;3:423–52.
5. Lichtenberger M, Orosz SE. Acute respiratory distress (ARD) - from anatomy through treatment. Providence (RI): Proc Assoc Avian Vet; 2007. p. 151–9.
6. Quesenberry KE, Hillyer EV. Supportive care and emergency therapy. In: Ritchie BW, Harrison GJ, Herrison LR, editors. Avian medicine: principles and application. Lake Worth (FL): Wingers Publishing Inc; 1994. p. 382–416.
7. King AS, McLelland J. Birds their structure and function. 2nd edition. East Sussex (England): Balliere Tindall; 1984.
8. Hawkins MG, Barron HW, Speer BL, et al. Birds. In: Carpenter JW, editor. Exotic animal formulary. St Louis (MO): Elsevier Saunders; 2013. p. 184–438.
9. Harrison GJ, Lightfoot TL, Flinchum GB. Emergency and critical care. In: Harrison GJ, Lightfoot TL, editors. Clinical avian medicine. Palm Beach (FL): Spix Publishing Inc; 2006. p. 213–32.
10. Antinoff N. Dyspnea from extraluminal tracheal compression in five birds. New Orleans (LA): Proc Assoc Avian Vet; 2014. p. 49.

11. Pees M, Krautwald-Junghanns ME. Cardiovascular physiology and diseases of pet birds. Vet Clin North Am Exot Anim Pract 2009;12:81–97.

12. Lumeij TJ. Gastroenterology. In: Ritchie BW, Harrison GJ, Herrison LR, editors. Avian medicine: principles and application. Lake Worth (FL): Wingers Publishing Inc; 1994. p. 482–521.

13. Hoefer HL. Diseases of the gastrointestinal tract. In: Altman RB, Club SL, Dorrestein GM, et al, editors. Avian medicine and surgery. Philadelphia: WB Saunders; 1997. p. 419–53.

14. Gelis S. Evaluating and treating the gastrointestinal system. In: Harrison GJ, Lightfoot TL, editors. Clinical avian medicine. Palm Beach (FL): Spix Publishing Inc; 2006. p. 411–40.

15. Joyner KL. Theriogenology. In: Ritchie BW, Harrison GJ, Harrison LR, editors. Avian medicine: principles and application. Lake Worth (FL): Wingers Publishing Inc; 1994. p. 748–804.

16. Speer BL. Urogenital disorders. In: Altman RB, Club SL, Dorrestein GM, et al, editors. Avian medicine and surgery. Philadelphia: WB Saunders; 1997. p. 625–44.

17. Boweles HL. Evaluating and treating the reproductive system. In: Harrison GJ, Lightfoot TL, editors. Clinical avian medicine. Palm Beach (FL): Spix Publishing Inc; 2006. p. 519–40.

18. Hadley TL. Management of common psittacine reproductive disorders in clinical practice. Vet Clin North Am Exot Anim Pract 2010;13:429–38.

19. Bowles JL. Reproductive diseases of pet bird species. Vet Clin North Am Exot Anim Pract 2002;5:489–506.

20. Krautwald-Junghanss ME, Kostka VM, Hofbauer H. Observations on the significance of diagnostic findings in egg binding of psittaciformes. Vet Rec 1998; 143:498–502.

21. Delk K. Clinical management of seizures in avian patients. J Exot Pet Med 2012; 21:132–9.

22. Atinoff J, Orosz SE. Don't be nervous! A clinician's approach to the avian neurological system. Louisville (KY): Proc Assoc Avian Vet; 2012. p. 121–33.

23. Platt SR. Evaluating and treating the nervous system. In: Harrison GJ, Lightfoot TL, editors. Clinical avian medicine. Palm Beach (FL): Spix Publishing Inc; 2006. p. 493–518.

24. Rosenthal K. Disorders of the avian nervous system. In: Altman RB, Club SL, Dorrestein GM, et al, editors. Avian medicine and surgery. Philadelphia: WB Saunders; 1997. p. 461–74.

25. Beaufrere H, Nevarez J, Gaschen L, et al. Presumed acute ischemic stroke in an African grey parrot (Psittacus erithacus erithacus): diagnosis and seizure management. San Diego (CA): Proc Assoc Avian Vet; 2010. p. 327.

26. Corboni DA, Nevarez JG, Tully TN, et al. West nile virus in a sun conure (Aratinga solstitialis). Monterrey (CA): Proc Assoc Avian Vet; 2005. p. 357–9.

27. Powers LV, Brofman P. Managing brain and spinal cord trauma in birds. Providence (RI): Proc Assoc Avian Vet; 2007. p. 59–65.

28. Degernes LA. Trauma Medicine. In: Ritchie BW, Harrison GJ, Harrison LR, editors. Avian medicine: principles and application. Lake Worth (FL): Wingers Publishing Inc; 1994. p. 417–33.

29. Worell AB. Dermatological conditions affecting the beak, claws, and feet of captive avian species. Vet Clin North Am Exot Anim Pract 2013;16:777–99.

30. Bennett AR. Surgery of the avian beak. Seattle (WA): Proc Assoc Avian Vet; 2011. p. 191–5.

31. Jenkins JR. Hospital techniques and supportive care. In: Altman RB, Club SL, Dorrestein GM, et al, editors. Avian medicine and surgery. Philadelphia: WB Saunders; 1997. p. 232–52.
32. Lightfoot TL, Yeager JM. Pet bird toxicity and related environmental concerns. Vet Clin North Am Exot Anim Pract 2008;11:229–59.

Emergencies and Critical Care of Commonly Kept Fowl

Mikel Sabater González, LV, CertZooMed, DECZM(Avian)[a],*,
Daniel Calvo Carrasco, LV, CertAVP, MRCVS[b]

KEYWORDS

- Emergency • Critical care • Fowl • Chicken • Waterfowl • Backyard poultry

KEY POINTS

- Fowl are stoic patients that commonly mask signs of illness in the early stages of disease and are not commonly presented as emergencies unless the acute or chronic condition is severe.
- An understanding of intraspecific and interspecific anatomic and physiologic variations is crucial to the successful management of critically ill fowl.
- Stabilization of the patient should be prioritized over diagnostic procedures.
- Clinicians treating fowl should be aware of infectious and noninfectious conditions considered emergencies in fowl.

INTRODUCTION

Fowl are birds belonging to one of the 2 biological orders, the game fowl or land fowl (Galliformes) and the waterfowl (Anseriformes). Studies of anatomic and molecular similarities suggest these two groups are close evolutionary relatives.[1]

Multiple fowl species, including chicken (eg, *Gallus gallus*), quails (eg, *Coturnix japonica* and *Colinus virginianus*), ring-necked pheasants (*Phasianus colchicus*), turkeys (eg, *Meleagris gallopavo*), Guinea fowl (eg, *Numida meleagris*), peafowl (*Pavo cristatus*), ducks (eg, *Anas platyrhynchos*), geese (eg, *Anser anser* and *Anser cygnoides*), and swans (eg, *Cygnus olor*) have a long history of domestication for socioeconomic reasons (eg, food, game, feather, or display).[2]

Fowl are stoic patients that commonly mask signs of illness in the early stages of disease and are not commonly presented as emergencies unless the acute or chronic condition is severe.

Disclosure: The authors have nothing to disclose.
[a] Exoticsvet, Marqués de San Juan 23, Valencia 46015, Spain; [b] Great Western Exotics, Vets-Now Referrals, Unit 10 Berkshire House, County Business Park, Shrivenham Road, Swindon SN1 NR, UK
* Corresponding author.
E-mail address: exoticsvet@gmail.com

Fowl are considered food-producing animals in most countries and clinicians should be aware and follow specific legislation when dealing with these patients, even if they are considered by the owners as pets.

This article reviews aspects of emergency care for most commonly kept fowl, including triage, patient assessment, diagnostic procedures, supportive care, short-term hospitalization, and common emergency presentations.

TRIAGE

Triage is the evaluation and allocation of treatment to patients according to a system of priorities designed to maximize the number of survivors. All stages of emergency evaluation are important to successfully manage critically ill birds because their low physiologic reserve does not allow them to tolerate errors of omission or commission.[3] A trained receptionist should be able to recognize an emergency during the initial phone call and to provide accurate and concise guidance about first aid treatment and transport. Before the bird arrives to the clinic, everything should be ready to attempt to stabilize it and achieve a diagnosis that guides the therapeutic plan because prompt and accurate treatment is vital for a favorable outcome.

On arrival to the clinic, a member of the medical team familiar with avian medicine should triage the patient, determining whether it requires immediate treatment or is stable enough to wait if necessary. Birds presenting with hemorrhage, head trauma, fractures, dyspnea, seizures, or toxicoses, or are unconscious or in extreme pain should be examined immediately. Critically ill patients should be isolated from other patients and other potential stressors until a complete assessment of their health status is made. Because fowl species are potential sources of infectious agents, precautions should be taken to prevent their transmission. Zoonotic pathogens reported in fowl include *Salmonella* spp, *Chlamydia psittaci*, *Mycobacterium* spp, *Campylobacter* spp, *Erysipelothrix coli*, *Listeria monocytogenes*, *Staphylococcus* spp, *Streptococcus* spp, *Enterococcus* spp, *Erysipelothrix rhusiopathiae*, avian influenza, Newcastle disease, eastern and western equine encephalomyelitis, West Nile virus, *Histoplasma capsulatum*, *Cryptosporidium* spp, *Microsporum gallinae*, *Ornithonyssus sylviarum*, *Dermanyssus gallinae*, *Toxoplasma gondii*, *Cryptosporidium* spp, and *Strongyloides avium*.[4]

PRIMARY SURVEY

The primary survey amplifies the information obtained during the triage in order to determine the stability of the patient, identify and treat immediate life-threatening conditions, decide the level of monitoring needed, and anticipate and prevent potential complications.

A brief anamnesis combined with an initial evaluation of the cardiovascular, respiratory, and nervous systems may allow clinicians to classify patients as stable or unstable.[3]

Cardiovascular monitoring is designed to ensure appropriate tissue perfusion. Auscultation of the heart allows monitoring heart rate and rhythm. The large pectoral muscle mass of fowl reduces transmission of cardiac sounds. Auscultation may be improved by placing the stethoscope diaphragm on the dorsal thorax, lateral thorax, or thoracic inlet. Alternatively, an electronically amplified esophageal stethoscope may be used. Pulses may be palpable at the tibiotarsal or deep radial artery.[5,6] A weak or thready pulse can be a sign of shock, whereas an absent pulse can indicate cardiac asystole, peripheral vasoconstriction, hypovolemia, or hypotension.[7] The basilic vein or cutaneous ulnar vein can be digitally pressed to examine capillary refill time (CRT). Normally, when the finger is removed from the vein, refilling cannot be witnessed visually. If it can be witnessed visually the bird is considered approximately 5% dehydrated, and if 1 second can be counted, then the bird is about 10% dehydrated or in shock.[8] In chickens, the comb should be firm and red. A CRT can be assessed on the comb. It should refill within 2 seconds.[8] Mucous membrane color can be assessed by everting the vent or the eyelid.

Respiratory monitoring includes auscultation of the upper and lower respiratory tracts, assessing breathing frequency and quality, as well as detection of signs of dyspnea (eg, orthopneic gait or tail bobbing).

The levels of brightness, alertness, and response should be evaluated as part of a first neurologic examination.

Birds showing depression or severe weakness should be placed immediately in a prewarmed incubator with 50% to 80% humidified oxygen and complete physical examination or diagnostic procedures may be delayed until the bird is stable enough to tolerate them.

SECONDARY SURVEY

Secondary survey includes obtaining a complete medical history, a full physical examination, assessment of the response to initial therapy, and more diagnostic procedures, which may provide a comprehensive diagnostic and therapeutic plan as well as orientate the owner about the potential economic costs and prognosis.[3]

A complete anamnesis should include, but is not restricted to, species; breed; age; gender; presenting complaint; source of the bird; diet; number of birds in the household; open or closed flock; acquisition date; date of the last addition to the flock; number and species of animals affected; potential exposure to toxins; length of illness; changes in behavior; history of previous diseases, treatments, and outcomes; reproductive history; and clinical signs, including their duration and progression.

Physical examination in fowl is similar to that of other avian species. Careful observation of the bird before handling is mandatory in order to determine the length and depth of the physical examination and further diagnostics that the patient is likely to tolerate. All equipment and supplies are readied before removing the bird from the holding container or the intensive care unit. If the patient is debilitated, examination can be performed in a stepwise fashion with small breaks given to the bird between handling, examination, diagnostics, and treatments.

HANDLING AND RESTRAINT

In general, fowl species may be handled without chemical restraint. Precautions should be taken in order to avoid physical injuries to the bird or the handler (bites, scratches [eg, from tarsal spurs], or blows from the wings [larger species]).

Fowl should be grasped across the back with or without a towel to avoid wing flapping. Then, the legs should be firmly grasped placing 1 finger between them to prevent pressure damage. The bird should then be restrained close to the handler's body or against a hard, nonmovable surface. Fractious birds may benefit from having their heads covered with a cloth.[9] Smaller species of waterfowl may be held single-handedly by restraining the animal with the wings folded or with fingers of one hand under each wing supporting the proximal humerus and the other hand supporting the bird's abdomen. Larger species, such as geese and swans, are typically restrained keeping the wings folded and facing backward under the arm of the handler. Large, calm species may also be straddled on the floor[10] (**Fig. 1**).

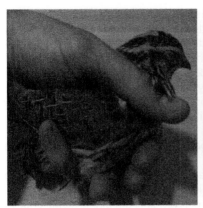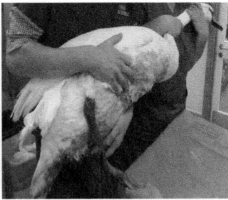

Fig. 1. Handling of a quail (*left*) and a swan (*right*).

The position of the bird during physical examination, diagnostic procedures, and therapeutic procedures may affect its cardiorespiratory function. Dorsal recumbency in conscious chickens decreases tidal volume by 40% to 50% and increases breathing frequency by 20% to 50%.[11] Birds showing signs of respiratory distress should be held upright. Respiratory compromise may be worsened in fowl by the inertial resistance of the large pectoral muscle mass to respiratory excursions of the keel. Enlarged viscera, excessive intracoelomic fat, or fluid within the coelom may compress the air sacs, reducing their effective volume and potentially leading to hypercapnia, respiratory acidemia, and death.[12]

Cloacal or body core temperature can be measured. Cloacal temperature depends on body temperature and cloacal activity over time.[13] Normal range for body temperature in waterfowl is 40°C to 42°C. To read body core temperature, the probe of a thermistor thermometer should be inserted along the esophagus until it passes the thoracic inlet.[6] Normal range for core body temperature in chickens is 40.6°C to 43.0°C.[8]

The body condition should be assessed and an accurate weight obtained on a gram or appropriately sized scale in order to correctly calculate potential drug dosages or to compare with previous or future weights (**Fig. 2**).

VASCULAR ACCESS AND FLUID THERAPY IN UNSTABLE PATIENTS

The patient's needs must be prioritized. Despite preferring that samples for hematologic and biochemical analysis be obtained before treatment for the best diagnostic ability, fowl in shock must be stabilized before extensive diagnostic sampling. A conservative minimum database includes determination of packed cell volume, total solids, and estimated white blood cell count. There is intraspecies variation in blood volume (67 ± 3 mL/kg for common pheasants and 111 ± 3 mL/kg for redhead and canvasback ducks).[14] In healthy patients, the amount of blood that can be removed without deleterious effects is 3% of body weight in ducks, 2% in chickens, and 1% in pheasants.[14] In compromised patients, this should be reduced to 0.5% of body weight. Reference values for multiple avian species can be found in the literature.

Intravenous or intraosseous fluid administration is essential when treating critical patients.

Catheters can be placed under general anesthesia if necessary. Sites for intravenous catheterization include the medial metatarsal vein, the ulnar vein, and the jugular vein (**Fig. 3**). Intraosseous catheters can be placed in the distal ulna or proximal tibiotarsus. Pneumatic bones, such as the femur or humerus, should be avoided.

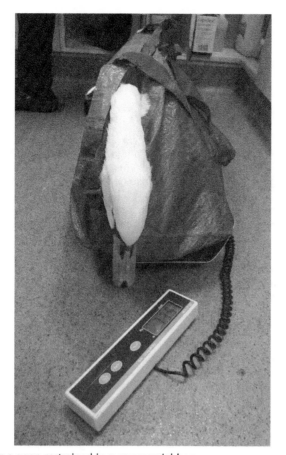

Fig. 2. Weighing a swan restrained in a commercial bag.

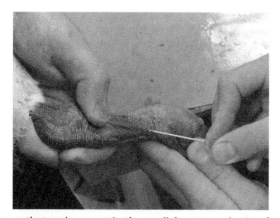

Fig. 3. Intravenous catheter placement in the medial metatarsal vein of a swan.

Most birds benefit from intravenous or intraosseous administration of warmed crystalloids at 3 mL/100 g body weight. Because fluid resuscitation in critically ill birds is difficult, administration of 1 bolus of crystalloids with Oxyglobin to hypovolemic birds may be beneficial.[15] Different types of colloids may be used as an alternative to oxyglobin.

ADDITIONAL MONITORING AND DIAGNOSTIC TECHNIQUES USED IN CRITICALLY ILL PATIENTS

Capnography, direct and indirect blood pressure, electrocardiography, and blood gas analysis are additional monitoring techniques that may be useful in assessing unstable patients. Deciding the instrumentation to use depends on practicality and procedure length.

Capnography measures end-tidal carbon dioxide concentrations in expired air and is a useful indicator of arterial carbon dioxide concentrations. The use of capnographs with sidestream sensors is recommended for small avian patients.

Pulse oximetry has not yet been validated for birds. The characteristics of oxygenated and deoxygenated avian and human hemoglobin are different, resulting in underestimation of hemoglobin saturation.[16]

An ultrasonic Doppler flow detector is most commonly used for cardiac monitoring but can also be used for indirect blood pressure measurement. Indirect blood pressure measurement techniques used in fowl include Doppler, photoplethysmographic/photoacoustic probes with a sphygmomanometer, and oscillometric monitors.[17] Systolic blood pressure determination via ultrasonic Doppler flow detection correlates well with direct blood pressure measurements in ducks (A platyrhynchos).[18] Diastolic, and therefore mean, blood pressure cannot be obtained with this method.[18] Direct arterial pressure measurement is ideal but not commonly used because of the need for specific technical skill, the invasive nature of the procedure, and the cost of equipment.[18] For medium to large birds (>200 g), the deep radial artery is the preferred site for arterial catheter placement, whereas for smaller birds (<200 g) the superficial ulnar artery is preferred. For waterbirds or long-legged birds, the cranial tibial or dorsal metatarsal arteries are acceptable sites for catheterization. Catheterization of the external carotid artery usually requires a cut-down for proper visualization.[19] A study performed on anesthetized Galliformes comparing glomerular filtration rate and blood pressure found that Galliformes were able to maintain their glomerular filtration rate when mean arterial pressure (MAP) ranged between 60 and 110 mm Hg. When MAP decreased to less than 50 mm Hg, chickens were unable to sustain glomerular filtration and urine output ceased.[19] Unlike chickens that have normal systolic, mean, and diastolic arterial blood pressures of 99 ± 13, 84 ± 13, and 69 ± 15 mm Hg, respectively, values for normotension are higher in other Galliformes (eg, turkeys).[18,19] If the definition of hypotension in humans (reduction of 30% from the baseline of conscious MAPs) is extrapolated to birds, the level of blood pressure at which birds are considered hypotensive would have a tendency to be higher than that recorded in mammals, with the exception of some Galliformes and Anseriformes species.[19] Hypovolemia is treated with intraosseous or intravenous bolus administration of crystalloids (10–20 mL/kg) or colloids (5 mL/kg) until systolic pressures are restored.[20,21] Reference blood pressure values have been determined for different species of fowl.[6,19]

Electrocardiography can be used to monitor cardiac rate and rhythm. Electrocardiographic parameters can be highly variable between fowl species, as shown by electrocardiographic studies published for several species including the chicken, turkey, quail, duck, swans, Muscovy ducks, Guinea fowl, and rock and chukar partridges.[22–34]

Arterial blood gasometry is the gold standard for assessing the acid-base status, ventilation, and tissue perfusion. It provides essential physiologic information for patients with critical illness or respiratory disease and is vital in the correction of any metabolic respiratory disorders.[19] Detailed information about blood gases in birds has been published.[19]

SEDATION AND ANESTHESIA

Sedation or anesthesia may minimize stress to fractious or painful patients. It also may aid in minimizing risk of capture myopathy in Canada geese or turkeys.[35,36] Midazolam is increasingly used in birds to produce sedation, hypnosis, anxiolysis, anterograde amnesia, centrally mediated muscle relaxation, and anticonvulsion activity.[37] The pharmacokinetics of midazolam hydrochloride following intravenous administration at 5 mg/kg were determined in broiler chickens, turkeys, ring-necked pheasants, and bobwhite quail.[38]

Several articles regarding fowl anesthesia and analgesia have been published.[5,6,39] Inhalation anesthesia with isoflurane or sevoflurane is the most common in-hospital method for anesthetizing fowl. Oxygen flow rates of 1 to 2 L/min allow rapid changes in anesthetic concentration if vaporizer setting is altered. Induction is typically via a face mask. The apnea and bradycardia that occur when an induction mask is placed over the beak and face are consequences of a stress response caused by stimulation of trigeminal nerve receptors.[40–42] Preoxygenation with 100% oxygen for several minutes reduced this response in dabbling but not diving ducks.[41] The isoflurane vaporizer is set to 3% to 4% for induction.[6] Intubation with a noncuffed endotracheal tube is recommended for anesthetic procedures lasting more than 15 minutes. Waterfowl females may require an endotracheal tube 0.5 to 1 full size larger than males of the same species.[6] If intubation is not feasible because of the nature of the procedure to be performed or anatomic structures preventing intubation (eg, presence of crista ventralis), ventilation can be achieved via air sac perfusion.[43] Airway patency should be regularly checked during waterfowl anesthesia because the thickening of mucus in the trachea or glottis may completely obstruct the endotracheal tube, leading to death of the patient. Anticholinergic drugs reduce pharyngeal and tracheal secretions but also increase their viscosity, and so are only recommended for treatment of bradycardia.[6]

In chickens and ducks, isoflurane has a minimum anesthetic concentration (MAC) of 1.32% and 1.3%, respectively.[5,6] Isoflurane produces dose-dependent cardiopulmonary depression in birds and in Pekin ducks induces tachycardia and hypotension.[44] In geese, an average Pa_{CO_2} of 53 mm Hg was necessary for spontaneous respiration to occur, and no respiration occurred with a Pa_{CO_2} less than or equal to 40 mm Hg.[45] Intermittent positive pressure ventilation may be used in anesthetized birds, even if some spontaneous breathing is present, to ensure adequate oxygenation of the blood.[46] Ventilation is assisted manually using the reservoir bag on the breathing system or a mechanical ventilator. A spontaneously breathing bird is given greater than or equal to 2 assisted beats per minute. If an anesthetized bird is apneic, the assisted ventilation rate is greater than or equal to 8 to 15 beats per minute depending on size (large birds require fewer breaths than small birds). Analysis of blood gases showed that effective gas exchange is achieved using mechanical ventilation.[5]

In chickens, sevoflurane MAC is 2.21%. At MAC, heart rate did not change significantly and cardiac arrhythmias were not observed at less than or equal to 2 times MAC. In another study in chickens, hypotension was observed during both spontaneous and controlled ventilation. However, this effect was only dose dependent during controlled ventilation. Tachycardia occurred during spontaneous ventilation, whereas heart rate remained unchanged during controlled ventilation.[5]

ANALGESIA

Species variability occurs because of differences in pain sensitivity, the conscious response to pain, and the physiologic response to analgesic therapy. Dosages and effects of opioids and nonsteroidal antiinflammatory drugs in fowl have been reviewed.[5,6,39]

HOSPITALIZATION

Many birds benefit from symptomatic treatment such as oxygen supplementation, nebulization, fluid therapy, broad-spectrum antibiotics, antifungals, and/or nutritional support and observation for 2 to 8 hours in a warmed incubator before diagnostic tests are performed.[15]

Separate equipment and housing should be used for birds with suspected contagious diseases and all equipment and cages should be thoroughly disinfected after use to minimize the risk of disease transmission.[15] The optimum temperatures for ill birds are 29.4°C to 32.1°C.

Administration of oral or subcutaneous fluids is reserved for stable fowl that are less than 5% dehydrated. Oral fluid administration requires a patient that can maintain an upright body position and has a functional gastrointestinal tract to avoid regurgitation and aspiration of fluids. Subcutaneous fluids may be administered in the inguinal web, interscapular area, axillary region, lateral flank, or midback.

Replacement fluid therapy is critical before nutritional support is instituted. Diets for stable hospitalized fowl should ideally be selected according to the natural diet of the species.

Commercially available feeding formulas, such as a formulated critical care diet Lafeber's Critical Care diet (Lafeber Company, Cornell, IL) or Hill's a/d diet (a/d Canine/Feline; Hill's Pet Nutrition, Topeka, KS) can be used on a short-term basis. The use of Emeraid exotic carnivore diet improves postsurgical recovery and survival of long-tailed ducks[47] (**Fig. 4**).

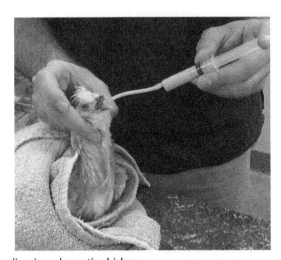

Fig. 4. Forced feeding in a domestic chicken.

COMMON CLINICAL EMERGENCY PRESENTATIONS
Hemorrhage

The most common causes of blood loss in birds include traumatic injury and hemorrhagic lesions of internal organs. The LD50 (lethal dose, 50%) for acute blood loss in mallard ducks was 60% of total blood volume. After chronic blood loss, the LD50 of mallard ducks was reached when 70% of blood volume was removed, compared with an LD50 in pheasants and chickens of 40% to 50% loss of total blood volume. Recommendations for fluid resuscitation after severe blood loss in birds have included the administration of crystalloids, colloids, and whole blood. Although no statistical difference in mortality was appreciated among the 3 fluid resuscitation groups (crystalloids, hetastarch, or a hemoglobin-based oxygen-carrying solution [HBOCS]) in the acute blood loss study, a trend of decreased mortality was observed in the HBOCS group. An early regenerative response was apparent following acute blood loss.[48]

Trauma

Traumatic injuries occur fairly frequently in fowl kept outdoors, either as a result of predator attack, gunshot, electrocution, or as a result of inappropriate housing. A thorough physical examination is essential to determine the extent of trauma and the best approach for treatment. Prioritize therapy (oxygen therapy, fluid therapy, and analgesia), control active hemorrhage, cleanse wounds, and stabilize fractures initially until patient stabilization allows a more specific treatment. Any animal that has a bite wound should be provided with antibiotics after a sample has been taken for microbiological culture and sensitivity.

Clinical signs of head trauma may include, but are not restricted to: anisocoria, head tilt, depression, or other neurologic signs, skull fractures, retinal detachment, or hemorrhage from the nares, oral cavity, ears, and/or anterior chamber of the eye. Mentation, pupil symmetry and size, and pupillary light reflex should be constantly monitored. Changes in pupil size to dilated and loss of pupillary light reflex along with mentation progression to stupors or coma indicate neurologic deterioration.[7]

Soft tissue injuries in the head and neck are commonly seen, and may require surgical repair.[49] Posttraumatic exposed epibranchial bones, part of the hyoid apparatus, can be surgically excised without significant postsurgical impairment, allowing easier surgical repair of wounds in the crown.[49] Fractures of the skull bones (eg, mandible, quadrate, jugal arches, palatine, pterygoid, and maxilla) can also occur. If the animal is able to groom and feed, healing by second intention can create a false joint allowing normal function.[49] Surgical repair of the beak and the use of prostheses have been reported.[50,51]

Anseriformes are prone to foreign body injuries. Ingestion of fishing hooks and lines is common in swans (**Fig. 5**). Lesions can be observed in the rhamphotheca, tongue, skin of the neck, and gastrointestinal tract. Management varies depending on the severity of the injuries. Endoscopy can be attempted, but sometimes surgery is required. Management of a neck injury caused by a nail shot from a pneumatic nail gun in a young Muscovy duck (*Cairina moschata*) has been reported.[52]

Ocular injuries can also be seen after head trauma. If the eye is not visual and is severely damaged, enucleation may be considered.

Injuries over the coelomic cavity should always be assessed to make sure no penetrating injuries are present. In such cases the prognosis is poor. Skin and muscle injuries can be surgically repaired when indicated, or managed medically to allow healing by second intention.

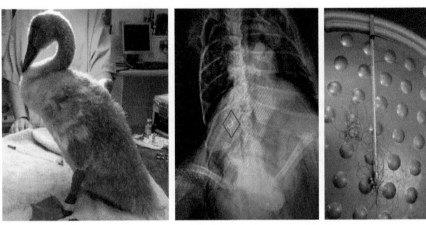

Fig. 5. Fishing line and hook (*red outline*) in a juvenile swan.

Fracture repair follows the same principles as in other avian species. In laying hens, pathologic fractures caused by hypocalcemia and metabolic bone disease might occur, and calcium status should be assessed and deficiencies corrected before surgical repair. Vitamin C deficiency can also cause secondary fractures.[53] Emergency care for bone fractures should align the fracture as fully as possible so further damage of the surrounding tissues and pain are minimized, and weight bearing can occur as soon as possible, avoiding excess stress and load on the unaffected limb. Luxations should be reduced as soon as possible to provide the best chance for joint mobility. Bandaging includes soft bandage material and splints applied for temporary support or permanent fixation of fractures. Bandaging techniques commonly used in other avian species (tape splint, football-type bandage, plastic spica bandage, modified Robert Jones bandage, Schroeder-Thomas splint, Ehmer-type bandage, and figure-of-eight bandage) can be also used in fowl[54] (**Figs. 6** and **7**).

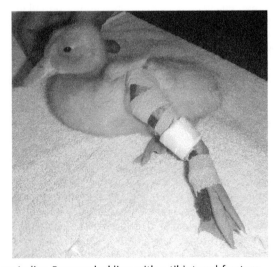

Fig. 6. Splint on an Indian Runner duckling with a tibiotarsal fracture.

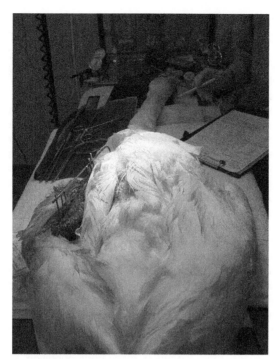

Fig. 7. Tie in a fixator for humeral fracture in a swan.

Damage to the cervical air sac can cause emphysema because of the leakage of air into the subcutaneous space. This condition is often self-limiting. A cauterized skin defect can also be created over the swelling to allow the air to escape. The cauterized hole takes longer to heal than the air sac lesion, preventing recurrence.[49]

Hypothermic Shock

Older hens quickly run for shelter when the weather conditions are not desirable. However, juvenile animals may stand on the wet ground, becoming hypothermic rapidly, especially those with thin skulls and crest, such as Polands and those with wooly feathering, such as silkies.[55] Nevertheless, adequate shelter must be always provided. Hypothermic patients may be warmed externally and via infusion of warmed fluids.

Heat Stress

Poultry experience heat distress when high temperatures accompanied by high humidity increase beyond their comfort zone. When the environmental temperatures are between 28°C and 35°C, birds use nonevaporative cooling in 2 ways: (1) increasing the surface area by relaxing the wings and hanging them loosely at their sides, and (2) increasing the peripheral blood flow. As the environmental temperature approaches the body temperature of the bird (41°C), the rate of respiration increases and the bird open-mouth breathes in order to increase evaporative cooling or water evaporation. If panting fails to prevent body temperature from increasing, birds become listless, comatose, and finally die of respiratory, circulatory, or electrolyte imbalances.[56]

Dyspnea and Respiratory Disease

Respiratory disease is a common presentation in avian practice. Clinical signs are often unspecific, and hardly ever pathognomonic. Respiratory signs are not only seen with primary respiratory disease but also with any organomegaly or distended coelom as a result of the pressure to the air sacs, or secondary to other disorders, such as cardiovascular disease.

Sinusitis is a common presentation in chickens and waterfowl, and often presents because of swelling of the periocular sinuses.[49] Different agents could cause sinusitis, such as *Mycobacterium* spp, *Pasteurella* spp, *Escherichia coli*, *Pseudomonas* spp, and some viral agents, such as avian influenza and Newcastle disease (both reportable diseases in the United Kingdom, European Union [EU], and United States (US); **Fig. 8**). However, Newcastle disease, avian influenza, and infectious laryngotracheitis are all rare in backyard poultry, and the most common causative agent of sinusitis in fowl in the US is *Mycoplasma*.[57–59] Different agents are often isolated from the nasal cavity, aggravating the clinical presentation. In such cases, the authors recommend performing an initial sinus flush with sterile saline, in order to obtain samples for culture and polymerase chain reaction (PCR) identification. Sinus flush should be performed under general anesthesia with an uncuffed endotracheal tube placed, to avoid fluid going into the respiratory tract. Once samples have been obtained, F10, enrofloxacin (not to be used in the USA and only to be used on label in egg laying chickens and turkeys in Europe), amikacin or gentamicin flush could be performed, and repeat it as necessary. If purulent material is present in the sinus, the author recommends surgical access to remove as much purulent material as possible, because antibiosis alone is unlikely to resolve it.

Mycoplasmosis is the most common respiratory condition seen in backyard poultry.[57,60] Poultry is mainly affected by 4 species of *Mycoplasma*: *Mycoplasma gallisepticum*, *Mycoplasma synoviae*, *Mycoplasma meleagridis*, and *Mycoplasma iowae*. *M gallisepticum* is often the pathogen causing respiratory signs, although *M synoviae* can also cause respiratory signs (sneezing, foamy nasal and ocular discharge, conjunctivitis, sinusitis, and/or purulent aural discharge). *Mycoplasma* spp can be latent within the flock and often causes disease when there is immunosuppression, stressful factors, and concomitant infections. Tylosin is the recommended treatment because it is licensed (at least in the United Kingdom/EU and United States). Antibiotic therapy does not eliminate *Mycoplasma*, but it can resolve clinical signs; equally important is to assess and treat any other stressful factors (ammonia and dust

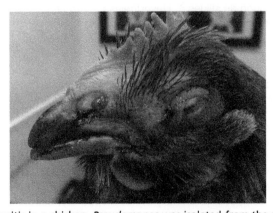

Fig. 8. Severe sinusitis in a chicken. *Pseudomonas* was isolated from the sinus.

levels, densities, overall hygiene, food and water quality). However, if symptoms persist despite treatment, euthanasia should be considered for the well-being of the flock.

Anseriformes are an important reservoir for avian influenza, often being asymptomatic carriers even from some of the high-pathogenic strains. Avian influenza or fowl plague is a rare disease in wild waterfowl, with few records in the wild.[59] Despite being uncommon, in particular in mixed flocks or flocks exposed to wild waterfowl, avian influenza should be considered and investigated in cases with compatible clinical signs, such as mucopurulent or caseous sinusitis.[59] Important management factors to control this disease, such as hygiene and density levels, should be assessed in captive waterfowl showing clinical signs.

Newcastle disease or avian paramyxovirus can also present with signs of upper respiratory disease, such as conjunctivitis or tracheitis, and it can also cause central nervous system and gastrointestinal signs.[49,61] Zoonosis can also occur, although this only causes mild conjunctivitis in humans. It is a relevant disease given the high economic losses it can produce in the commercial poultry industry, because there is no effective treatment. Vaccinations are available to reduce the likelihood of outbreaks. Vaccination against Newcastle disease is not currently allowed in the UK, but seems to be standard practice in the US.

Infectious laryngotracheitis (ILT) is caused by a herpesvirus, as well as Marek disease. ILT can affects chickens (mainly meat breeds) as well as pheasants, and is similar in presentation to other respiratory diseases. It is characterized by the formation of a diphtheritic membrane in the trachea that can cause obstruction; animals can present gasping. Vaccination can be attempted in an outbreak to reduce morbidity and mortality. Early vaccination prevents clinical manifestation, but not latent infection. Modified live vaccines are available in the UK, EU, and US.

Aspergillosis is a common condition affecting waterfowl, although it can also affect gallinaceous birds, such as chickens. As in other avian species, *Aspergillus fumigatus* is the main isolated pathogen, although others species of the genus *Aspergillus* can also cause disease.[61,62] In chickens, despite most healthy birds coping with a moderate exposure to the *Aspergillus* conidia, infection may occur in immunocompromised birds or when exposed to an overwhelming quantity of spores. Common sources of *Aspergillus* are contaminated food and moldy substrates. Clinical signs might include dyspnea, but it can present as lethargy, anorexia, and significant weight loss. Diagnosis and treatment present similar challenges to those faced in other avian species. Treatment is based in antifungal therapy, often an azole drug, together with supportive care.

Infectious bronchitis is caused by a highly infectious coronavirus and is characterized by having 2 main presentations depending on the age of the infected animals; in young chicks, respiratory disease is the predominant manifestation, whereas salpingitis and the subsequent decrease in egg production is most commonly seen in older laying hens. Soft, irregular, or rough-shelled eggs are often seen. In certain animals the lesions caused might impair normal laying for the rest of the animal's life, or even cause secondary problems, such as egg coelomitis.

C psittaci is a well-known pathogen among avian practitioners worldwide, not only relevant for its high prevalence but also for its zoonotic potential.[63] More than a 100 species have been shown to be infected, including galliformes.[64] Because of its very wide infection range, many different species can act as a reservoir, such as pigeons and waterfowl.[65] A recent study in pigeons showed a prevalence of 15% in adult animals, which was twice as high in juvenile birds.[66] Outbreaks in fowl occur only occasionally. In poultry, infection is often systemic, and occasionally fatal. Clinical signs, incubation periods, morbidity, and mortality vary widely depending on the virulence of the strain infecting the flock. Common clinical signs observed with chlamydiosis are sinusitis, rhinitis, diarrhea, and weakness. Postmortem findings in affected birds include splenomegaly, hepatomegaly, airsacculitis, pericarditis, and peritonitis.[67,68] In turkeys, the disease pattern differs from other species and tends to present as an explosive outbreak.[69] Clinical signs can be aggravated by concurrent infections, such as *Salmonella* or *Pasteurella*. Ideally, a combination of serology and PCR identification is used to diagnosis chlamydia. However, after adequate therapy, there is no currently available test to ascertain whether affected birds are no longer carriers; therefore, treatment should be carefully considered, because of its zoonotic risk, especially in collections open to the public.[61] Chlortetracycline (1000 ppm; ie, 18.2 g/kg food daily for 45 days) has been recommended in turkeys, although doxycycline (25 mg/kg PO twice a day or 240 ppm in food daily for 45 days; or 50–100 mg/kg IM weekly on 6 occasions) is also used in outbreaks to reduce mortality in turkeys as well as in other species.[64,70]

Avian tuberculosis can present as a respiratory emergency when lesions are localized in the pharynx or trachea.

Certain parasites can also cause respiratory disease in fowl, such as *Syngamus trachea* (commonly known as gapeworm), duck leeches (*Theromyzon tessulatum*), streptocariasis, (*Streptocara* spp), and air sac mites (*Cytodites nudus*).[71–73] If upper airways are affected, animals present gasping for air or open-mouth breathing, coughing, or retching. Diagnosis is based on identification of the parasites (adult forms, ova, or larvae).

Riemerella anatipestifer can cause a peracute infection in ducklings, which might present with upper respiratory clinical signs, such as dyspnea, or nasal or ocular discharge.[74] This condition evolves quickly and can cause sudden death. Samples should be obtained for culture and sensitivity, to allow adequate antibiotic therapy.

Neurologic Disease

Neurologic disease is common in fowl. Clinicians must be vigilant and aware of the reportable diseases that can present with neurologic signs, such as Newcastle disease, avian influenza, and chlamydiosis. Marek disease is common in unvaccinated chickens, and heavy metal poisoning should always be considered in waterfowl. Other possible causes are trauma, nutritional deficiencies, central nervous system ischemia, vascular insult, and other intoxications (**Fig. 9**).

Marek disease is caused by gallid herpesvirus 2, and has recently been described as the most common disease diagnosed in backyard poultry.[57] The disease is characterized by the presence of T-cell lymphoma as well as mononuclear infiltration of nerves, organs, reproductive tract, internal viscera, iris, muscle, and skin.[75] The mononuclear infiltration of peripheral nerves, in particular the sciatic nerve, causes paralysis. However, there is no treatment of affected birds and euthanasia should be considered in unvaccinated suspicious cases. Early vaccination (within the first

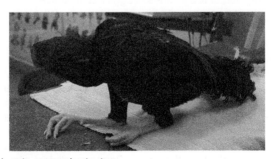

Fig. 9. Cockerel showing neurologic signs.

3 days of hatching) does not stop infection (the virus is considered ubiquitous world-wide) but achieves more than 90% protection under commercial conditions.[76]

Lead poisoning is thought to be one of the most significant causes of neurologic disease in waterfowl.[77] A recent report estimated between 50,000 and 100,000 (approximately 1.5%–3.0% of the wintering population) wildfowl deaths each winter are caused by lead poisoning. That number represents a quarter of all recorded deaths regarding migratory swans.[78] Not only waterfowl are affected by this, because other terrestrial game birds and fowl may ingest lead pellets that they mistake for grit or food; lead pellets may be buried in mud, in areas where fishing or hunting has previously taken place. Animals can experience chronic intoxication when ingesting small numbers of lead pellets intermittently, but can also present acutely and in the form of an outbreak when reduced water levels or other circumstances expose lead that was previously unavailable. In the United Kingdom, the sale and use by fishermen of lead leger weights and split shot weighing less than 28 g has been banned since 1987.[79] Since then, the incidence of lead poisoning has reduced significantly.[80] However, the environmental contamination will still have an effect for many years.

Characteristic clinical signs of lead toxicity include weight loss, weakness, and green faces; weakness of the neck muscles causes a typical posture with the head resting on the bird's dorsum.[81] Whole-body radiographs might reveal the presence of metallic objects in recent cases; however, the grinding action and pH of the ventriculus dissolves the lead pellets within a few days. Other common findings in chronic cases on radiographs are dilatation and impaction of the proventriculus.[79] A blood sample should always be tested for lead levels to achieve a definitive diagnosis (normal, <0.4 ppm; diagnostic, 0.5–2.0 ppm; severe, >2.0 ppm). Moderate anemia (20%–38% hematocrit) can be observed.[82] Delta amino levulinic acid dehydrase activity has been suggested as a more sensitive diagnostic indicator for lead intoxication.[83] Early treatment of lead toxicosis should include stopping any further lead absorption; lead particles within the gastrointestinal tract can be removed by lavage under general anesthesia with warm fluid via a gastric tube.[82] Some investigators recommend repeating gastric lavage within 24 to 48 hours if lead particles are still present in postlavage radiographs, because fragments of lead can be trapped in crevices in the koilin. Those particles precipitate when muscle activity has restarted.[84] Chelation therapy should be started in all affected animals. Sodium calcium edetate (10–40 mg/kg intramuscularly every 24 hours for 10 days, with a 5-day break at day 5) is the recommended treatment of lead and zinc toxicosis. Penicillamine can be used as an alternative if sodium calcium edetate (NaCaEDTA) is not available, or at the same time in severe cases.

Zinc toxicosis is less common in animals housed outdoors, and is similar in diagnosis and treatment to lead intoxication.[85]

Botulism occurs when animals are kept in water with anaerobic conditions, particularly in warm, dry periods. *Clostridium botulinum* overgrows and produces toxin type C, causing flaccid paralysis. Other clinical signs are similar to other heavy metal poisoning, such as weakness. A good anamnesis and water analysis allows a presumptive diagnosis.[86]

Other intoxications are common in fowl, such as coccidiostats in waterfowl (found in chicken-formulated commercial diets) or pesticides (dimetridazole and organophosphorus pesticides).[87,88]

Diarrhea

Diarrhea can have many different causes; after physical examination, clinicians should perform a direct observation, flotation, and Diff-Quik examination of a fresh fecal sample. Samples should also be taken for viral identification.

Duck plague or duck viral enteritis is caused by a herpesvirus, and can cause significant losses in waterfowl collections. Presentation can be peracute, including sudden death without previous obvious signs. Other described clinical signs are cloacal lethargy, diarrhea, hemorrhage, prolapse of the penis, photophobia, ataxia, and tremors.[49,89] Outbreaks are often seasonal (May to June in the United Kingdom). It can cause morbidities between 10% and 100% in unvaccinated collections.[90] In affected animals, the prognosis is very poor with no effective treatment. Annual vaccination is recommended in endemic areas.

Avian or fowl cholera, caused by *Pasteurella multocida*, is the most common pasteurellosis in poultry. Chickens, duck, geese, and turkeys can be affected. Outbreaks in turkeys can cause up to 65% mortality.[91] Clinical signs include oral and nasal discharge, dyspnea, diarrhea, and sudden death. This condition seems to be less frequent in the United Kingdom than in North America, where annual outbreaks can cause significant mortalities.[92]

Gastrointestinal Impactions

Impaction of the crop, proventriculus, or gizzard has occasionally been reported in poultry and waterfowl. Affected birds commonly present showing lethargy, emaciation, and esophageal or crop distension. Despite the crop/esophagus, proventriculus, and/or gizzard being full of a solid mass of interwoven fibrous material, the intestines of birds with this condition are frequently empty.[56] Poultry have been known to ingest poorly digestible items (eg, grass, newspaper, sawdust shavings/wood chips, and feathers) out of curiosity or as a response to stress, causing crop impaction. Crop impaction is most frequently seen in spring, when chickens ingest long stems of grass that get impacted in the crop. Captive waterfowl, especially geese, suddenly exposed to new environments may ingest nondigestible items like newspaper or plant products, like grasses. Ingestion of grains that have low moisture content with concurrent exposure to water can lead to grain swelling and result in impaction of the esophagus.[93] Gizzard impaction can cause high mortality during the first 3 weeks of life in turkey flocks.[56] Although rehydration of the impaction, gentle massage or flushing (only for crop or esophageal impactions), and liquid paraffin may help to resolve the impaction in early cases, surgical intervention might be necessary (**Fig. 10**).

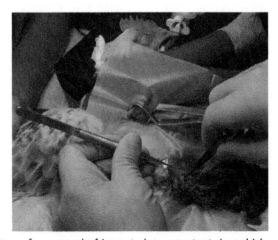

Fig. 10. Ingluviotomy for removal of impacted crop contents in a chicken.

Intussusception and Volvulus

These conditions occur sporadically in domestic fowl. Intussusception occurs most frequently in the intestine, but it has also been reported in the proventriculus. In young birds volvulus of the small intestine may be caused by twisting around the yolk sac. Intussusception and volvulus have been reported in chickens secondary to enteritis or abnormal peristalsis caused by nematode or coccidial infection. Intestinal torsion has also been associated with pedunculated neoplastic stalks. Clinical signs are anorexia and progressive weight loss, which may lead to death within a few days. Diagnosis may be achieved by ultrasonography, radiography, or endoscopy. If an early diagnosis is made, resection of the affected intestine can be performed.[56]

Coelomitis

Coelomitis is an occasional cause of morbidity and mortality in waterfowl and a common condition in chickens, particularly seen in laying or ex-battery hens.[94] Infection of the coelom can become established following infection of the respiratory system, penetrating injuries, neoplasia, heavy parasitism, or reproductive diseases. In chickens, *E coli* is often responsible of the oviduct infections. *Salmonella pullorum* or infectious bronchitis can also cause lesions in the reproductive tract.[60] Diagnosis may be achieved by aspiration of coelomic fluid (ultrasonographically guided if possible). Powerful antibiotic therapy is recommended (**Fig. 11**).

Egg Coelomitis

Egg coelomitis may occur because of an ectopic ovulation, when the follicle or yolk misses the infundibulum, or when the follicle in the oviduct moves back in a retroperistaltic manner. This condition can be caused by an underlying disorder or can occur

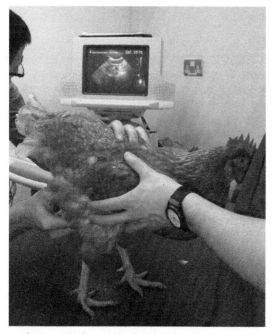

Fig. 11. Ultrasonography in a chicken with distended coelom.

after a stressful event while the egg was forming within the oviduct. In both situations the yolk reaches the coelomic cavity causing a coelomitis. Secondary bacterial colonization can occur. Often this occurs because of pathologic changes in the oviduct, with either infectious or neoplastic causes, or because of oviductal damage in battery hens. A recent study performed in backyard poultry in the United States revealed that the most common condition diagnosed was Marek disease.[57] In that study, the most common finding observed in gross postmortem was the presence of tumors affecting internal organs or carcinomatosis, which can affect the ovaries. Equally, non–viral-induced reproductive neoplasia, despite having significantly different findings in the 2 different institutions involved in the study, is also considered common. Salpingitis was one of the most common presentations in 1 of the institutions, with 7.8% of the presented cases.

Initial treatment can include coelomoentesis when dyspnea is observed; this technique, although not free of risk, also helps in achieving a diagnosis by analyzing the fluid drained. Fluid therapy, antibiosis, analgesia, and assisted feeding are required at initial stabilization. Salpingohysterectomy is likely to be required for long-term treatment because this condition is likely to reoccur.

Prolapsed Oviduct

Stress, age, obesity, and poor nutrition can contribute to the presentation of this condition, and good layers seem to have a higher predisposition.[60] This condition can be seen in animals with egg binding. Often animals had experienced trauma of exposed tissue from the other animals in the flock. Medical management is often unsuccessful and salpingohysterectomy is the preferred treatment option according to the investigators. Alternatively, a gonadotrophin-releasing hormone agonist implant (deslorelin acetate) can be used, once the prolapsed tissue has been repositioned and infection and inflammation controlled. Repeated applications are required long-term, and in certain animals the duration of the implant seems to decrease after repeated applications.

Egg Bound

This condition may result from inflammation of the oviduct, partial paralysis of the muscles of the oviduct, or production of an egg so large that it is physically impossible for it to be laid. Young pullets laying an unusually large egg are most prone to the problem.[56] As in other avian species, this condition is often linked to calcium imbalance, caused by a combination of dietary deficiencies, stress, and other husbandry-related problems. Treatment includes fluid therapy, calcium, and oxytocin administration. If initial medical management is unsuccessful, ovocentesis (either directly into the egg shell or via the coelomic wall) should be the next step. The egg should not be manually broken or pulled, because iatrogenic damage to the oviduct may occur. If the shell of the egg is not eliminated within 24 hours, salpingohysterectomy is indicated because the remnants of the shell might adhere to the oviduct, inevitably causing further complications in future oviposition.

Phallus Prolapse

Phallus prolapse is occasionally seen in Anseriformes associated with mechanical damage, infection (ie, *Cryptosporidum* spp., *Mycoplasma* spp, *Neisseria* spp…), hypersexuality or immunosuppression. Frostbite and bacterial infection may occur as a sequela of phallus prolapse.[56] Treatment may include analgesics, local and/or systemic antibiotherapy, and decongestive and lubrifying local therapies which allow reposition of prolapsed healthy tissues. Severe cases may require amputation of the phallus.

EUTHANASIA

Euthanasia might be required in cases with a poor prognosis and when certain infectious diseases have been confirmed. Euthanasia should always be performed in a humane manner. The authors' preferred method is intravenous administration of barbiturates, but other methods can be used.[95]

SUMMARY/DISCUSSION

Fowl are stoic patients that commonly mask signs of illness in the early stages of disease and are not commonly presented as emergencies until the acute or chronic condition is severe. An understanding of intraspecific and interspecific anatomic and physiologic variations is crucial to the successful management of critically ill fowl. Stabilization of the patient should be prioritized over diagnostic procedures. Clinicians treating fowl should be aware of infectious and noninfectious conditions causing emergencies in fowl.

REFERENCES

1. Sibley CG, Ahlquist JE, Monroe BL. A classification of the living birds of the world base on DNA-DDNA hybridization studies. Auk 1988;105:409–23.
2. Eo SH, Bininda-Emonds ORP, Carroll JP. A phylogenetic supertree of the fowls (Galloansera, Aves). Zool Scr 2009;38:465–81.
3. Brown AJ, Drobatz KJ. Triage of the emergency patient. In: King LG, Boag A, editors. BSAVA manual of canine and feline emergency and critical care. 2nd edition. Gloucester (UK): BSAVA; 2007. p. 1–7.
4. Grunkemeyer VL. Zoonoses, public health, and the backyard poultry flock. Vet Clin Exot Anim 2011;14:477–90.
5. Hawkins M, Pascoe P. Cagebirds. In: West G, Heard D, Caulkett N, editors. Zoo and wildlife immobilization and anesthesia. Ames (IA): Blackwell Publishing; 2007. p. 269–98.
6. Mulcahy DM. Free-living waterfowl and shorebirds. In: West G, Heard D, Caulkett N, editors. Zoo and wildlife immobilization and anesthesia. Ames (IA): Blackwell Publishing; 2007. p. 299–324.
7. Graham JE, Heatley JJ. Emergency care of raptors. Vet Clin Exot Anim 2007;10: 395–418.
8. Khamas W, Rutllant-Labeaga J, Greenacre CB. Physical examination, anatomy, and physiology. In: Greenacre CB, Morishita TY, editors. Backyard poultry medicine and surgery. A guide for veterinary practitioners. Ames (IA): Wiley-Blackwell; 2015. p. 95–117.
9. Morishita TY. Galliformes. In: Miller RE, Fowler ME, editors. Zoo and wild animal medicine. 8th edition. St. Louis (MO): Elsevier; 2015. p. 143–55.
10. Backues KA. Anseriformes. In: Miller RE, Fowler ME, editors. Zoo and wild animal medicine. 8th edition. St. Louis (MO): Elsevier; 2015. p. 116–26.
11. King AS, Payne DC. The maximum capacities of the lungs and air sacs of *Gallus domesticus*. J Anat 1962;96:495–503.
12. Phalen DN, Mitchell ME, Cavazos-Martinez ML. Evaluation of three heat sources for their ability to maintain core body temperature in the anesthetized avian patient. J Avian Med Surg 1996;10:174–8.
13. Edling T. Updates in anesthesia and monitoring. In: Harrison G, Lightfoot T, editors. Clinical avian medicine, vol. 2. Palm beach (FL): Spix Publishing; 2006. p. 747–60.

14. Lumeij JT. Avian clinical biochemistry. In: Kaneko JJ, Harvey JW, Bruss ML, editors. Clinical biochemistry of domestic animals. 6th edition. Cambridge (MA): Eds Academic; 2008. p. 839–72.

15. Bowles H, Lichtenberger M, Lennox A. Emergency and critical care of pet birds. Vet Clin Exot Anim 2007;10:345–94.

16. Schmitt PM, Gobel T, Trautvetter E. Evaluation of pulse oximetry as a monitoring method in avian anesthesia. J Avian Med Surg 1998;12:91–9.

17. Wagner AE, Brodbelt DC. Arterial blood pressure monitoring in anesthetized animals. J Am Vet Med Assoc 1997;210:1279–85.

18. Lichtenberger M. Determination of indirect blood pressure in the companion bird. Semin Avian Med Exot pet Med 2005;14(2):149–52.

19. Schnellbacher R, Da Cunha A, Olson EE, et al. Arterial catheterization, interpretation and treatment of arterial blood pressures and blood gases in birds. J Exot Pet Med 2014;23:129–41.

20. Lichtenberger M. Principles of shock and fluid therapy in special species. Semin Avian Exot Pet Med 2004;13:142–53.

21. Valverde A, Bienzle D, Smith DA, et al. Intraosseous cannulation and drug administration for induction of anesthesia in chickens. Vet Surg 1993;22:240–4.

22. Kadono H, Okada T. Physiological studies on the electrocardiogram of the chicken I: bipolar leads. Res Bull Fac Agric Gifu Univ 1959;11:164–72.

23. Kadono H, Okada T, Ohno K. Physiological studies on the electrocardiogram of the chicken III: on the normal values of the electrocardiogram of laying hens. Res Bull Fac Agric Gifu Univ 1962;16:173–81.

24. Kisch B. The electrocardiogram of birds (chicken, duck, pigeon). Exp Med Surg 1957;9:103–24.

25. Mukai S, Machida N, Nishimura M, et al. Electrocardiographic observation on spontaneously occurring arrhythmias in chickens. J Vet Med Sci 1996;58:953–61.

26. Sawazaki H, Hirose H, Matsui K, et al. Comparative electrocardiographical studies on the wave form of QRS complex in vertebrates. Nihon Juigaku Zasshi 1976;38:235–40.

27. Szabuniewicz M, McCrady JD. The electrocardiogram of the chicken. Southwest Vet 1967;20:287–94.

28. Boulianne M, Hunter DB, Julian RJ, et al. Cardiac muscle mass distribution in the domestic turkey and relationship to electrocardiogram. Avian Dis 1992;36:582–9.

29. McKenzie BE, Will JA, Hardie A. The electrocardiogram of the turkey. Avian Dis 1971;15:737–44.

30. Amend JF, Eroschenko VP. Scalar electrocardiographic measurements in unrestrained young Japanese quail. Lab Anim Sci 1976;26:190–4.

31. Andersen HT. Hyperpotassemia and electrocardiographic changes in the duck during prolonged diving. Acta Physiol Scand 1965;63:292–5.

32. Hassanpour H, Khadem P. Normal electrocardiogram patterns and values in Muscovy ducks (Cairina moschata). J Avian Med Surg 2013;27(4):280–4.

33. Hassanpour H, Zarei H, Hojjati P. Analysis of electrocardiographic parameters in helmeted Guinea fowl (Numida meleagris). J Avian Med Surg 2011;25(1):8–13.

34. Uzun M, Yildiz S, Onder F. Electrocardiography of rock partridges (Alectoris graeca) and chukar partridges (Alectoris chukar). J Zoo Wildl Med 2004;35(4):510–4.

35. Chalmers GA, Barret MW. Capture myopathy. In: Hoff GL, Davis JW, editors. Noninfectious diseases in wildlife. Ames, Iowa (USA): Iowa State University Press; 1982. p. 84–94.

36. Spraker TR, Adrian WJ, Lance WR. Capture myopathy in wild turkeys (*Meleagris gallopavo*) following trapping, handling, and transportation in Colorado. J Wildl Dis 1987;23(3):447–53.

37. Sanchez-Migallon D. Advances in avian clinical therapeutics. J Exot Pet Med 2014;23:6–20.

38. Cortright KA, Wetzlich SE, Craigmill AL. Plasma pharmacokinetics of midazolam in chickens, turkeys, pheasants, and bobwhite quail. J Vet Pharmcol Ther 2007; 30:429–36.

39. Hawkins MG, Paul-Murphy J. Avian analgesia. Vet Clin Exot An 2011;14:6–80.

40. Butler PJ. The exercise response and the 'classical' diving response during natural submersion in birds and mammals. Can J Zool 1988;66:29–39.

41. Jones DR, Furilla RA, Heieis MRA, et al. Forced and voluntary diving in ducks: cardiovascular adjustments and their control. Can J Zool 1988;66:75–83.

42. Woakes AJ. Metabolism in diving birds: studies in the laboratory and the field. Can J Zool 1988;66:138–41.

43. Wilson D, Pettifer GR. Anesthesia case of the month. J Am Vet Med Assoc 2004; 225(5):685–8.

44. Goelz MF, Hahn AW, Kelley ST. Effects of halothane and isoflurane on mean arterial blood pressure, heart rate, and respiratory rate in adult Pekin ducks. Am J Vet Res 1990;51:458–60.

45. Pizarro J, Ludders JW, Douse MA, et al. Halothane effects on ventilatory responses to changes in intrapulmonary CO2 in geese. Respir Physiol 1990;82:337–48.

46. Edling TM, Degernes LA, Flammer K, et al. Capnographic monitoring of anesthetized African grey parrots receiving intermittent positive pressure ventilation. J Am Vet Med Assoc 2001;219:1714–8.

47. Olsen GH, Ford S, Perry M, et al. The use of Emeraid exotic carnivore diet improves postsurgical recovery and survival of long-tailed ducks. J Exot Pet Med 2010;19(2):165–8.

48. Lichtenberger M, Orcutt C, Cray C, et al. Comparison of fluid types for resuscitation after acute blood loss in mallard ducks (*Anas platyrhynchos*). J Vet Emerg Crit Care 2009;19(5):467–72.

49. Waine JC. Head and neck problems. In: Forbes NA, Harcourt-Brown NH, editors. BSAVA manual of raptors, pigeons and waterfowl. Cheltenham (United Kingdom): British Small Animal Veterinary Association; 1996. p. 299–304.

50. Calvo Carrasco D, Dutton TAG, Shimizu NS, et al. Distraction osteogenesis correction of mandibular ramis fracture malunion in a juvenile mute swan (*Cygnus olor*). Proceedings of the Association of Avian Veterinarians Annual Conference. 2014. p. 339–40. Available at: http://www.vetexotic.theclinics.com/article/S1094-9194(15)00084-5/abstract).

51. Smith S, Rodriguez Barbon A. Waterfowl: medicine and surgery. In: Roberts V, Scott-Park F, editors. BSAVA manual of farm pets. Gloucester (United Kingdom): British Small Animal Veterinary Association; 2008. p. 250–73.

52. Maldonado N, Larson K. What is your diagnosis? J Avian Med Surg 2004;18(2): 112–5.

53. Butcher GD. Management of Galliformes. In: Harrison GJ, Lightfoot LT, editors. Clinical avian medicine volume II. Palm Beach (FL): Spix Publishing; 2006. p. 861–79.

54. Chavez W, Echols S. Bandaging, endoscopy, and surgery in the emergency avian patient. Vet Clin Exot Anim 2007;10:419–36.

55. Roberts V. Galliform birds: health and husbandry. In: Roberts V, Scott-Park F, editors. BSAVA manual of farm pets. Gloucester (United Kingdom): British Small Animal Veterinary Association; 2008. p. 190–212.

56. Crespo R, Shivaprasad HL. Developmental, metabolic, and other noninfectious disorders. In: Saif YM, editor. Diseases of poultry. 12th edition. Ames, Iowa (USA): Blackwell Publishing; 2008. p. 1150–6.

57. Crespo R, Senties-Cue G. Postmortem survey of disease conditions in backyard poultry. J Exot Pet Med 2015;24:156–63.

58. Madsen JM, Zimmermann NG, Timmons J, et al. Prevalence and differentiation of diseases in Maryland backyard flocks. Avian Dis 2013;57:587–94.

59. Olsen JH. Anseriformes. In: Ritchie BW, Harrison GJ, Harrison LR, editors. Avian medicine: principles and application. Lake Worth (FL): Wingers Publishing; 1994. p. 1237–70.

60. Roberts V. Galliform birds: medicine and surgery. In: Roberts V, Scott-Park F, editors. BSAVA manual of farm pets. Gloucester (United Kingdom): British Small Animal Veterinary Association; 2008. p. 215–36.

61. Brown MJ, Forbes NA. Respiratory diseases. In: Forbes NA, Harcourt-Brown NH, editors. BSAVA manual of raptors, pigeons, and waterfowl. Cheltenham (United Kingdom): British Small Animal Veterinary Association; 1996. p. 315–6.

62. Beernaert LA, Pasmans F, Van Waeyenberghe L, et al. Aspergillus infections in birds: a review. Avian Pathol 2010;39(5):325–31.

63. Laroucau K, Aaziz R, Meurice L, et al. Outbreak of psittacosis in a group of women exposed to *Chlamydia psittaci*-infected chickens. Euro Surveill 2015; 20(24) [pii:21155].

64. Woldehiwet Z. Avian chlamydophilosis (chlamydiosis/psittacosis/ornithosis). In: Pattison M, McMullin PF, Bradbury JM, et al, editors. Poultry diseases. 6th edition. Philadelphia: Saunders Elsevier; 2008. p. 235–43.

65. Vorimore F, Thébault A, Poisson S, et al. *Chlamydia psittaci* in ducks: a hidden health risk for poultry workers. Pathog Dis 2015;73(1):1–9.

66. Teske L, Ryll M, Rubbenstroth D, et al. Epidemiological investigations on the possible risk of distribution of zoonotic bacteria through apparently healthy homing pigeons. Avian Pathol 2013;42(5):397–407.

67. Page LA. Experimental ornithosis in turkeys. Avian Dis 1959;3:67–79.

68. Tappe JP, Andersen AA, Cheville NF. Respiratory and pericardial lesions in turkeys infected with avian or mammalian strains of *Chlamydia psittaci*. Vet Pathol 1989;26:385–95.

69. Andersen AA, Grimes JE, Wyrick PB. Chlamydiosis (Psittacosis, Ornithosis). In: Calnek BW, Barnes HJ, Beard CW, et al, editors. Diseases of poultry. 10th edition. Ames (IO): Mosby-Wolfe; 1997. p. 333–49.

70. Van Droogenbroeck C, Dossche L, Wauman L, et al. Use of ovotransferrin as an antimicrobial in turkeys naturally infected with *Chlamydia psittaci*, avian metapneumovirus and *Ornithobacterium rhinotracheale*. Vet Microbiol 2011;153:257–63.

71. Trauger DL, Bartonek JC. Leech parasitism of waterfowl in North America. Wildfowl 1977;28:142–52.

72. Mason RW. Laryngeal streptocariasis causing death from asphyxiation in ducks. Aust Vet J 1988;65:335.

73. McOrist S. *Cytodites nudus* infestation of chickens. Avian Pathol 1983;12(1): 151–5.

74. Turbahn A, De Jackel SC, Greuel E, et al. Dose response study of enrofloxacin against *Riemerella anatipestifer* septicaemia in Muscovy and Pekin ducklings. Avian Pathol 1997;26(4):791–802.

75. Calnek BW, Witter RL. Marek's disease. In: Calnek BW, Barnes HJ, Beard CW, et al, editors. Diseases of poultry. 10th edition. Ames (IO): Mosby-Wolfe; 1997. p. 369–413.
76. Witter RL. Protective synergism among Marek's disease vaccine viruses. In: Kato S, Horiuchi T, Mikami T, et al, editors. Advances in Marek's disease research. Osaka (Japan): Japanese Association on Marek's Disease; 1985. p. 398–404.
77. Goode DA. Lead poisoning in swans. Report of the Nature Conservancy Council working group. London: NCC; 1981.
78. Pain DJ, Cromie R, Green RE. Poisoning of birds and other wildlife from ammunition-derived lead in the UK. In: Delahay RJ, Spray CJ, editors. Proceedings of the Oxford Lead Symposium. Oxford (United Kingdom): University, Oxford; 2015. p. 58–84.
79. Forbes NA. Neonatal diseases. In: Forbes NA, Harcourt-Brown NH, editors. BSAVA manual of raptors, pigeons and waterfowl. Cheltenham (United Kingdom): British Small Animal Veterinary Association; 1996. p. 330–3.
80. Owen M. Progress on lead-free shot in the UK. Wildfowl 1992;43:223.
81. Ochiai K, Jin K, Itakura C, et al. Pathological study of lead poisoning in whooper swans (*Cygnus cygnus*) in Japan. Avian Dis 1992;36:313.
82. Degernes LA, Frank RK, Freeman ML, et al. Lead poisoning in trumpeter swans. In: Harisson LR, editor. Proceedings of the Association of Avian Veterinarians, Meeting location: Seattle, WA, US, p 144–55 (AAV office: Teaneck, New Jersey (USA)).
83. Degernes LA. Toxicities in waterfowl. Semin Avian Exot Pet Med 1995;4(1):15.
84. Forbes NA. Treatment of lead poisoning in swans. In Pract 1993;15(2):90.
85. Lichtenberger M, Richardson JA. Emergency care and managing toxicoses in the exotic animal patient. Vet Clin Exot Anim 2008;11:211–28.
86. Panto B. Triage of botulism in wild birds. In: Molenaar F, Stidworthy M, editors. Proceedings of the British Veterinary Zoological Society. Loughborough (UK): British Veterinary Zoological Society; 2015. p. 29.
87. Riddell C. Toxicity of dimetridazole in waterfowl. Avian Dis 1984;28(4):974–7.
88. Jiang Y, Liu X, Li S, et al. Identification of differentially expressed proteins related to organophosphorus-induced delayed neuropathy in the brains of hens. J Appl Toxicol 2014;34(12):1352–60.
89. Sandhu T. Duck, geese, swans, and screamers: infectious diseases. In: Fowler ME, editor. Zoo and wildlife medicine. 2nd edition. Philadelphia: WB Saunders; 1986. p. 333–64.
90. Wang G, Qu Y, Wang F, et al. The comprehensive diagnosis and prevention of duck plague in northwest Shandong province of China. Poult Sci 2013;92(11): 2892–8.
91. Alberts JO, Graham R. Fowl cholera in turkeys. North Am Vet 1948;9:24–6.
92. Blanchong JA, Samuel MD, Goldberg DR, et al. Persistence of *Pasteurella multocida* in wetlands following avian cholera outbreaks. J Wildl Dis 2006; 42(1):33–9.
93. Morishita TY, Porter RE. Gastrointestinal and hepatic diseases. In: Greenacre CB, Morishita TY, editors. Backyard poultry medicine and surgery. A veterinary guide for veterinary practitioners. Ames, Iowa (USA): Wiley-Blackwell; 2015. p. 181–203.
94. Brown MJ, Cromie RL. Weight loss and enteritis. In: Forbes NA, Harcourt-Brown NH, editors. BSAVA manual of raptors, pigeons, and waterfowl. Cheltenham (United Kingdom): British Small Animal Veterinary Association; 1996. p. 322–9.
95. Report of the American Veterinary Medical Association Panel on Euthanasia. J Am Vet Med Assoc 1993;202:229–49.

Approach to Reptile Emergency Medicine

Simon Y. Long, MS, VMD

KEYWORDS

- Reptile • Physiology • Anatomy • Emergency room veterinarians

KEY POINTS

- A basic understanding of reptile physiology and anatomy is essential in assessing, diagnosing, and treating reptile patients even in emergency room situations.
- Since reptiles are ectotherms, their physiology and anatomy is driven and determined by core body temperature derived from the environment.
- The general body systems of reptiles are similar but different from higher vertebrates with important differences even between reptilian species of the same family.
- Understanding these unique differences is key in properly medically managing and treating reptiles in an emergency room clinic.

INTRODUCTION

Over the last 20 years, there has been a steady increase in reptiles kept as pets, increasing the chances of a reptilian patient eventually entering a veterinary emergency clinic.[1]

A clinician should be familiar with basic reptile physiology and anatomy and understand the unique features of reptilian cardiovascular, respiratory, and metabolism predominantly affected by temperature in order to diagnose and determine what treatment is immediately necessary. Companion animal techniques and applications are commonly used in reptiles with the importance of temperature and a slower metabolism kept in mind. The class Reptilia is a diverse group made up of 4 orders: Crocodilia (crocodiles, gavials, caimans, and alligators), Rhynchocephalia (tuatara), Squamata (lizards, snakes, and worm lizards) and Chelonia/Testudines (turtles, terrapins, and tortoises), totaling more than 10,000 species in the world.[2] The wide diversity within this

Disclosure: The author has nothing to disclose.
Department of Molecular and Comparative Pathobiology, Johns Hopkins University School of Medicine, 733 North Broadway, Baltimore, MD 21205, USA
E-mail address: sylong@jhmi.edu

class with anatomic and physiologic adaptations to specific environmental niches produces a wide range of body conformations, behaviors, dietary requirements, and husbandry requirements that can be daunting, especially to clinicians who are not routinely exposed to these animals.

The purpose of this chapter is to provide a cursory overview of reptile anatomy and physiology for emergency room veterinary clinicians, while common reptile emergencies is covered later in this issue (See Music and Strunk: Reptile Critical Care and Common Emergencies, in this issue). It is beyond the scope of this chapter to cover each body system in detail, as each system alone deserves a chapter. Complete reviews of anatomy,[3–10] physiology,[11–13] clinical medicine,[1,10,14–23] and pathology[10,24–27] have been published. *Reptile Medicine and Surgery, 2nd edition*,[28] covers in depth every aspect of reptile anatomy, physiology, pathology, and clinical medicine. The recent *2014 Current Therapy in Reptile Medicine and Surgery*[29] contains some of the most recent updates in reptile medicine. The author recommends having these sources on hand if clinicians expect to consistently care for reptile patients as well as up-to-date information through professional organizations such as the Association of Reptilian and Amphibian Veterinarians (ARAV), veterinary medical journals, continuing education (CE), scientific meetings, and online resources.

HISTORY AND PHYSICAL EXAMINATION

Before accepting reptile patients, certain safety parameters such as excluding venomous or dangerous species is strongly recommended. The wide diversity of reptiles can be daunting to the uninitiated when first seeing a reptile patient. Properly identifying the species using information provided by the owner and confirming species utilizing an Internet search can also quickly provide essential information on a patient's physiology, anatomy, behavior, husbandry, and nutritional requirements. De la Navarre[2] provides a set of history questionnaires to obtain a thorough history of the patient and husbandry care. Obtaining a complete history for a reptile patient should also include husbandry care and nutritional history. Improper husbandry care is frequently the cause of disease, which needs to be reviewed with the rest of the clinical findings to determine the medical diagnosis. Husbandry deficiency in environmental, nutritional, and/or sanitation requirements are the common causes for an underlying chronic pathological disease.

Having a basic understanding of typical behavior of the commonly kept reptile species can help determine the normal versus abnormal behaviors (**Table 1**)[30], taking into account the effects of ambient temperature on a reptile's activity and responsiveness. As expected, cold reptiles clinically can be dull and lethargic with decreased (depressed) biological parameters. The physical examination of reptiles otherwise involves applying the same fundamental concepts of a physical examination of any domestic animal to reptiles with anatomical and physiological variations described below.[31]

PHYSIOLOGY
Thermoregulation

Reptiles are ectotherms deriving heat from the environment to maintain their body temperature with anatomic adaptations and behavioral adjustments to select the preferred optimal temperature range (POTR). The evolutionary advantage for

Table 1
Behaviors in reptiles

Behavior	Species	Comments
Catalepsy, death feigning, tonic immobility	Many: hog-nosed snakes, false spitting cobras, chameleons, leaf-tailed geckos, caiman	Behavior reduced or absent with time in captivity
Squirting blood	Horned lizards, Tropidophis sp (dwarf boas), long-nosed snakes	Accurate up to 2 m (6 ft)
Tail display	Many: Aniliidae (pipe snakes), Uropeltidae (shield-tailed snakes), ring-necked snakes, sand boas, rubber boas, coral snakes	Often waves or strikes with tail; mimics head
Tail vibrating	Many: kingsnakes, pine snakes, rat snakes, racers, coach-whip snakes	Can be mistaken for rattlesnake
Tail loss/autonomy	Some species in most families	Costly in terms of energy; may not reproduce first breeding season after tail loss
Caudal luring	Viperids (vipers/pit vipers)	Can be mistaken for neurologic disease
Hemipenial eversion	Many: blood pythons, coral snakes, monitors	Must differentiate from prolapse
Bluffs/threats	Many: Uromastyx (spiny-tailed agama), bearded dragons, chameleons, Monitors, Asian rat snakes	Can resemble respiratory disease
Fragile skin	Various gecko species	Usually no treatment necessary for skin defect
Balling behavior	Ball python, African burrowing python, rosy boas, rubber boas	—
Thermoregulation Reproductive behavior	Most species	Most common behaviors seen: head bobbing in lizards and chelonians, neck biting in snakes and lizards
Squamates	Most common species	—
Chelonians	Tortoises, box turtles	—
Incubation behavior	Pythons	Can resemble neurologic disease
Spectacle cleansing	Geckos	—
Stargazing	Boas, pythons, rattlesnakes	Able to assume normal posture
Circulation	Bearded dragons, Asian water dragons	—

From Lock BA. Behavioral and morphologic adaptations. In: Mader DR, editor. Reptile medicine and surgery, 2nd edition. St. Louis: Saunders Elsevier; 2006; with permission.

ectotherms by maintaining a body temperature that relies on the environment reduces the resource requirements needed to maintain physiologic homeostasis compared with mammals of a similar size. Heat transfer in reptiles can be achieved by radiation, convection, conduction, and evaporation based on species. The core body temperature is the major driving force determining metabolism, heart rate, stroke volume, oxygen consumption, systemic blood flow, and blood pressure.

Table 2
Preferred optimum temperature ranges for commonly housed captive reptiles

| Common Name | Scientific Name | Preferred Optimum Temperature Range (°F) | | | Buried Hot Rock or Under Enclosure with Heat Tape Necessary | 50-W to 75-W Sun Spotlight Bulb Necessary | Natural Spectrum Lighting Necessary |
		Day	Night	Winter Cool-down[a]			
Snakes							
Boa constrictor	Boa constrictor	Mid-80s	70-80	60-70	Yes	Optional	No
Rosy boa	Lichanura trivirgata	80-85	70-75	58-60	Yes	No	No
Ball python	Python regius	Mid-80s	70-80	60-70	Yes	Optional	No
Burmese python	Python molurus	Mid-80s	70-80	60-70	Yes	Optional	No
Green tree python	Morelia viridis	75-82	70-75	60-64	Yes	Optional	Optional
Carpet python	Morelia spilota	80-85	70-75	60-64	Yes	Optional	Optional
Corn snake	Elaphe guttata	77-84	67-75	55-60	Yes	Optional	No
Yellow rat snake	Elaphe obsoleta	77-84	67-75	55-60	Yes	Optional	No
Gopher/bull snake	Pituophis melanoleucus	77-84	67-74	50-60	Yes	Optional	No
Common kingsnake	Lampropeltis getula	78-84	68-74	55-60	Yes	Optional	No
Mountain kingsnake	Lampropeltis zonata	78-84	66-74	55-60	Yes	Optional	No
Gray-banded kingsnake	Lampropeltis alterna	79-84	70-75	58-60	Yes	Optional	No
Garter snakes	Thamnophis sp	75-80	65-72	54-59	Yes	Optional	No
Lizards							
Green iguana	Iguana iguana	84-90	67-77	64-69	Optional	Yes	Yes
Basilisks	Basiliscus sp	82-87	75-77	68-70	No	Yes	Yes

Leopard gecko	Eublepharis macularius	77–85	65–75	None	Yes	No	No
African fat-tailed gecko	Hemitheconyx caudicinctus	78–85	67–75	None	Yes	No	No
Day geckos	Phelsuma sp	85	75	None	No	Yes	Yes
Madagascar leaf-tailed gecko	Uroplatus sp	81–84	72–78	None	No	No	Optional
Chameleons (montane)	Chamaeleo sp	77–84	55–67	None	No	Yes	Yes
Chameleons (lowland)	Chamaeleo sp	80–84	70	None	No	Yes	Yes
Bearded dragons	Pogona sp	84–88	68–74	62–69	Optional	Yes	Yes
Blue-tongued skinks	Tiliqua sp	80–85	67–75	60–65	Optional	Yes	Optional
Monitor lizards	Varanus sp	84–88	74–78	66–70	No	Yes	Optional
Tegus	Tupinambis sp	80–86	70–78	60–70	No	Yes	Optional
Turtles							
Semiaquatic turtles	Most species	80–84	65–70	Optional	No	Yes	Optional
Tropical turtles	Most species	82–86	74–80	None	Optional	Yes	Yes
Box turtles	Terrapene sp	Outdoors in backyard for late spring, summer, early fall 78–89	70	50–65	No	Yes	Yes
Tortoises	Most species	Outdoors in backyard for late spring, summer, early fall 82–88	70–76	Temperate climate species only	No	Yes	Yes

[a] With no food in gut.

From Rossi JV. General husbandry and management. In: Mader DR, editor. Reptile medicine and surgery, 2nd edition. St. Louis: Saunders Elsevier; 2006; with permission.

Reptile patients should be evaluated based on understanding the effects of core temperature on these parameters. Mader and Rossi[32] list a table (**Table 2**) showing the wide ranges of POTR between the different reptile species. Inadequate POTR in husbandry settings is a common problem seen in reptile care. Cold reptiles cannot maintain an active metabolism and other associated parameters (heart rate, stroke volume, oxygen consumption, systemic blood flow, and blood pressure) resulting in a downstream cascade of clinical disease. Generally, healthy reptiles can withstand short-term inadequate temperature periods. However, long-term inadequate temperature range can result in more severe diseases, such as respiratory infection or nutritional secondary hyperparathyroidism (metabolic bone disease) in some species. A reptilian patient exposed to chronic long-term inadequate temperature can also result in decreased food and water intake that may lead to suppression and dehydration which in itself may be a factor resulting into an infection or renal failure.[33]

Metabolism

The reptilian metabolic rate is approximately one-tenth to one-third lower than similar-sized mammals with variation based on species, body size, behavior, and size.[3] The metabolic rate can vary between reptilian orders with the generalized category of ambushing predators (boa constrictors and pythons) having a lower rate than active foraging predators (varanid lizards). The core body temperature directly affects the metabolic rate, which in turn affects and is influenced by food procurement, digestion, absorption of nutrients, and metabolic rate.[33] Therefore, temperature and metabolism should be factored together when evaluating and choosing a treatment plan for a patient.

In addition to temperature range requirements for metabolism, there are species-specific physiologic and anatomic adaptations allowing these species to survive or take advantage of their native environment and habitats. Andersen and colleagues[34] reported that Burmese pythons (*Python bivittatus*), after a consumption of a meal, are able to increase metabolic rate 40-fold relative to starved rate, increase oxygen consumption up to 7-fold, and increase their cardiac ventricle mass by 40% lasting up to 14 days. On the opposite end of this spectrum, some reptile species can slow their metabolic rate for starved and dormant periods to avoid heat, cold (brumation), drought, or lack of food.[33] Aquatic turtles such as Red-eared sliders (*Trachemys scripta elegans*) in the temperate climates can go into brumation during cold weather submerged underwater with a reduction of metabolic rate to 10% of normal.[33] Reptiles also have a buffering mechanism allowing switching from aerobic to anaerobic metabolism to withstand high levels of lactic acid accumulation, especially noted in diving species. Jackson and colleagues[35,36] reported that freshwater turtles are able to store lactate in their shells and skeletons as calcium lactate, allowing them to survive their months-long hibernation period.

Anatomy

The overarching theme of the reptile body systems (**Figs. 1–5**)[37–39] is a generalized layout of anatomic elements similar to higher vertebrates with variations from higher vertebrates, between reptile orders, and even within reptile families allowing species to adapt to specific environmental habitats.

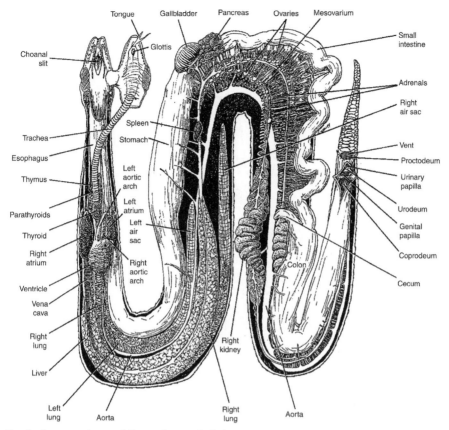

Fig. 1. Gross anatomy of the snake, ventral view.

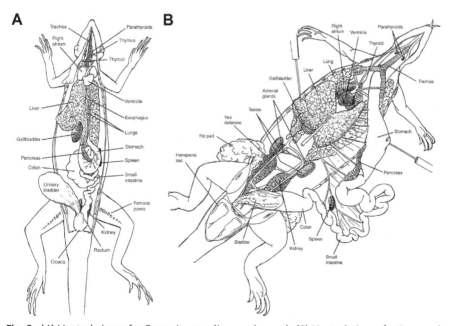

Fig. 2. (*A*) Ventral view of a Green Iguana (*Iguana iguana*). (*B*) Ventral view of a Savannah Monitor Lizard (*Varanus exanthematicus*).

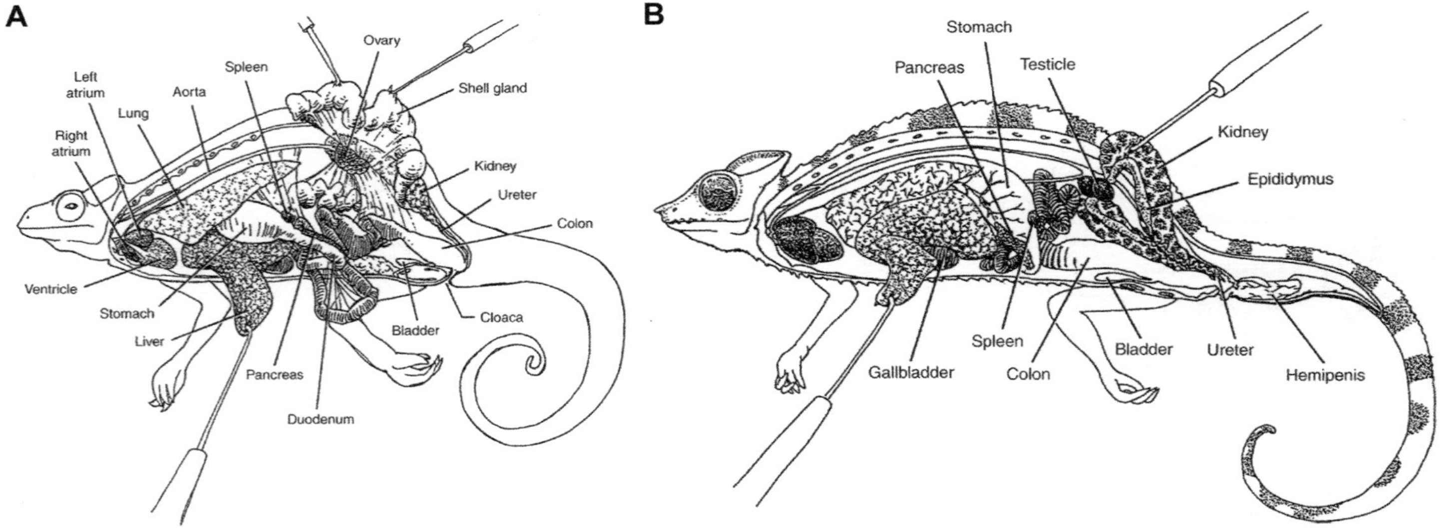

Fig. 3. (*A*) Lateral, midsagittal view of female chameleon. (*B*) Lateral, midsagittal view of male chameleon.

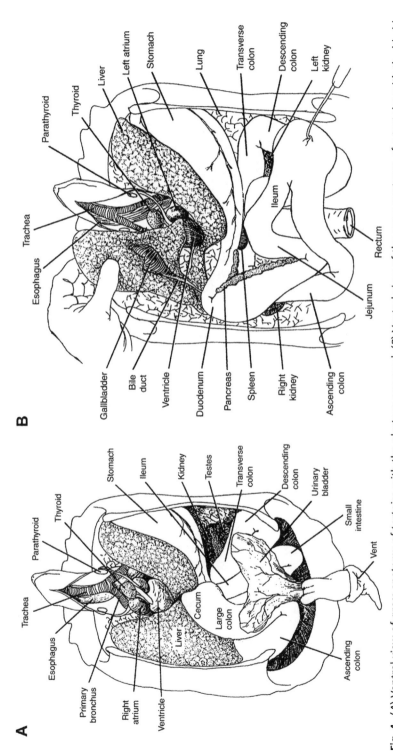

Fig. 4. (A) Ventral view of gross anatomy of tortoise with the plastron removed. (B) Ventral view of the gross anatomy of a tortoise with the bladder removed. The right lobe of the liver is reflected to expose the gallbladder. (C) Ventral view of the gross anatomy of a tortoise with the liver and intestinal tract removed. In this male, the testicles are attached to the ventral aspect of kidneys. (D) Midsagittal view of gross anatomy of the tortoise.

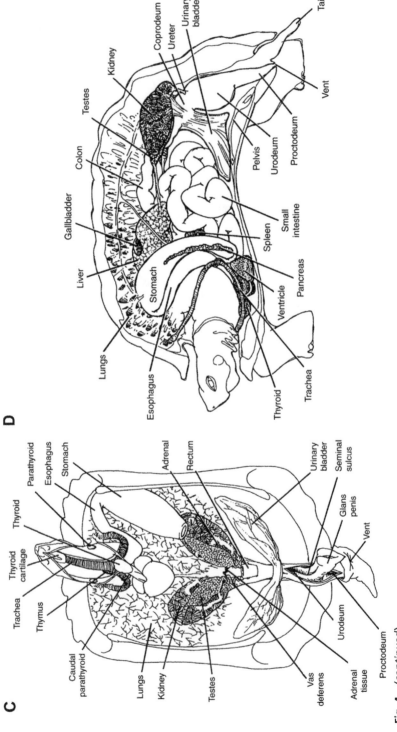

Fig. 4. (*continued*)

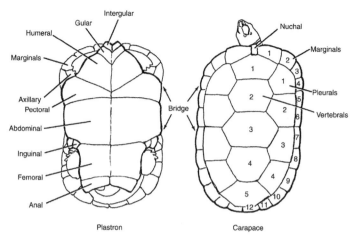

Fig. 5. Nomeclature of plastron and carapace scutes.

Nervous System

As in higher vertebrates, the nervous system is divided into the central and peripheral nervous systems. The central nervous system (CNS) consists of the brain and spinal cord. The peripheral nervous system is composed of all the nerves outside the CNS. Reptiles have 12 cranial nerves arising from the brain and spinal nerves arising from the spinal cord. The brain is housed in a tubular braincase and is divided into forebrain (telencephalon and diencephalon), midbrain (mesencephalon), and hindbrain (metencephalon and myelencephalon)[4] (**Fig. 6**).

The forebrain is responsible for smell, taste, rhythms, and sensory-motor integration and mediation.[4] The midbrain is responsible for visual processing and neuroendocrine roles.[4] The hindbrain is responsible for hearing, balance, and physiologic homeostasis (respiratory center, heart rate, and gastrointestinal mobility/secretion).[4] The reptilian CNS is different from that of higher vertebrates with the cerebral hemisphere lacking sulcus and gyrus[4] and the reptilian spinal cord lacking defined functional regionalization.[4]

The parietal eye–pineal complex contributes to behavior, gonadal activity, thermoregulation, and color change,[3] arising from the roof of the diencephalon in lizards. The parietal eye (also called pineal eye or third eye) is a single epithelial vesicle with a dorsal lens and ventral retina that functions as a sensory photoreceptor,[3,37] lacking both muscle and eyelid. The parietal eye is found in chelonians and some lizards on the dorsal aspect of the head but is absent in snakes. Chelonians, snakes, and some lizards have a pineal gland. The complex is absent in crocodilians.

Snakes and some lizards (Gekkonidae) lack eyelids. During development in these species, a transparent spectacle is formed by the fusion of the eyelids protecting the eye and is shed with the rest of the skin during ecdysis.[3] In snakes, the spectacle covering the cornea acquires a dull to deep blue discoloration, which is part of the normal ecdysis cycle. A normal behavior in geckos lacking eyelids is spectacle cleansing with their tongue. Crocodilians have a third eyelid, the membrana nictitans, covering the eye for protection while diving underwater.

The auditory sensory system in reptiles are limited to lower frequencies and seismic vibrations.[4] Lizards and crocodilians have external ears, which are absent in both snakes and chelonian. Snakes lack external ears, tympanic membrane, tympanic cavity, and auditory canals.

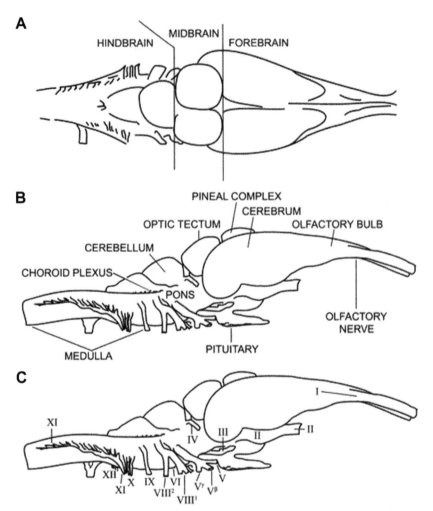

Fig. 6. Gross structure of a reptilian brain (generalized from turtles and lizards). (*A*) Dorsal view showing major regions. (*B*) Lateral view with major external components identified. (*C*) The cranial nerves, labeled by Roman numerals, in a nonsquamate reptile. Rostrum is toward the right. (*From* Wyneken J. Reptilian neurology: anatomy and function. Vet Clin North Am Exot Anim Pract 2007;10(3):837–53; with permission.)

The vomeronasal organ (Jacobson organ) is a chemoreceptive structure located on the roof of the mouth in lizards and snakes. This organ is highly developed in varanid lizards and snakes. The tongue is used to collect aerosolized particles, which are deposited into the duct of the vomeronasal organ for olfaction.

Snake species in the families Boidae, Pythonidae, and Viperidae subfamily Crotalinae have infrared receptors (pit organs) for prey location.[3] These pit receptors can be either multiply located in the supralabial and infralabial scales (Boidae and Pythonidae) or a single pit receptor located between the external nares and eyes (crotalids). Heat sensing of the pit receptor is accomplished with a free nerve ending within a concave sensory membrane suspended within the cavity.[3]

As reptile medicine continues to grow and develop, more research on pain perception and analgesia is being done. Studies have shown that reptiles have the neuroanatomical components for nociception[38,39] and similar neurotransmitters to mammals for nociceptive modulation.[40] However, establishing whether reptiles can feel pain is still difficult.[20] Though the question is still undecided, it is the professional responsibility of veterinarians to assume that reptiles can feel pain and to provide adequate pain relief and management when appropriate. Therefore, people are changing their views of whether reptiles are capable of sensing pain and learning how to recognize reptiles in pain.[19] Assessing pain in reptiles can be extremely difficult in this nonverbal group in which behavioral assessment is the best indicator of pain.[20] Mosley[20] offers a comprehensive approach to assessing pain in reptiles (**Box 1**). Comprehensive tables of drug formulary and delivery methods for analgesia commonly used in reptiles have already been published.[19,29]

Box 1
An approach to pain assessment in reptiles

Behavior

Species considerations

Requires proper species identification and familiarity with species-specific behaviors. Basic species differences affect behavioral patterns and these are important when attempting to differentiate normal from abnormal behaviors.
  Predominant activity pattern (diurnal, nocturnal)
  Predated or predator species
  Habitat (arboreal, aquatic, terrestrial, fossorial)

Individual patient considerations
  Stage of ecdysis
    Some may become more aggressive during this time
  Hibernation status
    Hibernating animals or those inclined to hibernate may be more docile and less responsive than normal
  Socialization
    Altered response to human interaction (ie, a normally docile animal biting or poor response to caregiver)
  Concurrent illness
    Patient may be incapable of showing behaviors associated with pain, or behaviors associated with disease may be mistaken for pain behaviors
  Owner assessment
    Owners are often more familiar with their animals' normal behavior; however, owners may also be biased based on their own understanding and belief regarding their animals conditions

Environmental considerations
  Enclosure
    Home enclosures often more complex, compared with hospital enclosures, providing animal with plenty of opportunity to show normal behaviors
  Preferred optimal body temperature observer
    Ambient environmental temperature is one of the main determinants of metabolic rate in resting reptiles and consequently normal behavior may be influenced by alterations in metabolic rate

Locomotor activity
  Posture
    Hunched, guarding of affected body area, not resting in normal posture

Gait
Must differentiate neurologic and mechanical dysfunction from pain-induced lameness
Other
Excessive scratching or flicking foot, tail, or affected area
Unwillingness to perform normal movements (look up, step up, thrash with tail)
Exaggerated flight response

Miscellaneous
Appetite
Reduced appetite may be related to underlying disease but may also be related to pain
Eyes
Species with eyelids may close lids when painful or ill
Color change
Species capable of color change may do so in response to stress and/or pain
Abnormal respiratory movements
May be associated with primary respiratory disease but also pain affecting the muscles and tissues involved in respiration

Anticipated level of pain
The anticipated level of pain is commonly used to evaluate pain in reptiles and is based on the likelihood and severity of tissue trauma associated with a particular procedure or condition. This is a well-accepted approach in veterinary medicine, particularly when dealing with less familiar species.[22,23] However, in addition to significant species differences, significant individual differences in response to therapy and response to tissue trauma can be seen.

Physiologic Data
Most physiologic parameters have been shown to be poor indicators of pain in most species. Physiologic parameters can be influenced by disease and excitement. In addition, the physiologic parameters of reptiles may be influenced by several metabolic processes, such as activity level, temperature alterations, and feeding.

Response to palpation
In some species a negative response to palpation can be a useful indicator of pain. However, in reptiles this may be less sensitive because most reptiles withdraw from touch regardless of whether the animal is experiencing pain.

From Mosley C. Pain and nociception in reptiles. Vet Clin North Am Exot Anim Pract 2011;14(1):45–60; with permission.

Cardiovascular System

The reptile heart can be divided into 2 categories: noncrocodilian hearts and crocodilian hearts. The noncrocodilian 3-chambered heart consists of the sinus venosus, a right and left atrium, and a single ventricle with an incomplete interventricular septum.[5] The crocodilian 4-chambered heart is similar to the noncrocodilian heart but with a complete ventricular septum forming a right and left ventricular chamber, preventing mixture of oxygenated and nonoxygenated blood. The anatomic location of the heart varies in the coelomic cavity between and within the orders: within the thoracic girdle in most lizards; in close proximity to the liver in chelonians, crocodilians, and some lizards[3]; cranial to the liver in snakes.[3] There are other variations in cardiac morphology based on behavioral physiology (active foraging versus ambush prey) and allowing species to adapt to specific habitats (aquatic, terrestrial, or arboreal).

The flow of blood in the 3-chambered heart flows from the systemic vasculature to the sinus venosus, to the right atrium, to the ventricle, to the pulmonary artery, to the lungs, returning to the heart through the pulmonary vein to the left atrium, into the ventricle, and returning to the systemic vasculature by either the left or right aorta (**Fig. 7**).[41] The noncrocodilian ventricle can be further divided into 3 compartments from right to left: cavum pulmonale, cavum venosum, and cavum arteriosum.[41–43] The cavum arteriosum and cavum venosum are connected by an interventricular canal,[41,42] whereas a muscular ridge[8] separates the cavum pulmonale from the cava arteriosum and venosum.[41,42] The muscular ridge and a 2-phased ventricular heart contraction allow the 3-chambered model to function as a 4-chambered model without the mixture of oxygenated and nonoxygenated blood.[43] In pythons and varanid lizards, there is an additional structure called the bulbuslamelle abutting the muscular ridge during cardiac contraction and forming a pressure-tight closure between the different pressured compartments, allowing mammal-like blood pressure[8] that has been documented and confirmed on high-resolution angioscope study.[12]

The lower cardiac output of reptiles compared with mammals is consistent with the 10-fold lower metabolism of reptiles.[44,45] The low cardiac output is caused by the lower heart rate[46] but the stroke volume of the pulmonary and systemic circulation is similar to that of mammals and birds.[8,44,47]

Heart rate is determined by body temperature, body size, metabolic rate, respiratory rate, and sensory stimulation.[48] At lower temperatures, the cardiac output is maintained by increasing the stroke volume.[49,50] Heart rate increases during active

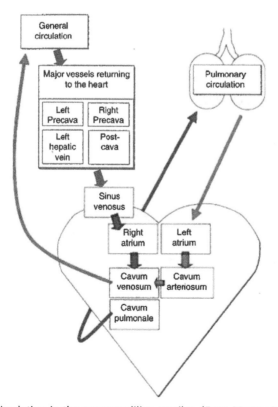

Fig. 7. General circulation in the noncrocodilian reptiles. (*From* Murray MJ. Cardiopulmonary anatomy and physiology. In: Mader DR, editor. Reptile medicine and surgery, 2nd edition. St. Louis: Saunders Elsevier; 2006; with permission.)

respiration, decreasing pulmonary resistance and increasing pulmonary blood flow for maximum gas exchange.[41,42] During periods of apnea, the heart rate decreases.

In the noncrocodilian heart, the cardiac output from the ventricle contraction is determined by the resistance differences between the pulmonary and systemic circulations. This difference between the resistances can result in cardiac shunts with blood returning from the pulmonary circulation to reenter the pulmonary circulation (left-to-right shunt) or oxygen-poor blood from the systemic circulation reentering the systemic circulation (right-to-left shunt).[8] Cardiac shunting is predominantly controlled by the autonomic nervous system.[8] Apnea, bradycardia, diving, or lung disease can increase pulmonary resistance, inducing the right-to-left cardiac shunting and directing blood flow from the right to left ventricles, bypassing the lungs. The physiologic advantage of shunting is that it allows the continual circulation and delivery of oxygen to the tissues during apnea. Cardiac shunting can also result in clinical challenges such as (1) a decrease in respiration and perfusion, (2) the need to rule out lung disease, (3) difficulties monitoring anesthetic depth and maintaining gas anesthesia due to apnea, and (4) the difficulty of monitoring the degree of shunting.

Some unique features of the reptile cardiovascular system involve or pertain to thermoregulation and physiologic hypertrophy. The cardiovascular system plays a major role in thermoregulation by governing the circulation of warmed and cooled blood to adjust core body temperature by using vasodilation or vasoconstriction of cutaneous vessels during basking and cooling. Studies have also shown that Burmese pythons can increase their ventricle muscles by 40% with normal physiologic hypertrophy via increased gene expression of muscle-contractile proteins within 48 hours of meal ingestion with the heart returning to normal size after the complete digestion of the prey.[34]

The renal portal circulation system is responsible for venous blood return from the tail and hind legs being filtered by the kidneys and the liver. This system allows continuous perfusion of the kidneys even in water-deprived conditions.[41,42] Veterinarians are commonly taught to avoid administrating drug injections in the hind legs or tail because some medications are either nephrotoxic or excreted/metabolized by the kidney before reaching the systemic circulation, although recent pharmacokinetic studies with certain drugs in reptiles have contradicted these claims.[51,52] As noted by Mader and Murray,[41] it is generally recommended to give injections into the cranial half of the body until further studies are done.

Respiratory System

Key differences between the reptile and mammalian respiratory system include the lack of a functional diaphragm (except in some crocodilians), saclike lungs with or without caudal air sacs, the ability to physiologically withstand prolonged periods of apnea by switching to anaerobic metabolism, and evolved specialized adaptations by aquatic species to perform extrarespiratory carbon dioxide elimination. As in other systems, there are variations in both pulmonary anatomy and physiology between reptiles within orders and families.[53]

Respiration in reptile species can be propelled by diaphragmaticus (only crocodilians), glottis (chelonians), intercostal (squamates and crocodilians), pectoral (chelonians), and abdominal (squamates) musculature[11,53] controlled by spinal or cranial nerves (X or XII).[11] Respiratory airflow in reptiles in general moves from the external nares to the nasal sinuses/nasal cavity, to the internal nares into the glottis, into the trachea, and into the lungs. Variations in this include glottis location, incomplete versus complete tracheal rings, location of trachea bifurcation, the presence and absence of intrapulmonary bronchi, paired versus single lung (most snakes), lung anatomic location, and lung types based on partitions and parenchyma. In most snakes and carnivorous lizards, the glottis is easily located rostrally in the oral cavity, making intubation relatively easy. In herbivorous lizards and chelonians, the glottis is located caudal to the base of the fleshy tongue. In crocodilians, the epiglottal flap seals the glottis for swimming. Snakes and lizards tend to have incomplete cartilaginous tracheal rings, whereas chelonians are complete.[3]

Chelonians, crocodilians, lizards, and boid (pythons and boa constrictors) snakes have paired lungs, whereas most snakes have a dominated (functional) right lung lobe with a vestigial left lung lobe. The lungs are categorized based on partitioning: unicameral (single chamber), paucicameral (central lumen dived by a small number of septa), multicameral (multiple chamber), and transitional.[54] Snakes have a unicameral lung. Families of lizards such as chameleons, agamids, and iguanids have a paucicameral lung. Crocodilians, varanids, and chelonians have a multicameral lung type. Additional classification of the lungs is based on the parenchyma: trabecular, edicular, and faveolar. In some lungs there is a gradual transitions into air sacs in the caudal lung region,[3] which can act as oxygen reservoirs or buoyancy organs in aquatic species.[3] Additional specialized adaptation by aquatic turtles and snakes provide the ability to eliminate carbon dioxide across the pharynx (softshell turtles), cloacal mucosa, and skin (softshell turtles).[3,53]

Some unique physiologic aspects of reptile respiration need to be considered when performing a physical examination, monitoring for anesthesia, and planning treatment. Reptiles in general have a 10% to 20% greater lung volume[55] compared with mammals of similar weight but with a comparably lower oxygen consumption rate matching their lower metabolic rates. Reptile lungs have a higher compliance value[53] and thinner lungs with diminished exterior muscular support[19] compared with mammalian lungs, which can lead to damage from overexpansion/inflation during inhalant anesthetic administration and ventilation.[19] Reptile respiration is largely driven by hypoxia, hypercapnia, and environmental temperature.[11,53] It is commonly thought that reptiles will stop spontaneously breathing or delay return of spontaneous respiration during recovery on a high percent of oxygen. Therefore ventilation with room air is often recommended using an Ambu bag attached to the endotracheal tube with IPPV performed till spontaneous breathing returns for recovery.[19] Schumacher[53] writes that "The increase in hypercapnia will lead to an increase in tidal volume while hypoxia will lead to an increase in respiratory rate," and that "increase in temperature or prolonged diving periods in aquatic species is met by increased tidal volume instead of increasing respiratory rate"[53] with the predominant stimulus to breathe coming from low blood oxygen concentration.[41] Cardiac shunting and the unique buffering system described earlier helps maintain tissue perfusion, and conversion to anaerobic metabolism both increases the tolerance for long periods of apnea for diving species.

Digestive System

The reptile digestive tract is similar to that of higher vertebrates starting from the oral cavity and ending at the cloaca with both macroscopic and microscopic variation in different anatomic locations depending on diet. Diet can be carnivorous, herbivorous, or omnivorous depending on the species, which can also make fulfilling nutritional requirements challenging in a clinical setting.

The oral cavity is lined by a mucous membrane moist from saliva production from multiple salivary glands (lingual, sublingual, and labial glands).[3] Teeth types and locations vary from crocodilians (thecodont teeth- "socket-teeth") to lizards (acrodont-[teeth attached to the edge of the jawbone without sockets] or pleurodonts) to snakes (thecodont). Venomous snakes (families Colubridae, Elapidae, and Viperidae) and helodermatid lizards have modified teeth and poison glands for venom delivery. Chelonians lack teeth and instead have keratinous jaw sheaths[43] or rhamphothecas. The tongue varies in morphology based on feeding behavior, ranging from keratinized (monitors and crocodilians) to long, forked, muscular, and aglandular in snakes,[3] to a fleshy tongue with numerous taste buds in chelonians. The paired vomeronasal organs mentioned earlier are chemosensory organs located at the base of the nasal cavity above the palate. Paired internal nares/choanae are present in the hard palate in snakes, chelonians, and lizards.

The esophagus delivers and stores ingested food from the oral cavity to the stomach. The esophagus in most snakes has a thin and highly distensible cranial portion with increasing musculature caudal to the heart.[3,12] Esophageal muscularis mucosa is lacking in most chelonians but is present in tortoises and sea turtles prominently in the caudal portion.[3] The stomach is where most of the digestions occurs, with variations in shape between the subgroups. The stomachs of chelonians have a greater and lesser curvature, whereas lizards have an ovoid shape, crocodilians have a saccular stomach, and snakes a linear and elongated stomach that fulfills their linear body plan.[3] The stomach is divided into 2 regions: corpus (fundus) and pars pyloric.[56] The stomach terminates in the pylorus, a muscular sphincter that controls movement of food from the stomach into the small intestines.

The small intestine is where digestion continues with nutritional absorption and allows the mixture of ingesta with gastric, bile, pancreatic, and intestinal enzymes.[3] Small intestinal length and convolutions is dependent on diet, with increased length and volume capacity in herbivores. The colon length and volume vary similarly to the small intestine and based on diet. The colon has mucosal folds.[3] Some herbivorous species have partitions in the cranial colon dividing it into compartments to aid in hindgut fermentation of plant material.[57] The cecum is located between the small intestine and colon. The cloaca is the terminal chamber for both the digestive and urogenital tract.

The liver in reptiles is frequently bilobed and dark brown, and lined by a connective tissue capsule, with the gallbladder residing in the right liver lobe and with a bile duct delivering bile to the duodenum.[3] The snake gallbladder tends to be located caudal to the liver and closely associated with the pancreas and spleen.[3] The reptilian pancreas ranges from trilobed in lizards to being consolidated in snakes to have both endocrine and exocrine components, with varying distributions of these components between the orders.[58]

The gastrointestinal physiology is determined by the environmental and core body temperature affecting the digestion rate, passage rates of food through the gastrointestinal tract, motility, and absorption rate.[3] Digestion has been reported to cease at 7°C and is extremely slow at 10 to 15°C in reptiles in general.[3] Digestion has also been noted to slow down near the highest temperature tolerated by species.[3] When at the upper range of the POTZ, general metabolism and secretion of digestive juices are increased.[3]

Urogenital System

Reptiles produce nitrogenous excretions (ammonia, urea, or uric acid) with a urinary system made up of paired kidneys, paired ureters, the presence or absence of a urinary bladder, cloaca, and a vent. Reptile kidneys vary in location (caudal coelomic to pelvic canal), slightly lobulated to lobulated, symmetric to asymmetrical (crocodilians), with slight moderation of the vascular pattern between the groups.[59] Squamate kidneys may be sexually dimorphic with males having an enlarged portion called sexual segments located between distal renal segments and collecting tubules during breeding seasons[60] giving a creamy pale coloration to the kidney from hypertrophy, which may be confused with renal gout.[3]

Predominantly, chelonians and most lizards have urinary bladders, which are absent in crocodilians and snakes. However, the urinary bladder is used for storage of water, as the ureters empty into the cloaca. The cloaca is the common chamber into which urinary, digestive, and reproductive tract contents exit. The cloaca is defined by 3 regions: coprodeum (anterior), urodeum (middle), and proctodeum (caudal). The coprodeum is where digestive waste from the rectum is received. The urodeum is where the ureters, urinary bladder, and genital ducts are connected to receive content. The proctodeum is proximal to the vent.

Aquatic species excrete mostly ammonia (crocodilians and marine turtles) or urea (freshwater turtles).[3] Ammonia is the simplest form of excreted waste but requires large amounts of water, therefore this method of excretion is predominantly used by aquatic species.[59] Terrestrial reptile species excrete primarily uric acid.

The reptile kidney consists of nephrons that lack the loop of Henle therefore producing only isosthenuric urine. Water retention is maintained by using uric acid for nitrogenous waste elimination. Special protein complexes with urea or uric acid, either sodium (carnivores) or potassium (herbivores), forms a suspension containing spheres composed of 65% uric acid.[59] Additional glycoproteins or mucopolysaccharides from the kidney aids in the sphere formation and prevents the urates from clogging the renal ducts.[59] Once this suspension reaches the cloaca, the proteins are reabsorbed and recycled by the cloacal mucosa and the presence of hydrogen ions acidifying the urine promotes the precipitation of uric acid.[59] The reptile kidney not only removes nitrogenous waste from the blood but also synthesizes vitamin C[61] and converts 25-hydroxycholecalciferol to the active forms 1,25-dihydroxycholecaliferol or 24,25-dihydroxycholecalciferol.[62]

An additional difference between mammalian and reptile renal physiology are that only 30% to 50% of water is absorbed by the proximal tubules in reptiles compared with 60% to 80% in mammals.[59] Downstream sites absorb the remaining water in reptiles: the distal renal tubules, colon, bladder, and cloaca. The urinary bladder also absorbs sodium and bicarbonate. Reptiles in general have a lower reduced glomerular filtration rate caused by the lower 20-mm Hg diastolic blood pressure compared with the 120 mm Hg of diastolic birds.[63]

The decrease of glomerular filtration when an animal is dehydrated is controlled by the posterior pituitary gland releasing arginine vasotocin, causing the afferent arteriole to constrict.[59] Cessation of blood flow through the glomeruli is a major concern because it can result in ischemic necrosis of the kidneys, which is prevented by the renal portal blood system allowing continual circulation of blood through the kidneys.

The reptilian testes and ovaries are paired, located in the coelomic cavity near the cranial poles of the kidneys (crocodilians, chelonians, and many lizards) or caudal to the gallbladder (snakes). In squamates, the right testicle is cranial to the left while they are symmetrically arranged in crocodilians and chelonians. Testes can increase in size because of spermatogenesis during breeding season. Lizards and snakes have paired hemipenes inverted in the base of the tail. The penises of chelonians and crocodilians is located cranial to the cloacal opening. Females have paired ovaries and paired oviducts, with fertilization occurring internally near the cranial aspect of the oviduct. Reptiles can be either oviparous (egg layers) or viviparous (live bearers).[64]

Integument System

As in other animals, the role of the integument is integral in (1) protection from the external environment, (2) retention and prevention of the loss of body fluid, and (3) prevention of pathogen entry. The integument is composed of the epidermis (outer) and the dermis (inner). Scales are formed from the folding of the epidermis,[3] with snake skin having the greatest folding capability with flexible hinges located between adjacent scutes.[3]

The reptilian epidermis is continuously renewed with growth and replacement cycles called ecdysis (shedding). There are 2 types of ecdysis: continuous (turtles and crocodilians) and discontinuous (lizards and snakes). The cycle of ecdysis consists of periods of the formation of new inner epidermal layer and loss (shedding). Snakes and some lizards shed the entire whole body skin, whereas some lizards shed in portions over periods of 1 to 2 weeks. Shedding frequency is also affected by age, frequency, food consumption, and temperature.

Chelonia is the reptile group that is known for having a shell composed of the carapace (dorsal) and the plastron (ventral) connected[65] by the bridges. The shell is covered by scutes formed by specialized, hard epidermal parts.[3] The junction between the scutes forming the seams is where keratin is formed. Hirasawa and colleagues[66] reported that the chelonian carapace consists of coastal plates that are continuous with the thoracic ribs and neural bony plates that are continuous with the vertebrae. Most of the carapace is formed from the endoskeletal ribs and not from dermal origins as previous hypothesized.

Additional accessories to the reptile skin present in some species include musk glands in the cloaca, mental or chin of chelonians, the dentary bone of crocodilians located on the inside of each half of the mandible, and specialized glands associated with the angle of the jaw in chameleons. Some lizards, especially noted in male iguanids, have femoral pores that are holocrine secretory glands on the ventral aspect of their thighs, releasing pheromones for attracting mates or marking territory.[65] In addition, many reptile species have a wide variety of horns, dewlaps, beards, armor, sails, as well as color variations (eg, albino and melanistic), which makes these species popular with reptile enthusiasts.

Musculoskeletal System

The musculoskeletal system in reptiles has been adapted for many different environments and subenvironmental niches and for aquatic to terrestrial to arboreal to fossorial locomotion. Crocodilians, chelonians, and lizards are the quadrupeds of the group, with both pectoral and pelvic girdles supporting limbs for location. The chelonians have lost the sternum element with both their pectoral and pelvic girdle surrounded by the ribs. Snakes lack the pectoral girdle and pelvic girdle, whereas some pythons still have a vestigial pelvic girdle with bilateral pelvic spurs. Ribs contribute to respiration in most reptiles, except the chelonians, in which they have evolved to be within the order's characteristic shell.[3] In snakes, the ribs are anchored with connective tissue, and are continuous with enlarged ventral scales.[3]

Certain lizard species have tail autotomy as a predatory defensive mechanism, allowing the loss of the tail with minimum blood loss and trauma to adjacent tissue. Alibardi[67] showed putative stem cells residing in the cartilaginous region of the vertebra that are responsible for the cartilaginous tube replacement in tail regeneration.

Stress

When first exposed to reptiles, clinicians often overlook stress. Martínez Silvestre[21] writes that, "Stress is an adaptive response of any animal to a stimulus that presents a threat to homeostasis." It is commonly used by herpetoculturists to explain the failure to thrive or the cause of death in reptiles; however, clinicians should determine the cause of stress based on a complete history and physical examination. Martínez Silvestre[21] lists the 4 responses altered by stress: (1) behavior changes, (2) alterations in the functioning of the autonomic nervous system, (3) altered

Table 3	
Time to response after stressor	
Stressor	**Time**
Capture	3 min to 6 h
Exposure to cold and heat	15–25 min
Hyperosmotic saline injection	30 min
Intermittent change of environment	30 min
Repeated blood sampling	1–4 h
Severe restraint	4–8 h
Hypotonic fluid injection	8 d
Exposure to salt water	1–4 wk
Hierarchy with dominating males	10–30 d
Overcrowding	10–14 d
Low relative humidity	3 wk

The time to response is the time to stimulation of corticosteroid release.
From Martínez Silvestre A. How to assess stress in reptiles. J Exot Pet Med 2014;23(3):240–3; with permission.

neuroendocrine responses, and (4) altered immune responses.[21] Stress activation of the neuroendocrine response of the hypothalamus-pituitary-adrenal axis, which is essential for regulation of physiologic function, derails its control over immune competence, metabolism, and behavior.[21] Causes of stress in reptiles can include inappropriate husbandry, nutritional deficiency, cohoused hierarchy conflict, and restraint and handling. Martínez Silvestre[21] provides correlating causes of stress and the time for corticosterone release after stressors (**Table 3**).[21] Clinicians should be aware that reptilian patients are already stressed from their underlying medical conditions. The physical examination, sample collecting, and treatment plan should be planned and executed with efficiency to minimize the extent to which handling and restraint add additional stress to the patient. Housing patients in a hospital setting to reduce stress should also be considered by providing species-specific husbandry requirements with special emphasis on hide boxes, avoiding housing in high-traffic areas, and isolating patients from clinic patients that are considered predators to reptiles.

SUMMARY

This article summarizes the physiology and anatomy of reptiles, highlighting points relevant for emergency room veterinarians. The purpose of this chapter is not simply to provide an overview but also to encourage clinicians to seek additional species specific information to better medically diagnose and treat their reptile patients. Given the thousands of reptile species kept as pets, and our limited knowledge about their natural habitat requirements making husbandry care a challenge, caring for reptiles as veterinarians will continue to be a great challenge. Educating ourselves about their unique features and husbandry needs is the beginning to providing the best possible veterinary care.

REFERENCES

1. de la Navarre BJS. Common procedures in reptiles and amphibians. Vet Clin North Am Exot Anim Pract 2006;9(2):237–67, vi.

2. Abraham S. Reptile database surpasses 10,000 reptile species. 2014. Available at: http://phys.org/news/2014-08-reptile-database-surpasses-species.html.

3. Jacobson E. Overview of reptile biology, anatomy, and histology. In: Infectious diseases and pathology of reptiles. CRC Press; 2007. p. 1–130.

4. Wyneken J. Reptilian neurology: anatomy and function. Vet Clin North Am Exot Anim Pract 2007;10(3):837–53.

5. Kashyap HV. The reptilian heart. Proc Natl Inst Sci India 1959;234–54.

6. Jensen B, Nyengaard JR, Pedersen M, et al. Anatomy of the python heart. Anat Sci Int 2010;85:194–203.

7. Webb GJW. Comparative cardiac anatomy of the Reptilia. J Morphol 1979;161: 221–40.

8. Jensen B, Moorman AFM, Wang T. Structure and function of the hearts of lizards and snakes. Biol Rev Camb Philos Soc 2014;89(2):302–36.

9. Kik MJL, Mitchell MA. Reptile cardiology: a review of anatomy and physiology, diagnostic approaches, and clinical disease. Semin Avian Exot Pet Med 2005; 14(1):52–60.

10. Mitchell MA, Diaz-Figueroa O. Clinical reptile gastroenterology. Vet Clin North Am Exot Anim Pract 2005;8:277–98.

11. Taylor EW, Leite CAC, McKenzie DJ, et al. Control of respiration in fish, amphibians and reptiles. Braz J Med Biol Res 2010;43:409–24.

12. Jensen B, Nielsen JM, Axelsson M, et al. How the python heart separates pulmonary and systemic blood pressures and blood flows. J Exp Biol 2010;213:1611–7.

13. Hicks JW. The physiological and evolutionary significance of cardiovascular shunting patterns in reptiles. News Physiol Sci 2002;17:241–5.

14. Martinez-Jimenez D, Hernandez-Divers SJ. Emergency care of reptiles. Vet Clin North Am Exot Anim Pract 2007;10(2):557–85.

15. Sykes JM, Greenacre CB. Techniques for drug delivery in reptiles and amphibians. J Exot Pet Med 2006;15(3):210–7.

16. Mariani CL. The neurologic examination and neurodiagnostic techniques for reptiles. Vet Clin North Am Exot Anim Pract 2007;10(3):855–91.

17. Sladky KK, Mans C. Clinical anesthesia in reptiles. J Exot Pet Med 2012;21(1): 17–31.

18. Hunt C. Neurological examination and diagnostic testing in birds and reptiles. J Exot Pet Med 2015;24(1):34–51.

19. Sladky KK, Mans C. Clinical analgesia in reptiles. J Exot Pet Med 2012;21(2): 158–67.

20. Mosley C. Pain and nociception in reptiles. Vet Clin North Am Exot Anim Pract 2011;14(1):45–60.

21. Martínez Silvestre A. How to assess stress in reptiles. J Exot Pet Med 2014;23(3): 240–3.

22. Sykes JM 4th, Klaphake E. Reptile hematology. Vet Clin North Am Exot Anim Pract 2008;11(1):481–500.

23. Mans C. Clinical update on diagnosis and management of disorders of the digestive system of reptiles. J Exot Pet Med 2013;22(2):141–62.

24. Infectious diseases and pathology of reptiles: color atlas and text. 2007.

25. Selleri P, Hernandez-Divers SJ. Renal diseases of reptiles. Vet Clin North Am Exot Anim Pract 2006;9(1):161–74.

26. Zwart P. Renal pathology in reptiles. Vet Clin North Am Exot Anim Pract 2006;9(1): 129–59.

27. Montali RJ. Comparative pathology of inflammation in the higher vertebrates (reptiles, birds and mammals). J Comp Pathol 1988;99(1):1–26.

28. Mader DR. Reptile medicine and surgery. Elsevier; 2006.
29. Mader DR, Divers SJ. Current therapy in reptile medicine and surgery. Elsevier; 2014.
30. Mader DR, Lock BA. Reptile medicine and surgery. Elsevier; 2006.
31. Wilkinson SL. Guide to venomous reptiles in veterinary practice. J Exot Pet Med 2014;23(4):337–46.
32. Mader DR, Rossi JV. Reptile medicine and surgery. 2nd edition. Elsevier; 2006.
33. Mader DR, Donoghue S. Reptile medicine and surgery. Elsevier; 2006.
34. Andersen JB, Rourke BC, Caiozzo VJ, et al. Physiology: postprandial cardiac hypertrophy in pythons. Nature 2005;434(7029):37–8.
35. Jackson DC, Ramsey AL, Paulson JM, et al. Lactic acid buffering by bone and shell in anoxic softshell and painted turtles. Physiol Biochem Zool 2000;73(3):290–7.
36. Jackson DC, Crocker CE, Ultsch GR. Bone and shell contribution to lactic acid buffering of submerged turtles Chrysemys picta bellii at 3 degrees C. Am J Physiol Regul Integr Comp Physiol 2000;278(6):R1564–71.
37. Eakin RM. Further observations on the fine structure of the parietal eye of lizards. J Biophys Biochem Cytol 1960;8:483–99.
38. Liang YF, Terashima S. Physiological properties and morphological characteristics of cutaneous and mucosal mechanical nociceptive neurons with A-delta peripheral axons in the trigeminal ganglia of crotaline snakes. J Comp Neurol 1993;328(1):88–102.
39. Stoskopf MK. Pain and analgesia in birds, reptiles, amphibians, and fish. Invest Ophthalmol Vis Sci 1994;35(2):775–80.
40. de la Iglesia JA, Martinez-Guijarro FI, Lopez-Garcia C. Neurons of the medial cortex outer plexiform layer of the lizard Podarcis hispanica: golgi and immunocytochemical studies. J Comp Neurol 1994;341(2):184–203.
41. Mader DR, Murray MJ. Reptile medicine and surgery. Elsevier; 2006.
42. Mitchell MA. Reptile cardiology. Vet Clin North Am Exot Anim Pract 2009;12(1):65–79.
43. Vitt LJ, Caldwell JP. Herpetology. Elsevier; 2014.
44. Burggren W, Farrell A, Lillywhite H. Vertebrate cardiovascular systems. In: Comprehensive physiology. John Wiley; 1998. p. 215–308.
45. Hulbert AJ, Else PL. Basal metabolic rate: history, composition, regulation, and usefulness. Physiol Biochem Zool 2004;77(6):869–76.
46. Lillywhite HB, Zippel KC, Farrell AP. Resting and maximal heart rates in ectothermic vertebrates. Comp Biochem Physiol A Mol Integr Physiol 1999;124(4):369–82.
47. Seymour RS, Blaylock AJ. The principle of Laplace and scaling of ventricular wall stress and blood pressure in mammals and birds. Physiol Biochem Zool 2000;73(4):389–405.
48. Cooper JE, Jackson OF. Diseases of the Reptilia, vol. 1. London: Academic Press; 1981.
49. White F, Dawson W. Biology of the Reptilia. 1976.
50. Sykes JM, Klaphake E. Reptile Hematology. Clin Lab Med 2015;35(3):661–80.
51. Holz P. The reptilian renal-portal system: influence on therapy. 1999.
52. Holz P, Burger J, Pasloske K, et al. Effect of injection site on carbenicillin pharmacokinetics in the carpet python, Morelia spilota. J Herp Med Surg 2002;12–6.
53. Schumacher J. Reptile respiratory medicine. Vet Clin North Am - Exot Anim Pract 2003;6:213–31.
54. Perry S. Reptilian lungs: functional anatomy and evolution. 2013.

55. Perry S. Lungs: comparative anatomy, functional morphology, and evolution. Biol Reptil 1998;1–92.
56. Luppa H. Histology of the digestive tract. In: Gans C, Parsons CS editors. Biology reptilia. 1977.
57. Gross and anatomy of the heart of the lizard. 1055.
58. Stahl SJ. Diseases of the reptile pancreas. Vet Clin North Am Exot Anim Pract 2003;6:191–212.
59. Mader DR, Holz P. Reptile medicine and surgery. Elsevier; 2006.
60. Bishop JE. A histologic and histochemical study of the kidney tubule of the common garter snake, *Thamnophis sirtalis*, with special reference to the sexual segment in the male. J Morphol 1959;104:307–57.
61. Gillespie DS. Overview of species needing dietary vitamin C. Journal of Zoo Animal Medicine 1980.
62. Ullrey D, Bernard J. Vitamin D: metabolism, sources, unique problems in zoo animals, meeting needs. In: Fowler's zoo and wild animal medicine current therapy. 4th edition. WB Saunders; 1999.
63. Rodbard S, Feldman D. Relationship between body temperature and arterial pressure. Proc Soc Exp Biol Med 1946;63(1):43.
64. Packard GC, Tracy CR, Roth JJ. The physiological ecology of reptilian eggs and embryos, and the evolution of viviparity within the class Reptilia. Biol Rev 1977; 52(1):71–105.
65. Pianka ER, Vitt LJ. Lizards: windows to the evolution of diversity. University of California Press; 2003.
66. Hirasawa T, Nagashima H, Kuratani S. The endoskeletal origin of the turtle carapace. Nat Commun 2013;4:2107.
67. Alibardi L. Original and regenerating lizard tail cartilage contain putative resident stem/progenitor cells. Micron 2015;78:10–8.

Reptile Critical Care and Common Emergencies

Meera Kumar Music, BVM&S, MRCVS*, Anneliese Strunk, DVM, DABVP (Avian)

KEYWORDS

- Emergency • Reptile • Monitoring • Fluid therapy • Euthanasia

KEY POINTS

- The physical examination and methods of monitoring a critical patient are vital when providing supportive care in an emergency situation and will aid in diagnosis and targeted treatment.
- Common emergency presentations for review include acute pathologic changes and illness sustained from chronic husbandry deficiencies and dietary insufficiency.
- In the case of patients with guarded to poor prognoses, humane and compassionate euthanasia may be required.

INTRODUCTION

Reptile emergencies are an important part of exotic animal critical care, both true emergencies and those perceived as emergencies by owners. Although most cases in later discussion are typically chronic in nature, they may present acutely, such as a reptile with poor husbandry presenting for a pathologic fracture, egg binding, or respiratory issues.[1] When approaching a reptile emergency, keep in mind that whatever underlying medical issue causing the clinical signs has taken a long time to occur, and an immediate fix is unlikely to be possible.

PHYSICAL EXAMINATION AND MONITORING

The physical examination of a reptile is a valuable tool in diagnosing and treating medical emergencies. The physical examination of a reptile should include, but is not limited to the following:

- Assessment of mentation and response to handling/awareness of surroundings
- Musculoskeletal/neurologic examination, including observation of posture:
  - Can the lizard or chelonian hold its entire body off of the examination table when ambulating? Assess "knuckling" (conscious proprioception) response

The authors have nothing to disclose.
The Center for Bird and Exotic Animal Medicine, 11401 NE 195th Street, Bothell, WA 98011, USA
* Corresponding author.
E-mail address: drmusic@theexoticvet.com

of all 4 limbs. When placed in dorsal recumbency, lizards should attempt to right themselves head first. Chelonians will often move their head and legs all together to attempt righting; this is an excellent time to assess limb movement.

- o Some lizards (like iguanas) have a menace response that can be assessed.[2]
- o Can the snake right itself if placed in dorsal recumbency? Does the snake have a jerky motion when moving through substrate or across the examination table?[2]
  - ■ NOTE: when performing a reptile neurologic examination, be aware that the patient will become increasingly less responsive the longer the examination continues. Less responsiveness is not necessarily an indication of neurologic dysfunction.
- • Hydration: Look for sunken eyes, a skin tent, or increased creasing when a snake curls up (creasing in snake skin can also occur in cases of weight loss). On oral examination, dehydrated reptiles may also exhibit "ropy" saliva.
- • Palpation:
  - o With large lizards, like iguanas, rectal examinations should be performed in order to assess the kidneys.
  - o Full-body palpation is possible with snakes. Diagrams of snake anatomy demonstrate the relative locations of organs within the coelom.[3]
  - o The prefomoral fossa should be palpated in chelonians. Often if the animal is reproductively active, you can palpate follicles or eggs; enlarged organs may also be palpable. Be careful when palpating to prevent crushed fingers when the leg is forcefully withdrawn.
- • Auscultation
  - o Auscultation can be challenging in the reptilian patient; however, the heart can be ausculted in most lizard patients, as can the lungs in most reptile species. Moist gauze can be used as an aid by decreasing airspace between scales when placed between the stethoscope and skin.
  - o A Doppler unit may also be used to take a heart rate during a physical examination and monitor an anesthetized or debilitated reptile.[4] The probe can be placed over the heart in snakes. In lizards, the heart can usually be detected with a Doppler when placed in the axillary region aiming toward the chest, or directly over the heart in the cranial coelom.[5] Keep in mind species variations; monitor lizard hearts are more caudally located than other lizard species. With lizards and chelonians, the carotid can be monitored using a probe in the cervical region. With chelonians, angling a cervically placed probe toward midline will allow for cardiac monitoring.

Reptiles often present with low body temperatures on emergency, which may affect the physical examination findings. It is ideal to reassess the patient after restoring the appropriate body temperature in order to get the most accurate information.

DIAGNOSTICS

Different diagnostics that will help to target treatment with reptile patients are largely similar to mammalian and avian patients, though reptile venipuncture can be challenging in some species (**Table 1**). These diagnostics include the following:

1. Complete blood count (CBC): reptile red blood cells contain a nucleus, requiring manual evaluation of blood slides. In-house estimated white blood cell counts may be performed in emergency cases, but ideally, samples should be sent to a laboratory with personnel comfortable with evaluating a reptile hemogram.

Table 1			
Venipuncture sites			
Species	Venipuncture Site	Sedation Needed	Notes
Lizards	Ventral coccygeal vein	No	—
	Cranial vena cava[7]	Yes	Iso induction or alfaxalone 5–15 mg/kg IM[8]
	Femoral vein	Maybe	Not commonly performed
Snakes	Cardiocentesis	No	—
	Ventral coccygeal vein (large snakes)	No	—
Chelonia	Jugular	Not usually	Unless very large and head cannot be extended
	Brachial vein/plexus	Not usually	Unless very large and arm cannot be extended
	Dorsal midline tail vein	Not usually	Unless very large and tail cannot be extended
	Subcarapacial (subvertebral) venous sinus	No	Usually this site is accessible regardless of how cooperative the chelonian is; however, use only as a last resort. Paresis has been reported from simple venipuncture (Paul Gibbons, personal communication, 2015)

Data from Refs.[9–11]

2. Chemistry panel: often very small amounts of blood can be submitted to external laboratories for a full panel. A chemistry panel can help determine reproductive status as well as liver and kidney function. Consult individual laboratories to determine the minimum amount of blood required to run the desired panel.
3. Ionized calcium: a bench top analyzer (i-STAT handheld; Abbott Point of Care Inc, Princeton, NJ) can provide an ionized calcium level in minutes and can help to determine the extent of hypocalcemia and level of intervention needed.
4. Blood culture: helps with antibiotic determination in the septic patient. Indications of sepsis are discussed later in the article.
5. Radiographs: used to visualize the presence of follicles or eggs in the coelom, evaluate the respiratory and gastrointestinal (GI) tracts, assess bone density and conformation, and screen for fractures.
6. Ultrasound: helpful in cases of coelomic effusion and reproductive disease.
7. Anaerobic and aerobic culture and sensitivity of lesions: ideal for targeted antibiotic therapy. When submitting cultures, request the sample be held for 2 weeks at room temperature to best grow bacteria. Certain reptile bacteria may not grow in the temperatures that many avian and mammalian cultures are processed.[6]

FLUID THERAPY

Maintenance fluid requirements in reptiles range from 10 to 30 mL/kg/d.[4,12] Before fluid administration, warm fluids to the patient's optimal body temperature. Be careful to avoid rates in excess of 40 mL/kg/d to minimize the risk of fluid overload.[13]

Most isotonic parenteral crystalloid solutions are acceptable for use in reptiles (the authors use 0.9% sodium chloride solution).[13] Although lactated Ringer's is commonly used in most cat and dog practices, it has been suggested that the level of lactate present may place an added burden on the metabolism of the compromised reptile and is not ideal for rehydration.[14] However, reptiles have a buffer system that allows them to deal with high levels of lactate. The level of lactate in lactated crystalloid solutions appears to not be clinically relevant unless the patient has severe (end-stage) hepatic compromise.[13]

There are several routes of fluid administration available for the reptile patient:

1. Orally: ideal administration in order to promote absorption and quick rehydration. However, this depends on the reptile having an appropriate body temperature and a functional gastrointestinal tract, which may not be possible in an emergent situation.[12]
2. Subcutaneous: large boluses are not always possible due to the decreased elasticity of reptile skin, but are ideal in the case of a moderately stable reptile at its appropriate body temperature. Plan to instill subcutaneous fluids in multiple small boluses where loose skin is seen. Regions to use for subcutaneous fluids include the flank region and along the epaxial muscles in lizards, prefemoral fossa (or axillae) in chelonians, and areas of loose skin when snakes are curled up.
3. Intravenous/intraosseous (IV/IO): in the critically ill patient, IV or IO catheter placement allows for more direct fluid administration and critical rehydration (**Table 2**).

Table 2
Sites for intravenous and intraosseous catheter placement

Species	IV Catheter	Placement Notes	IO Catheter	Placement Notes
Chelonia	Jugular	Generally straightforward; may require cut down	Cranial or caudal aspect of the bony bridge (connection between plastron and carapace)	Very small medullary cavity present
			Proximal tibia	Difficult to maintain if the leg can withdraw into the shell
			Distal femur	Try to avoid (involves stifle, may lead to articular cartilage damage); difficult to maintain if the leg can withdraw into the shell
Snakes	Cardiac	Sedation required to maintain catheter	No acceptable IO sites	
	Jugular	Surgical approach required for jugular; only good in short term		
Lizards	Cephalic	Requires cut down	Proximal tibia	
	Jugular	Requires surgical approach	Distal Femur	Try to avoid (involves stifle, may lead to articular cartilage damage)
	Ventral coccygeal vein	Difficult to maintain in conscious patient		
	Ventral abdominal vein	For anesthetized patients only		

Data from Refs.[9–11,15]

Use sedation or anesthesia as well as local anesthesia to aid in placement. Orthogonal radiographs are required to assure appropriate placement of IO catheters. Catheters can be secured with a combination of tissue glue, sutures, tape and bandaging. Catheters may be difficult to maintain in reptiles once they are stabilized and regain strength.

4. Intracoelomic: although this method of fluid administration is described in many places, there are significant drawbacks. Mainly, when fluids are given via the intracoelomic route, there is no guarantee that the fluid will not be given directly into the lungs, bladder, or GI tract. There are safer methods of fluid administration that should always be considered before this one.[13]

COMMON EMERGENCY PRESENTATIONS
Bites/Trauma

Bites can occur from dogs, cats, outdoor predators like raccoons, or rodent prey fed to the reptile.[16] Wounds should be swabbed for culture and sensitivity and thoroughly explored. Any hemorrhage will need to be immediately stopped, and appropriate fluid therapy should be administered. Hemostasis can be achieved with pressure, cautery, or surgical ligation of vessels.[4] Wounds entering the coelomic cavity will likely require surgical attention, while surface wounds may be left to heal by second intention. Primary wound closure can be performed on noncontaminated wounds less than 12 hours old.[17] Antibiotics may be used, but debridement and copious flushing may be all that is needed for superficial wounds.[17]

In the case of traumatic wounds, screening radiographs should be considered to check for fractures. If there is concurrent evidence of poor husbandry, radiographs may help to rule out pathologic fractures. A CBC and chemistry panel may help discover electrolyte abnormalities or systemic infection.[4]

Chelonian Shell Fracture

Shell fractures for chelonian species can be particularly gruesome on presentation. However, even in cases of extreme trauma, it may be possible to fix the damage present. When the animal is being examined, if the lungs appear to be collapsed, the patient can be intubated and oxygenated before continuing the examination.[18] Be diligent about fully exploring the extent of soft tissue damage. Injury to the GI tract, lungs, and evaluation of blood loss is vitally important, both in terms of stabilizing the patient, and in determining long-term prognosis.

Supportive care is a vital part of addressing this critical patient. Although it can be tempting to try fixation immediately, it is far more important to provide analgesia, thoroughly clean the wounds, provide fluid support, and administer antibiotics than it is to fix the shell. The shell itself can wait until the patient is more stable; decontamination and support of the critical patient must be the first priority.

Before cleaning the wound, consider taking both bacterial and fungal cultures, particularly in the instance of exposed lung or coelomic organ tissue.[18] When cleaning the wounds, be very careful to physically remove as much debris as possible. Do not flush debris into the coelom and be extremely careful not to drown the patient by flushing fluid into the lungs. Even when dealing with aquatic species, do not place the patient back into water; these patients must be dry-docked, and additional fluid support must be part of the treatment plan.[18] While the chelonian is being stabilized and awaiting surgery, maintain a moistened sterile bandage to protect exposed bone and tissue. It is not necessary to place a patch or apply a fixation device in an emergency setting.

Focus on keeping the wounds clean and stabilizing the patient. Once the patient is stable, more definitive wound care and/or surgical fixation can be attempted. There are several excellent resources available for this type of procedure.[18–20]

If the patient is concurrently displaying neurologic signs, that is, the patient is unable to ambulate normally, rule out the possibility of back or pelvic fracture with radiography. If none is evident, warn owners that full return to function, if possible, can take anywhere from 6 to 12 months (or longer).[18,21]

In general, shell fractures carry an excellent prognosis, particularly if there is no spinal involvement and the fractures do not expose the coelomic cavity. When the pelvis or spine is involved, or where there are multiple fracture sites, including trauma and contamination of the coelomic cavity, the prognosis is much more guarded.[22]

Dystocia

Dystocia is often seen in relation to improper husbandry and dietary deficiencies. Difficulty ovipositing can be due to a lack of appropriate nesting space, lack of access to water, improper temperatures, lack of appropriate calcification of the egg, and weakness of the animal (hypocalcemia).[16]

In most instances of dystocia, decreased stool production and anorexia are frequently reported. In the case of bright, alert, and active patients, dystocia may not be a true emergency. However, if the reptile is presenting depressed and lethargic, the situation is likely emergent and requires immediate intervention.

Gentle palpation of the coelomic cavity or prefemoral fossa in chelonians may reveal the presence of ova or follicles. Radiographs or ultrasound is a more definitive way to determine if the reproductive stage is preovulatory (developing follicles), or postovulatory (shelled eggs/fetuses) (**Figs. 1** and **2**).[17] On radiographs, follicles will appear soft-tissue dense, and in these cases, ultrasound may be more helpful.[23]

Ultrasound is an important tool when investigating dystocia cases. The presence of fluid and uniformity of follicles should be noted. Fluid may suggest coelomitis, especially if it is flocculent.[24] Aspirates may be performed for cytology and culture. Variation in the appearance of follicles suggests that there may be a pathologic process occurring. These cases require supportive care and antibiotics due to concern for sepsis. Depressed, lethargic reptiles with coelomic/follicular abnormalities may require emergency surgery to undergo an ovariectomy ± salpingohysterectomy.[25] Blood culture, CBC, and chemistry panel are also useful in assessing the health status of the patient.

When reproductive activity occurs, and there is a history of insufficient husbandry, it is not uncommon for a female reptile to also exhibit signs of hypocalcemia due to the body's demand for calcium during egg production.[17] These signs can include weakness, muscle fasciculation, pathologic fractures, or even seizures, depending on the severity of the hypocalcemia. An ionized calcium level can quickly diagnose this problem. In healthy iguanas, mean ionized calcium concentration in blood is 1.47 ± 0.105 mmol/L.[26] Ionized calcium concentration in captive tortoises is 1.9 mmol/L.[27] In the case of dystocia with severe hypocalcemia, immediate correction of temperature, hydration, calcium, and electrolytes is required (see later section on renal failure).

Fractures (Pathologic vs Traumatic)

If fractures are present, a detailed history is important to help determine if the fracture is pathologic (generally secondary to husbandry deficiencies) or if it is traumatically induced.

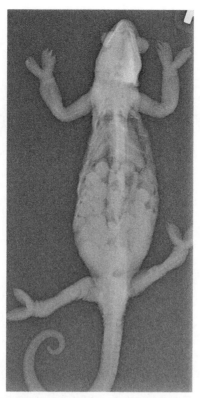

Fig. 1. Dorsoventral radiograph of a veiled chameleon (*Chamaeleo calyptratus*) with dystocia. Note follicles in the coelom, and pathologic fractures on long bones.

Radiographs are used to characterize the nature of the fracture and assess for the presence of bone loss. Radiographs can also reveal angular deformities of the long bones (more common in lizards), because these may influence clinical decisions on how best to address the fracture.[28] A chemistry panel and ionized calcium level should be used to determine the reptile's calcium status.

If the animal's bones appear to have appropriate bone density, and calcium levels are normal on blood work, fixation of the fracture can be performed via surgical techniques or external coaptation, once the patient is deemed stable for surgery.[29] Limb fractures may be stabilized in lizards by securing the limbs caudally along the body (thoracic limbs) or tail (pelvic limb). Chelonian limb fractures may be stabilized in some cases by returning the limb to its flexed position within the shell and using tape to prevent extension. Strict cage rest and analgesia should be provided in conjunction with any fixation technique.

If the bone density is decreased, even a light splint can lead to the development of further pathologic fractures at the fulcrum of the splint. Strict cage rest, analgesia, and supportive care, including hand feeding and calcium supplementation, are often the most appropriate recommendation in these cases.

Gastrointestinal Presentations

Reptiles with GI-related emergencies often present for regurgitation, vomiting, constipation, and inappetence.[17] GI issues can stem from primary GI disease,

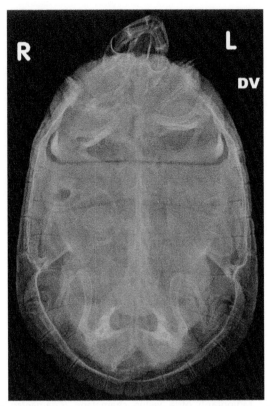

Fig. 2. African side-necked turtle (*Pelusios sinuatus*) dystocia. Note poorly calcified eggs in the coelom.

including infection, foreign body, neoplasia, torsion, or obstruction; or secondary causes, including metabolic disorders, dehydration, cardiac disease, neoplasia, and ovostasis. Workup for ovostasis is discussed in more detail in the dystocia section.

Physical examination may reveal the presence of ingested foreign bodies, presence of eggs or follicles, large amounts of gas within the GI tract, constipated feces, or obstruction. Both lizards and chelonians frequently ingest particulate substrates, which may be palpable within the digestive tract (**Fig. 3**). The likelihood of substrate consumption increases when the reptile is fed directly on the substrate in question (**Figs. 4** and **5**). Large boids have been reported to actually eat towels when consuming prey items.[16] Foreign body ingestion in snakes can cause the same kinds of severe complications as seen with other species, including complete obstruction of the GI tract, ulceration, or perforation, leading to life-threatening peritonitis.

Methods of feeding can also affect a reptile's ability to appropriately digest their diet. For example, feeding multiple prey items simultaneously can cause obstruction of the GI tract, and inappropriate owner handling after eating can cause regurgitation (**Fig. 6**).[16]

Chronic dehydration can cause constipation in all species (**Fig. 7**). Bearded dragons suffering from chronic dehydration can form large urate plugs that physically block feces from exiting. These plugs can usually be removed with soaking followed by gentle probing and manipulation of the plug out of the rectum.

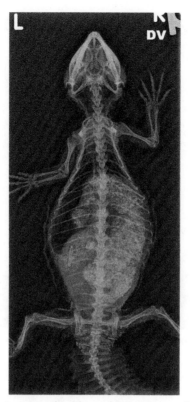

Fig. 3. Uromastyx (*Uromastyx ornata*) with sand impaction and several mineral dense GI foreign bodies in GI tract.

Organ enlargement can lead to narrowing of the intestinal lumen, causing signs of constipation. In snakes, this can be secondary to enlarged ovaries/testes or kidneys. This narrowing can also be seen in lizards with kidney enlargement, because the kidneys lie within the pelvic canal. Clinically, this can present as straining during defecation, or sometimes, a complete blockage of the GI tract.[30]

Rarely, palatability of the ingested item can cause snakes to violently heave and regurgitate (Music, personal observation, 2014); this has been noted in the clinical setting after oral administration of metronidazole and lactulose.

Diagnosis heavily depends on a detailed history as well as a thorough coelomic palpation. If substrate has been ingested, it may be palpable within the digestive tract. Radiographs, both with and without contrast, are also a helpful indicator of the underlying issue. A fecal examination should also be performed, including a direct (wet mount) and float.[31] A certain level of parasites is not uncommon in most reptile species. However, it is important to be familiar with what constitutes a "normal" parasitic load in a reptilian GI tract versus a population of parasites that may actually cause a problem.[31] Routine hematology and chemistry panel is helpful in order to determine if antibiotics are warranted, and if there are any other concurrent underlying issues that may be causing or contributing to this clinical presentation.

Often, medical management is sufficient to resolve the issue, including subcutaneous fluids, increasing soaking frequency, oral hydration, laxatives, coelomic massage,

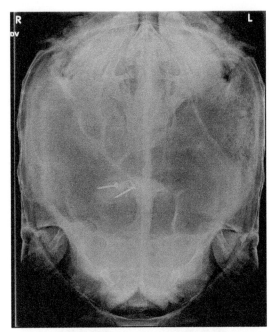

Fig. 4. Sulcata tortoise (*Centrochelys sulcata*) foreign bodies identified on radiographs.

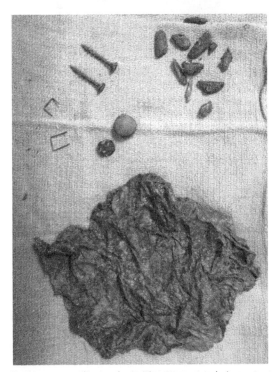

Fig. 5. Foreign bodies seen on radiographs in **Fig. 4**, removed via gastrotomy. 2 nails, 2 staples, wood chips, pebbles, and large cloth foreign body were removed.

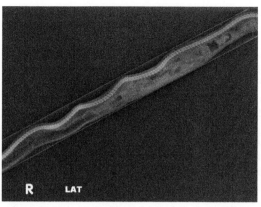

Fig. 6. Amethystine python (*Morelia amethistina*) with multiple impacted prey items.

and enemas.[16] Cooling of reptiles has also been described in an attempt to cause regurgitation of a large foreign body that would have otherwise required surgical removal, although the authors have not used this technique.[32]

In chelonian species with anorexia, an esophageal tube may need to be placed, to allow feeding of an appropriate critical care diet. The tube can be maintained in place for several months and is similar to placement of a tube within a dog or cat. This tube placement has been detailed in other texts.[12,33] Key differences in the placement include entry of the tube in the mid to lower cervical esophagus compared with the upper esophagus or pharyngeal region in the mammalian patient.[34] Also, remember to test the formula before placing the tube, to ensure that the tube diameter is sufficient to allow passage of the diet. The tube is secured using butterfly tape tabs, purse-string, and/or Chinese finger lock and can remain in place for several months until the patient is eating normally on their own.[18,34]

It is always important to set accurate expectations for the owner as far as how long resolution can take. In cases of severe constipation, a medical management approach can take several weeks before full evacuation of the bowels is seen and the patient is eating normally again. In unremitting cases, a surgical approach may be needed to resolve the issue. However, please note that if obstipation has been present for too long, surgical correction may not be able to resolve the problem, due to permanent stretching of the bowel walls.

Neurologic Presentations

Ataxia, paresis, and seizures are common reptile emergency presentations. Other presentations that may not immediately appear to be primary neurologic issues include general lethargy and depression.

Differentials include hypocalcemia related to Nutritional Secondary Hyperparathyroidism (from chronic inappropriate husbandry leading to dietary imbalances),

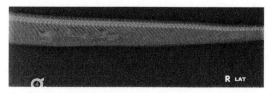

Fig. 7. Ball python (*P regius*) with constipation secondary to chronic dehydration.

reproductive activity, toxin exposure (particularly in the event of recent environmental parasitic treatments), infection, parasitic infestation, metabolic disorders (liver or kidney disease), and neoplasia.[17,35]

Diagnosis starts with obtaining a complete history with detailed information on husbandry. After the physical examination, the diagnostic workup should include a chemistry panel, ideally run concurrently with an ionized calcium level. Additional tests include a CBC, as well as fecal analysis, radiographs, and blood culture as warranted by the history and physical examination findings.

Treatments may include injectable and oral calcium supplementation, antibiotics, parasite treatment, correcting metabolic imbalances, and addressing organ dysfunction. If initial diagnostics do not reveal a cause for the clinical signs, more advanced diagnostics are warranted, including computed tomography (CT) or MRI.[36]

Nutritional Secondary Hyperparathyroidism (Commonly Referred to as "Metabolic Bone Disease")

Nutritional secondary hyperparathyroidism occurs when there is an imbalance of calcium, phosphorus, and vitamin D_3 in a reptile. Imbalances often result from improper husbandry, diet, and/or organ dysfunction. (Renal secondary hyperparathyroidism, a common concurrent issue, is discussed later in this article.) It can result in the types of common clinical signs that trigger an owner to bring their reptile in, including anorexia, lethargy, swollen eyes, pathologic fractures, thickening of the digits, limbs, and mandible (fibrous osteodystrophy).[12]

It is important to obtain a thorough, detailed history in order to spot gaps in husbandry, including, but not limited to: lack of ultraviolet B radiation, low temperatures, and nutritional deficiencies (inadequate calcium supplementation, inappropriate diet, or lack of gut loading prey).[17] An important piece of history is to know the reproductive status of the animal in question.[17,23,37] Remember that although diagnostic testing is undertaken to ascertain the extent of disease present, the owner must also be educated so they can properly address any husbandry deficits.

Important diagnostics include a chemistry panel and ionized calcium. Radiographs should be performed to assess bone density and to check for pathologic fractures. Concurrent infections can also be seen in cases with a severely compromised reptile. A CBC ± a blood culture may be warranted depending on the clinical assessment.

Treatment of this condition should concentrate on correcting husbandry deficiencies: correcting hydration, calcium supplementation, and attending to any concurrent underlying medical issues.

Although these cases may present on emergency, it is important that owners are given a clear indication of how long resolution of signs can take. Also include in the discussion that full resolution of symptoms may not necessarily be possible. It can be difficult to convey to an owner that mistakes made in the reptile's husbandry from years ago can still be affecting their adult animal, or that even a short period of inadequate husbandry in a young reptile may also have caused life-long problems.

Ocular Presentations

There are many ocular conditions that may present on emergency, though trauma is one of the most common (**Table 3**). Depending on the species of reptile, injuries to the eye can involve the spectacle (as in snakes and lizards with spectacles), or can be directly related to the cornea (lizards without spectacles and chelonians).[38] Specific findings can include pus beneath the surface of the spectacle (subspectacular abscess), anterior uveitis, buildup of debris under the lids (shed skin, purulent debris, substrate), corneal ulceration, and more. Damage may occur when a naturally wrinkled spectacle (seen in many wild-type ball pythons [*Python regius*]) is mistaken as a "retained spectacle." Aggressive debridement, or repeated attempts to remove the spectacle, can cause pain, scarring, or even globe rupture depending on level of trauma. Trauma may also be induced from a prey item, foreign bodies, and so forth.[38]

In general, diagnostic testing to help understand and treat the issues in the reptile eye includes the same basic testing that is recommended for mammalian patients: fluorescein staining, cytology/culture of any debris, or culture of material aspirated from the anterior chamber (under sedation), hematology, and chemistry panel.

Treatment includes both topical and systemic medication, supportive nutritional care in the case of dietary deficiencies, and analgesia as needed.[39]

Extensive discussion with and education of the client are also warranted, to ensure that any husbandry deficits are corrected immediately.

Prolapse

A cloacal prolapse of the snake, lizard, or chelonian is an emergency and should be seen immediately. Prolapses of the cloaca can be related to the reproductive, urinary, or GI systems.[17] It is important to identify which structures have actually prolapsed, in order to best plan how to replace them and help determine the underlying cause (**Table 4**). However, if the structures have been prolapsed for an extended period of time, tissue necrosis and devitalization may make identification difficult.

Prolapses can occur secondary to any underlying cause of excessive straining, such as egg binding/dystocia, hypocalcemia, urolithiasis, gastrointestinal disease (infection, impaction, parasitism, etc.), intracoelomic disease/mass, organ dysfunction, poor husbandry, and neoplasia. Routine hematology, chemistry panel, ionized calcium, radiographs, ultrasound, and fecal analysis are all important diagnostics to consider when dealing with a prolapse. The owner must be made aware the replacement of the prolapse is not a permanent solution if the underlying cause has not been identified and addressed.[11,17,23,40]

The tissues may be heavily engorged and turgid on presentation. Placing the reptile into a shallow bath of a saturated sugar solution for 20 to 30 minutes can help to decrease swelling of the tissues prior to attempting replacement. A sugar pack (granulated sugar mixed with water-based lubricant, like Surgilube (Savage Laboratories, Melville, NY)), held in place with Tegaderm Film (3M Health Care, St. Paul, MN), is also useful to help reduce swelling.

Once swelling has been reduced, gently manipulate the tissue back into its normal anatomic position using copious amounts of lubrication. Consider sedation or anesthesia before replacement of the prolapse. A conscious animal may struggle or strain against the replacement, causing itself damage, and re-prolapse of the tissue. This tissue is often extremely friable and must be handled with care. It is important to evenly apply pressure with probes, fingers, or cotton tipped applicators by using the largest surface area possible to place gentle pressure on the tissue, to avoid causing punctures.[11,23]

Sutures are placed to keep the replaced prolapsed tissue in place. Other surgical approaches may be required to replace tissue that will not return back through the vent. Detailed descriptions of this procedure may be found in other texts, but in general, placing 2 interrupted sutures on each side of the vent (perpendicular to the vent opening) is helpful in snakes and lizards. Chelonians have a more round vent opening; therefore, a purse-string suture to help decrease the diameter of the vent

Table 3
Common ocular presentations

Presentation	Species	Differential Diagnosis/Etiology	Treatments/Supportive Care	Additional Notes
Anterior uveitis (flare, hypopyon, hyphema), may be associated with conjunctivitis, episcleral injection	All	Infection (local or systemic), trauma, neoplasia; hypopyon may be present in chelonians after exposure to freezing temperatures	Antimicrobials, anti-inflammatories, correct husbandry	CBC and blood culture; consider aspirate of anterior chamber under anesthesia for culture
Corneal disease (corneal opacity, ulceration, debris in conjunctival sac); may be associated with discharge, blepharospasm, periocular swelling	Reptiles without spectacles	Trauma (including substrate, presence of retained shed within the conjunctival sac); infection (may lead to accumulations of purulent debris in conjunctival sac)	Copious lavage to remove debris, topical +/− systemic antimicrobials, non steroidal anti-inflammatories, lubricants, adjust husbandry (i.e. remove particulate substrate if cause of signs)	Fluorescein staining needed to assess cornea
Episcleral injection	Species with visible sclera	Suggests sepsis; distinguish from red color seen in some varanid lizard species	Assess for underlying systemic infection (hematology, blood culture) and treat with appropriate antimicrobials	Authors see this most commonly in green iguanas (Iguana iguana)
Ocular discharge	Leopard geckos (Eublepharis macularius)	Vitamin A deficiency, blocked nasolacrimal duct, infection	Vitamin A supplementation; Additional supportive care as warranted by presentation	May see concurrent hemipenal plugs or dysecdysis
Periocular swelling +/− discharge, conjunctival hyperemia, blepharospasm	Reptiles without spectacles	Vitamin A deficiency, infection (local vs. systemic), trauma/presence of substrate, parasites, neoplasia; Chelonians: primary respiratory pathogen (mycoplasma vs herpes vs other); may be accompanied by nasal discharge	Flush to remove any possible debris, address husbandry deficiencies, treat according to results of testing with antimicrobials, supportive care/nutrition, antiparasitic medications, etc.	Chelonians: if mycoplasma confirmed, look for other underlying disease processes (i.e. liver, reproductive, kidney disease)

Retained spectacle (tends to have thickened appearance with rough edges)	Reptiles with spectacles	Inadequate humidity or availability to soak, presence of mites (Ophionyssus natricis); distinguish from wild type ball pythons (Python regius) that may have a mild wrinkled appearance to the spectacles	Soak multiple times then gently attempt debridement with cotton tipped applicators	Attempting to remove adherent spectacles with forceps may lead to severe trauma to the underlying spectacle
Spectacle opacity	Reptiles with spectacles	White or blue coloration present prior to ecdysis, dark pigmentation may be present secondary to prior trauma	No treatment necessary	Avoid handling snakes prior to ecdysis to prevent damage to newly developing skin and subsequent dysecdysis
Spectacle swelling/ bulging	Reptiles with spectacles	Bullous spectaculopathy (pseudobuphthalmos) – if fluid behind spectacle is clear (obstructed nasolacrimal duct; rule out local vs. systemic infection, congenital obstruction) Subspectacular abscess – if fluid behind spectacle is opaque white/ yellow (rule out local vs. systemic infection)	Provide appropriate systemic antimicrobials, non steroidal anti-inflammatories, analgesics	CBC, blood culture, aspirate subspectacular space under sedation/ anesthesia for culture; look for stomatitis that could be contributing to nasolacrimal duct obstruction May require surgical wedge resection of spectacle for drainage
Trauma to globe (from prey)	Snakes and live rodent eaters	Diagnose based on history	Symptomatic care including topical +/- systemic antimicrobials, non steroidal antiinflammatories, analgesics	Enucleation may be necessary depending on extent of lesions

Data from Refs.[38,39,53]

Table 4
Different kinds of vent prolapses

Structures Prolapsed from the Vent	Characteristics	How to Identify	Note
Hemipenis/phallus	Can range in color from pink to red to black. No lumen opening present	Lizards and snakes may have one or both prolapsed, noted to extend from caudal aspect of vent. A chelonian phallus extends from cranially within the ventral aspect of the cloaca. A lubricated probe will reach a blind end ventrally and pass easily dorsal to a prolapsed phallus	If the structures have been prolapsed for an extended period of time, identification may not be possible. Hemipenal plugs of waxy material may protrude from vent opening and appear to be a prolapse
Salpinx prolapse	Tubular with a lumen opening present at its distal extent; striated longitudinally	A probe may stop lateral to the prolapsed tissue on the side from which the salpinx originates. The probe will extend medial to the salpinx. May be difficult to differentiate from GI tract. Radiographs or ultrasound demonstrating eggs or follicles may suggest that the salpinx is the prolapsed tissue.	
Rectal/colon prolapse	Tubular with a lumen opening at its distal extend; smooth surface, may be very edematous	Probing similar to evaluating a prolapse in mammals. If the prolapse originates from the cloaca or distal rectum, a probe will stop on all sides. A probe placed within the lumen will continue to pass	
Urinary Bladder prolapse	Fluid-filled sac, if ruptured, is thin, ragged; no lumen opening present	If fluid filled, will be evident; otherwise can be very difficult to identify	

Adapted from Hernandez-Divers SJ. Diagnostic techniques. In: Mader DR, Divers SJ, editors. Reptile medicine and surgery. 2nd edition. St. Louis: Saunders Elsevier; 2006; and McArthur S. Problem-solving approach to common diseases of terrestrial and semi-aquatic chelonians. In: McArthur S, WR, Meyer J, editors. Medicine and surgery of tortoises and turtles. Oxford: Blackwell; 2004.

opening may be more appropriate. If a phallus or hemipene is too traumatized or necrotic, it may require surgical removal, which will not impact the ability to urinate.

Chameleon patients may present with tongue prolapses. These prolapses are usually secondary to hypocalcemia. Reduction is very difficult, and treatment is generally amputation; special care is required to facilitate feeding for the rest of the chameleon's life.[41]

Renal Failure

Reptiles with renal failure may present on emergency for lethargy and anorexia. With iguanas, rectal examination may reveal a decrease in the diameter of the pelvic canal from renomegaly.[11] Very large kidneys may extend cranially from the pelvic inlet and be palpable on coelomic examination. In some cases, the enlarged kidney may actually be seen as a bulge along the lateral aspect of the coelom when seen from above. Kidneys are palpable within the pelvic canal at 10 and 2 o'clock, while the patient is standing in normal ventral recumbency. Marked renomegaly may occlude part or the entire distal colon and can cause constipation and obstipation in extreme cases.[30]

Kidney disease can result from several potential causes, including but not limited to chronic dehydration, improper diet (vitamin A deficient, high levels of protein), infection (bacterial or viral, including inclusion body disease), trauma, and fibrosis.[4,42] A chemistry panel and ionized calcium are important for diagnosis, and hematology is important to evaluate for underlying infection. Ultrasound and radiographs may also be useful for diagnosis of kidney disease.[24,28] Urinalysis in reptiles is described; however, renal function may not be accurately represented due to changes that occur within the bladder.[43]

A chemistry panel may reveal elevated uric acid, a calcium:phosphorous imbalance, elevated phosphorus alone, and in at least one case, hyperkalemia.[16,44,45] Hypocalcemia can result in seizures and muscle fasciculation and must be addressed immediately.

Emergency treatment of renal failure should include fluid therapy and nutritional support. Severe cases should receive IV or IO fluid therapy and hospitalization. Correction of diet and husbandry is also required. Phosphate binders and oral and injectable calcium supplementation should be considered in individual cases, ideally based on ionized calcium levels. Detailed protocols for renal failure treatment are beyond the scope of this article. The practitioner is advised to review renal failure treatment in other sources if the clinical presentation supports this diagnosis.[16,44,45]

Respiratory Presentations

Dyspnea must be differentiated from aggressive, open-mouthed posturing of animals. However, when an open mouth is accompanied with increased respiratory rate and effort, it is likely that there is a pathologic reason for the presentation. Snakes will often hold themselves vertically, along the sides of the enclosure, exhibiting increased respiratory rate and effort.

Differentials include poor husbandry with inappropriate ventilation, infectious (bacterial, viral, fungal, or parasitic causes), intracoleomic space-occupying masses (follicles, eggs, organomegaly), and neoplasia.[46]

Radiographs and blood work should be performed to try to help to determine the underlying cause of the respiratory symptoms. In chelonians, 3 radiographic views should be taken: (1) a dorsoventral view; (2) a standing, horizontal beam lateral view (to avoid organ shifting if the patient is placed on its side); and (3) a standing anterior-posterior view of the chelonian. All 3 views will allow full assessment of the chelonian respiratory tract, including any asymmetry of right and left lung fields. CT is a more accurate imaging tool for the reptile respiratory system, if available.

If pneumonia is suspected, the best way to diagnose the etiologic agent is via tracheal lavage for cytology and culture and sensitivity.[9]

Treatment includes antibiotic therapy for pneumonia, and as warranted by other diagnostics. Keep in mind that oxygen therapy may not be appropriate for a reptile with severe pulmonary disease. Stimulus for reptile ventilation is not an increase in carbon dioxide (Pco_2) as with mammals and avian patients, but a decrease of blood oxygen concentration. An oxygen-rich environment can actually suppress spontaneous respiration in a reptile.[47] In a situation where hypoxemia is suspected, oxygen may be administered, but the patient may need to be sedated and placed on a ventilator, or have intermittent positive pressure ventilation administered until the hypoxemia has been resolved.[47]

Thermal Burns

Reptile burns are a commonly presented emergency. Ventral burns can occur if a reptile has been resting on a heat source. Dorsal burns occur when the reptile has been basking too close to a heat source placed above the patient. Burns can occur when the heat source malfunctions, if there is not enough insulation over an under tank heater, if it is too powerful for the enclosure size, or if a heat source fails. Burns can present in 3 different ways: (1) first-degree (superficial or partial thickness), (2) second-degree (deeper partial thickness), or (3) third-degree (full thickness) (**Table 5**).[16,48]

Fluid support is critical when treating burn patients because of the fluid that is lost from the oozing wounds. In an emergency, collect a swab for culture, then clean the wounds using dilute iodine or dilute 2% chlorhexidine gluconate. Silver sulfadiazine 1% cream (Ascend Laboratories, LLC, Montvale, NJ) is an excellent topical choice after the wound has been thoroughly cleaned. To keep the ointment in place,

Table 5
Types of thermal burns

Category	Anatomy	Clinical Appearance	Time to Heal	Notes
First-degree (superficial or partial thickness)	Epidermis	Erythema, pain, wrinkling	Approximately 1 mo with ideal husbandry	—
Second-degree (deeper partial thickness)	Extending into middermis	Blisters, plasma ooze ± crust	>1 mo, variable	—
Third-degree (full thickness)	—	Dry/black ecshar or underlying muscle exposed	>1 mo, variable	Less common, less painful (nerves destroyed) "Fourth-degree" burns are third-degree burns that are full thickness and affect muscle and bones as well; this has a grave prognosis

Data from Boyer DH. Emergency care of reptiles. Vet Clin North Am Exot Anim Pract 1998;1(1):191–206, vii; and Mader DR. Thermal burns. In: Mader DR, Divers SJ, editors. Current therapy in reptile medicine and surgery. 2nd edition. Philadelphia: Elsevier; 2014.

Tegaderm Film (3M Health Care, St. Paul, MN) can be used to wrap the wound site. Elastikon elastic tape (Johnson and Johnson, New Brunswick, NH) can also be used to help keep the dressing in place. Bandages should be changed every 1 to 2 days, being careful not to cause additional trauma when removing bandages. After healing has progressed and there is a clear delineation between necrotic and live tissue, the burn area should be debrided under sedation. Healing will progress dramatically through each shed; however, full-thickness burns can take months before full resolution of the burn is achieved.[16] Treatment should also include systemic antibiotics.[4]

Keep in mind that burns can look very similar to septic changes (erythema and blistering) seen on the integument of reptiles.[4] Hematology will help when trying to distinguish between them by showing acute versus chronic changes, toxic change to the cells, and so on.

Sepsis

Sepsis is often seen secondary to inadequate husbandry. Clinical signs of sepsis include lethargy, anorexia, petechiation, episcleral injection, stomatitis, ventral erythema (snakes), skin sloughing, and seizures.[17,49] Chelonian sepsis can result in superficial to deep abscessation, known as septicemic cutaneous ulcerative dermatitis, or "shell rot."[50]

Diagnosing sepsis should include hematology, blood culture, and sensitivity before antibiotic administration, culture and sensitivity of any cutaneous or oral lesions, ± radiographs when osteomyelitis is suspected. A chemistry panel should be performed to evaluate organ function and electrolyte abnormalities.[4]

Treatment should be based on culture and sensitivity, if possible, and the spectrum should include wide coverage of gram-negative, anaerobic bacteria. Enrofloxacin has been long considered a "go-to" drug for the exotics practitioner, but repeat injections cause painful muscle necrosis, and the spectrum of coverage does not include anaerobes. Ceftazidime, 20 mg/kg intramuscularly (IM) every 72 hours, is a good choice for antibiotic coverage because of its less frequent dosage, relative lack of nephrotoxicity, broad anaerobic spectrum, and specific antipseudomonal coverage.[8]

Euthanasia

Euthanasia is a difficult decision for any reptile owner to make. Many owners want to be present for the passing of their animal, and this can be intimidating if reptile euthanasia has never been performed before. The authors prefer a "2-stage" approach to euthanasia. This 2-stage approach allows for the attached owner to be present during the initial stages of unconsciousness and be able to say their goodbyes in a meaningful way. Simultaneously, the reptile receives sedation and anesthesia, ensuring a humane passing.

"Two-stage" euthanasia entails first deeply sedating/anesthetizing the reptile patient using a combination of agents like tiletamine-zolazepam, butorphanol, and dexmedetomidine, or high doses of ketamine, dexmedetomidine, and midazolam.[51,52] Both options allow for IM administration, which is ideal for dehydrated or fractious patients, or for those with inaccessible peripheral veins. Warn owners before administration that the injection may sting. Once the combination has been given, the animal can remain with the owner, providing time for good-byes to be said.

When the owner is ready, and the reptile is completely nonresponsive, the euthanasia solution can be delivered directly via an intracardiac, IV, intracoelomic, or intracranial injection. Determination of death may be difficult, and pithing or freezing the patient should be considered once the heartbeat is no longer discernable.[51]

Carriage Return

It is very important to ensure that the reptile is supplied with heat support during the entire euthanasia process. Maintaining an appropriate body temperature allows for more predictable absorption and metabolism of the sedation agents and euthanasia solution. Without thermal support, the euthanasia process will likely be prolonged.

SUMMARY

When addressing a reptile emergency, remember that in general, safe, helpful medical practices are comparable across species. Hemostasis, thermal, nutritional, and fluid support, in particular, should always be addressed. From there, successful reptile medicine heavily depends on one's familiarity with different species husbandry and diet requirements. Helpful aids include *Carpenter's Formulary* (4th edition) to determine safe drug doses, and *Mader's Reptile Medicine and Surgery*, as well as the more recent *Current Therapies*, and should be part of the library of any practice that sees exotic species.

REFERENCES

1. Divers SJ. Clinical evaluation of reptiles. Vet Clin North Am Exot Anim Pract 1999; 2(2):291–331.
2. Bennet RA, Mehler SJ. Neurology. In: Mader DR, Divers SJ, editors. Reptile medicine and surgery. 2nd edition. St. Louis (MO): Elsevier; 2006. p. 239–50.
3. Funk RS. Snakes. In: Mader DR, Divers SJ, editors. Reptile medicine and surgery. 2nd edition. St. Louis (MO): Elsevier; 2006. p. 42–58.
4. James FX, Wellehan D, Cornelia I, et al. Emergent diseases in reptiles. Semin Avian Exotic Pet Med 2004;13(3):160–74.
5. Heard DJ. Critical care monitoring. Vet Clin North Am Exot Anim Pract 1998; 1(1):1–10.
6. Harr K. Reptile Cytology Masterclass. Proceedings of ExoticsCon 2015. San Antonio, Texas, August 29 - September 2, 2015.
7. Mayer J, Knoll J, Wrubel KM, et al. Characterizing the hematologic and plasma chemistry profiles of captive crested geckos (Rhacodactylus ciliatus). J Herpetol Med Surg 2011;21(2–3):68–75.
8. Gibbons PM. Reptiles. In: Carpenter JW, editor. Exotic animal formulary. 4th edition. St. Louis: Elsevier; 2013. p. 84–182.
9. de la Navarre D. Common procedures in reptiles and amphibians. Vet Clin North Am Exot Anim Pract 2006;9:237–67.
10. Hernandez-Divers SM. Reptile critical care in emergency practice. International Veterinary Emergency and Critical Care Symposium. Atlanta, GA, September 7–11, 2005.
11. Hernandez-Divers SJ. Diagnostic techniques. In: Mader DR, Divers SJ, editors. Reptile medicine and surgery. 2nd edition. St. Louis (MO): Elsevier; 2006. p. 490–532.
12. Donoghue S. Nutrition. In: Mader DR, Divers SJ, editors. Reptile medicine and surgery. 2nd edition. St. Louis (MO): Elsevier; 2006. p. 251–98.
13. Gibbons PM. Fluid therapy and transfusion medicine in reptiles. Proceedings of PacVet. San Diego, CA, June 19 - 22, 2014.
14. Prezant RM, Jarchow JL. Lactated fluid use in reptiles: is there a better solution? Proceedings of the Association of Reptilian and Amphibian Veterinarians Annual Conference. Houston, TX, October 26–30, 1997. p. 83–7.

15. Heard DJ. Reptile anesthesia. Vet Clin North Am Exot Anim Pract 2001;4(1): 83–117.
16. Boyer DH. Emergency care of reptiles. Vet Clin North Am Exot Anim Pract 1998; 1(1):191–206, vii.
17. Martinez-Jimenez D, Hernandez-Divers SJ. Emergency care of reptiles. Vet Clin North Am Exot Anim Pract 2007;10:557–85.
18. Barbara B, Bonner BB. Chelonian therapeutics. Vet Clin North Am Exot Anim Pract 2000;3(1):257–332.
19. Mitchell M. Diagnosis and management of reptile orthopedic injuries. Vet Clin North Am Exot Anim Pract 2002;5:97–114.
20. McArthur S, Hernandez-Divers S. Surgery. In: McArthur S, Wilkinson R, Meyer J, editors. Medicine and Surgery of Tortoises and Turtles. Blackwell: Oxford; 2004.
21. Mitchell MA, Diaz-Figueroa O. Wound management in reptiles. Vet Clin North Am Exot Anim Pract 2004;7:123–40.
22. Gregory J, Fleming D. Clinical technique: chelonian shell repair. Journal of Exotic Pet Med 2008;17(4):246–58.
23. McArthur S. Problem-solving approach to common diseases of terrestrial and semi-aquatic chelonians. In: McArthur S, Wilkinson R, Meyer J, editors. Medicine and Surgery of Tortoises and Turtles. Blackwell: Oxford; 2004. p. 309–77.
24. Claudia Hochleithner MH. Ultrasonography. In: Mader DR, Divers SJ, editors. Current therapy in reptile medicine and surgery. St. Louis (MO): Elsevier; 2014. p. 107–27.
25. Denardo D. Dystocias. In: Mader DR, Divers SJ, editors. Reptile medicine and surgery. 2nd edition. St. Louis (MO): Elsevier; 2006. p. 376–90, 787–92.
26. Dennis PM, Bennett RA, Harr KE, et al. Plasma concentration of ionized calcium in healthy iguanas. J Am Vet Med Assoc 2001;219:326–8.
27. Eatwell K. Effects of storage and sample type on ionized calcium, sodium and potassium levels in captive tortoises., Testudo spp. J Herpetol Med Surg 2007; 17:84–91.
28. Silverman S. Diagnostic imaging. In: Mader DR, Divers SJ, editors. Reptile medicine and surgery. 2nd edition. St. Louis (MO): Elsevier; 2006. p. 471–89.
29. Mader D, Bennett RA, Funk RS, et al. Surgery. In: Mader D, editor. Reptile Medicine and Surgery. 2nd edition. St. Louis (MO): Elsevier; 2006. p. 581–630.
30. Barten SL. Lizards. In: Mader DR, Divers SJ, editors. Reptile medicine and surgery. 2nd edition. St. Louis (MO): Elsevier; 2006. p. 59–77.
31. Greiner EC, Mader D. Parasitology. In: Mader D, editor. Reptile Medicine and Surgery. 2nd edition. St. Louis (MO): Elsevier; 2006. p. 343–64.
32. Rossi J. Quick tips for 5 common reptile problems. Proceedings of North American Veterinary Conference 11:755. 1997.
33. McArthur S. Feeding Techniques and Fluids. In: McArthur S, Wilkinson R, Meyer J, editors. Medicine and Surgery of Tortoises and Turtles. Blackwell: Oxford; 2004. p. 257–72.
34. Norton TM. Chelonian emergency and critical care. Semin Avian Exotic Pet Med 2005;14(2):106–30.
35. Divers SJ. Reptile critical care. Exotic Dvm 2003;5(3):81–7.
36. Wyneken J. Computed Tomography and Magnetic Resonance Imaging. In: Mader D, Divers S, editors. Current Therapy in Reptile Medicine and Surgery. St. Louis (MO): Elsevier; 2014. p. 93–106.
37. McArthur S, Barrows M. Nutrition. In: McArthur S, Wilkinson R, Meyer J, editors. Medicine and Surgery of Tortoises and Turtles. Blackwell: Oxford; 2004. p. 73–85.

38. Lawton MPC. Reptilian ophthalmology. In: Mader DR, Divers SJ, editors. Reptile medicine and surgery. 2nd edition. St. Louis (MO): Elsevier; 2006. p. 323–42.

39. Wiggins TK, Guzman DS-M, Reilly CM. Prevalence and risk factor of ophthalmic disease in leopard geckos. Proceedings of ExoticsCon 2015. San Antonio, Texas, August 29 - September 2, 2015.

40. Denardo D. Reproductive biology. In: Mader DR, Divers SJ, editors. Reptile medicine and surgery. 2nd edition. St. Louis (MO): Elsevier; 2006. p. 376–90.

41. E Klaphake. Chameleon Medicine. Proceedings of ABVP, 2013.

42. Miller H. Urinary diseases of reptiles: pathophysiology and diagnosis. Semin Avian Exotic Pet Med 1998;7(2):93–103.

43. Zwart P. Urogenital system. In: Beyon PH, Lawton MPC, Cooper JE, editors. Manual of reptiles. Cheltenham: British Small Animal Veterinary Association; 1992. p. 117–27.

44. Campbell TW. Clinical pathology of reptiles. In: Mader DR, Divers SJ, editors. Reptile medicine and surgery. 2nd edition. St. Louis (MO): Elsevier; 2006. p. 453–70.

45. Wilkinson R. Clinical pathology. In: McArthur S, Wilkinson R, Meyer J, editors. Medicine and surgery of tortoises and turtles. Blackwell: Oxford; 2004. p. 141–86.

46. Corcoran M. Protozoan pulmonary disease in a carpet python. Proceedings of ExoticsCon 2015, San Antonio, Texas, August 29 - September 2, 2015.

47. Murray MJ. Cardiopulmonary anatomy and physiology. In: Mader DR, Divers SJ, editors. Reptile medicine and surgery. 2nd edition. St. Louis (MO): Elsevier; 2006. p. 124–262.

48. Mader DR. Thermal Burns. In: Mader DR, Divers SJ, editors. Reptile medicine and surgery. 2nd edition. St. Louis (MO): Elsevier; 2006. p. 916–23.

49. Mader DR. Emergency and critical care. In: Mader DR, Divers SJ, editors. Reptile medicine and surgery. 2nd edition. St. Louis (MO): Elsevier; 2006. p. 533–48.

50. Barten SL. Shell damage. In: Mader DR, Divers SJ, editors. Reptile medicine and surgery. 2nd edition. 2006. p. 893–99.

51. Mader DR. Euthanasia. In: Mader DR, Divers SJ, editors. Reptile medicine and surgery. 2nd edition. St. Louis (MO): Elsevier; 2006. p. 564–8.

52. Ko JC, Berman AG. Anesthesia in shelter medicine. Top Companion Anim Med 2010;25(2):92–7.

53. Williams DL. The reptile eye. Ophthalmology of exotic pets. John Wiley & Sons; 2012. p. 159–96.

Wildlife Emergency and Critical Care

Jennifer Riley, DVM[a],*, Heather Barron, DVM, DABVP–Avian[b]

KEYWORDS

- Wildlife • Critical care • Emergency • Avian • Reptile • Small mammal

KEY POINTS

- To treat wildlife patients, it is essential that veterinarians know how to properly handle and restrain common species.
- As in domestic species, physical examination, blood work, and knowledge of common conditions are important in making a diagnosis and properly treating a patient.
- Pain can be difficult to assess in wildlife patients, and analgesics have not been studied in many species; however, there are an increasing number of studies and resources to assist veterinarians.
- It is important that veterinarians are aware of state and federal laws that relate to wildlife.

BIRDS

Patient Assessment

A visual examination should be done before handling any wildlife patient. This provides the veterinarian with the opportunity to see how the animal is breathing; standing; holding its head, body, and appendages; and how it is behaving. In some cases, it may be appropriate to observe the animal in an enclosure where free movement or flight is possible and gait, fitness, and other behaviors can be more easily assessed. This observational period is a crucial part of the initial examination.

Equipment necessary for handling should be chosen based on the patient's size, behavior, defense tactics, and planned diagnostics. If diagnostics such as venipuncture or radiographs are planned, be sure that necessary items and appropriate caging are set up before restraining the patient. Handling should be done in close proximity to the caging when possible.

Sedation and Anesthesia

If an animal is believed to be medically stable, but appears psychologically stressed, time to relax, sedation, or anesthesia are reasonable options. In cases of extreme

The authors have nothing to disclose.
[a] Lion Country Safari, 2003 Lion Country Safari Road, Loxahatchee, FL 33470, USA; [b] Clinic for the Rehabilitation of Wildlife, 3883 Sanibel-Captiva Road, Sanibel, FL 33957, USA
* Corresponding author.
E-mail address: jlr233@cornell.edu

stress or excessive pain, anesthesia or sedation may be necessary for a complete physical examination and will provide a stress-free opportunity to do diagnostics such as blood work and radiographs.

Avian Handling and Restraint

Many birds can be restrained and handled with an appropriately sized towel. For raptors, in addition to towels, leather gloves of various sizes, lengths, and thickness should be used as a level of protection from talons. A hood or other covering can be used to calm any bird. Even when hooded, care should be taken to control the head of a raptor and its potentially damaging beak. Some raptors, once hooded, may become more manageable if cast on their backs. Longer gloves should be used for birds with hooked beaks, such as vultures and cormorants. Eye protection is important when handling birds with stabbing beaks, such as large egrets, herons, and anhingas. When in doubt, be safe and use all forms of personal protective equipment.

Birds housed in larger aviaries may require nets to assist in capture. Once caught in the net, towels can be used to get the patient in hand.

When handling any bird, be careful with the feathers to prevent damage and be sure to allow for proper breathing by not pushing down on the sternum with excessive force. In birds that lack nares, such as pelicans, make sure the restraint allows them to breathe through their mouths. Stressed or fractious birds may also benefit from anxiolytics, such as midazolam or diazepam, given before a full examination.

Physical Examination

The carrier should be examined once the bird is in hand to check for any signs of blood and to look at feces and urates for color, volume, and consistency. If you cannot get a weight in the carrier, it is important to get a weight as part of the initial examination. Weights are necessary in dosing medications and determining feeding and fluid requirements in addition to measuring success of treatment. Raptors and other potentially dangerous birds can most easily be weighed in a box or carrier, but also can be wrapped in a towel with only the feet out and easily accessible to gloved hands.

Early in the examination, assess the patient for signs of shock:

- Depression
- Cyanosis
- Tachycardia, which can progress to bradycardia as the bird decompensates
- Hypothermia

A basic neurologic examination also should be done on all patients to look for signs of head trauma or signs of paresis or paralysis. A full ophthalmologic examination is imperative. Continue by examining the ears, nares, and oral cavity of the bird looking for any abnormalities including blood or discharge of any type. Palpate all bones to identify fractures. In a bird that is not flying, radiographs can be very important, as coracoid fractures can be difficult or impossible to identify by palpation.

Basic Diagnostics

In a stable bird, it is acceptable to take up to 1% of body weight in blood for a minimum database and any additional diagnostics, such as testing for toxins or infectious diseases. Fecal examinations (directs, floats, Gram stains) also can be helpful, and should be done on any new patient, as heavy parasitic burdens may impede recovery.

Radiographs are a valuable diagnostic tool important for looking at anything from broken bones, to enlarged organs, to metal or other foreign bodies in the bird.

Depending on the patient's level of cooperation or current mental state, high-quality radiographs can be taken with minimal manual restraint, hoods, and good positioning. Anesthesia or chemical sedation is often necessary for radiographs, especially if looking at organ size and position or symmetry in smaller bones. Well-positioned radiographs with orthogonal views should be taken whenever possible.

Fluid Therapy

Assessing the animal's hydration status is the first step in formulating a fluid therapy plan (**Table 1**). Fluid therapy can be initiated based on the following guidelines:

Severe dehydration or shock warrants the use of intravenous (IV) or intraosseous (IO) fluid replacement. IV catheters are always preferred over IO catheters because of the potential complications that may arise from the latter. IV catheters are most commonly placed in the medial metatarsal, cutaneous ulnar, or jugular veins. IO catheters often require analgesics and a local anesthetic block to place. Placement of IO catheters can be most easily accomplished with the use of an appropriately sized spinal needle into the plucked and sterilely prepared distal ulna or proximal tibiotarsus. The catheter should then be secured with taping and bandaging of the leg or of the wing in a figure of 8. Remember that medications given parenterally in the caudal half of the body may be filtered through the renal portal system, which may impact choice of catheter site or drugs given.

Drugs Used in Avian Wildlife Patients

Pain can be very difficult to assess in wildlife patients, as they tend to be very stoic despite severe and painful injuries. In general, it is best to assume that anything expected to be painful in other species should be considered painful to the avian patient. Analgesics commonly used in avian patients are described further in (**Table 2**).

Table 1
Fluid therapy guidelines

Level of Dehydration	Clinical Signs	Fluid Therapy Recommendations
<5% dehydration	Bright and alert, normal skin turgor, normal capillary refill time, bird appears normal, assume some level of dehydration	Oral rehydration is appropriate, maintenance requirement is approximately 75–150 mL/kg/d
5%–10% dehydration	Loss of skin elasticity/tenting, slightly tacky mucous membranes, slow capillary refill time	Subcutaneous fluids may be appropriate, add deficit and ongoing losses to maintenance requirements and replace deficit over at least 24 h, consider IV/IO catheter placement
>10% dehydration	Wrinkled skin with significant loss of turgor, stringy saliva, dry feces and urates, lethargic, cool extremities, shock	IV or IO catheter placement, replace deficits and provide maintenance fluids, may require boluses of crystalloid or colloid fluids at, (10 mL/kg) supplemental electrolytes or glucose may be added depending on blood values

Abbreviations: IO, intraosseous; IV, intravenous.

Table 2
Analgesics commonly used in avian patients

Drug Type	Recommended Dose	Related Information	Side Effects
Nonsteroidal anti-inflammatory drugs			
Meloxicam	0.5–2 mg/kg PO, IM q12h[1,2]	• Make sure patient is well hydrated • Limit use to inflammatory phase • Carprofen, ketoprofen, piroxicam, and so forth, have been used, doses can be found in formularies	• Renal toxicity • Gastrointestinal ulceration
Opioids			
Butorphanol	1–4 mg/kg IM q1–3h[3–6]	No sedation and respiratory depression seen	• Bradycardia • Respiratory depression • GI side effects/ileus • Sedation
Buprenorphine	IM or SC[7,8] 0.1–0.6mg/kg IM or SC q6-12h	Analgesia slightly longer lasting than butorphanol	
Hydromorphone	0.1–0.6 mg/kg IM[9]	—	
Fentanyl	—	Used as injection, CRI, or transdermal patch[3,8,10]	
Tramadol	5–30 mg/kg PO q6–12h[11,12]	—	
Dissociatives			
Ketamine	5–10 mg/kg IM[13]	Used alone or in combination with other drugs (xylazine, diazepam)	—
GABA agonist			
Gabapentin	11–82 mg/kg q12h PO[14,15]	Heavy sedation at higher doses can be prevented by gradually increasing the dose	—

Abbreviations: CRI, continuous rate infusion; GABA, gamma aminobutyric acid; GI, gastrointestinal; IM, intramuscular; PO, by mouth; q, every; SC, subcutaneous.

Anxiolytics

Stress associated with hospitalization can cause abnormal behaviors that can be confused with pain or can augment pain signals in the patient. Many avian patients will benefit from anxiolytics, such as diazepam, while in the hospital, as they may make the patient more likely to self-feed, prevent abnormal behaviors, and aid in more rapid healing. A dose of 1 mg/kg diazepam was successful when used orally in the passerine Hawai'i 'amakihi[16] and the authors have used doses between 0.5 mg/kg and 2 mg/kg every 12 in various avian species.

Antibiotics

Antibiotic selection in birds is similar to any other animal. Bite wounds, hook wounds, and skin or fecal contamination are common in wildlife patients, and appropriate antibiotics should be chosen with this is mind. Doses and/or dose frequencies are often higher in birds than those used in mammals. There are many articles and formularies from which doses may be found or extrapolated.

Antifungals

Antifungals should be given to any bird with diagnosed fungal disease. The authors would also recommend considering giving antifungals prophylactically to ocean-dwelling birds such as loons, gannets, osprey, shorebirds, and some species of raptors. These birds would be less likely to encounter fungal organisms in the wild and have a lower resistance to opportunistic fungal infection than other species. *Aspergillus* spp. are the most common fungal organisms causing respiratory disease in wildlife patients, and itraconazole or voriconazole are the most common antifungal medications used to treat or prevent a fungal infection. In very severe cases, physical endoscopic debulking of a fungal granuloma may be required before treatment is attempted. Itraconazole doses as low as 5 mg/kg orally (PO) every 24 can be used prophylactically and treatment doses of 10 mg/kg PO every 12 to 24 are common. There is a fairly narrow safety margin with itraconazole and the dose should be lowered or divided if side effects such as anorexia or liver value changes are seen. Because of its hepatic metabolism and subsequent effects on the liver, urates from birds on itraconazole should be monitored closely for yellow or green color changes.

Candidiasis is another fungal infection that maybe seen in wild avian patients, particularly neonates. Its overgrowth in the gastrointestinal tract, particularly the crop, can cause regurgitation, delayed crop emptying, or anorexia. Nystatin is commonly used to treat this infection, and must make contact with the yeast directly, as it is not absorbed systemically. It is best given by mouth (not using a feeding tube, as the tube will bypass the area affected by the yeast) before feeding. Amphotericin B is another option for treatment of yeast. Appropriate doses for antifungal drugs can be found in formularies.

Supportive Care

Caging

The type of caging chosen should be suitable for the size and species being hospitalized. All caging should be easily cleaned and safe and comfortable for the patient. Birds that are able to perch should be provided with appropriately sized, clean perches. Pelagic birds that spend most of their time on the water should be provided with soft net bottoms to their cages or extra cushioning and frequent cleanings. Keeping human noise to a minimum and blocking visual stimulation with the use of a towel on the cage door will help manage patient stress.

More critical patients who cannot thermoregulate properly or who are having respiratory difficulty may require housing with oxygen and heat supplementation. Incubators and oxygen cages are appropriate in these cases.

Seabirds should be provided with a source of saltwater to prevent atrophy of the salt glands, which would put them at risk of severe dehydration and electrolyte imbalances on release.

Nutritional support

Patients should always be rehydrated and have a normal body temperature before feeding at the hospital. Emaciated patients should have food introduced even more slowly than birds that come in at a reasonably normal body condition. The natural response to seeing an emaciated bird is to feed it as much as possible as quickly as possible, but this can lead to refeeding syndrome.

The ultimate feeding goal is to have the bird maintain weight by self-feeding and ingesting whole food. Whole foods should be offered only once the patient is well hydrated and electrolyte abnormalities are resolved. In raptors, prey items may be easier to digest initially if skin or parts that are tougher to digest are removed at first. In birds with injuries, prey items may need to be cut into bite-sized pieces if their bandaging or specific injury make manipulating and tearing prey difficult. Once the animal is eating whole prey, it is important to check daily for casts and feces to ensure that they are digesting their prey well.

Common Emergency Presentations

Trauma

Many types of trauma are seen in birds, including fractures, head trauma, wounds from predator attacks, gunshots, electrocutions, and many others. In general, wounds and fractures should be cleaned and bandaged until the patient can be stabilized for surgery. Patients presented with a history of predator attack should be started on antimicrobials even in the absence of visibly detectable wounds.

Patients with head trauma often present fluffed and depressed with head tilts, anisocoria, nystagmus, and often hemorrhage found in the eyes, ears, nares, or oral cavity. A complete ophthalmic examination should be performed on all patients, but especially birds with head trauma to determine the degree of damage. Birds affected by head trauma often require IV fluid therapy and support with heat, oxygen, and pain medications. As long as they are fairly well hydrated, they may benefit from a dose of mannitol to reduce intracranial swelling. Corticosteroids have not been shown to be beneficial in head trauma in other species and may in fact be harmful. An exception may be made in the case of retinal damage by giving one injection of a short-acting corticosteroid.

Spinal trauma is a top differential in birds that appear mentally appropriate, but have rear limb paresis or apparent paralysis. Radiographs can help in identifying clearly displaced fractures, but they are often not sufficient for more subtle spinal trauma. A complete neurologic examination, including assessment for superficial and deep pain, should be performed in these cases. Spinal injuries, especially those with loss of deep pain, carry a poor prognosis.

Electrocution can be difficult to diagnose on presentation, as many signs develop over the following days. A history of the bird being found beneath power lines or transformers is common. Dermal burns or a burnt smell can occasionally be seen on intake, as well as damage to feather barbs and barbules. If feather damage is the only issue, the patient can be supported until there is new feather growth. Pulmonary edema and pericardial effusion may develop in the 24 to 48 hours following admission, which can cause death. If signs of these problems are noted, oxygen therapy and furosemide may be indicated. Peripheral edema and ultimately loss of peripheral circulation and necrosis can develop in wings, legs, and other areas. Many electrocution injuries are severe enough to warrant euthanasia. If clinical signs are minimal, treat symptomatically, making sure to provide analgesia, until the signs improve or clearly worsen.

Anemia

Anemic birds often present as weak or ataxic and mentally depressed. They may be pale, tachypneic, and have delayed capillary refill time. If the etiology of the anemia is not obvious on intake, focus on looking for other causes during the physical examination. Look for blood in the oral cavity, in the feces, signs of coagulation disorders from rodenticide toxicity, and listen closely to the lungs. Emaciated animals, especially juveniles, often present with anemia and/or hypoproteinemia. Whenever anemia is suspected, blood should be collected for packed cell volume (PCV), total protein (TP), and blood smear. This will provide a starting point for treatment and allow tracking of progress. PCVs of birds are similar to those seen in mammals. TP is typically lower than in mammals and ranges from 3.5 to 5.5 g/dL. The blood smear should be examined for signs of red cell regeneration, signs of infection, thrombocytopenia, and parasitism. Avian red blood cells normally have a short life span of 28 to 45 days. This predisposes birds to develop anemia of chronic disease more quickly than reptiles or mammals.[17]

In patients that are clearly anemic from acute blood loss, treatment with fluids, iron dextran at 10 mg/kg intramuscularly (IM) every 7 days, and supportive care should help to correct the problem. If the PCV is less than 15%, a transfusion should be considered. Ideally the donor would be a healthy individual of the same species, but heterologous transfusions have been successfully performed. It is safe to take 1% of the donor's body weight in blood, assuming the donor's PCV and TP are within normal limits. Heparin can be used to prevent coagulation at 5 to 10 units/mL blood. Transfusion reactions can happen, but are not very common. Ideally, a crossmatch is performed before transfusion.[17]

Gunshot or other deliberate, human-inflicted wounds should be reported to the US Fish and Wildlife Service (FWS).

Euthanasia

Euthanasia can be performed via IV administration of euthanasia solution. If IV access is difficult to obtain for any reason, the bird can be anesthetized and euthanized via intracardiac or occipital sinus injection. The FWS should be contacted if the euthanasia of any threatened or endangered birds or native eagles is being considered.

REPTILES
Patient Assessment

As in any other wildlife species, visual examination should ideally be done before handling. In reptiles, observe their mental status, strength, symmetry, breathing, nasal discharge, ocular abnormalities, and walking or other movements. Body condition and signs of dehydration also can be assessed before handling. As some reptiles are venomous and require special precautions, it is important to know the species before handling the patient, and clinicians should familiarize themselves with venomous species in their area.

Reptiles rely on external heat, and each species has a preferred body temperature (PBT) at which they can best perform metabolic processes such as digestion, reproduction, and healing. For most species in South Florida, this temperature is between 75 and 85°F. The patient can be kept at this temperature until the PBT is found in a reference text or online. Medications will not be metabolized properly until the patient has reached its PBT, so when possible, medications should be administered after the patient is warmed. Hypothermic reptiles should be warmed slowly, at least over 4 to 6 hours or, in some cases, several days.

Sedation and Anesthesia

Sedation or anesthesia may be necessary for a complete examination on aggressive animals. Often times, the initial examination can be done awake with the plan to explore the head and oral cavity after the animal is sedated. Anesthesia can be induced using inhalant anesthetics in many reptilian species, but some, especially chelonians, may require injectable anesthetics due to breath holding.

Physical Examination

It is important to get a weight on each patient, both for the purpose of dosing medications correctly and for monitoring hydration.

The body should be examined and palpated for evidence of fractures, joint swellings, and wounds. In chelonians, the carapace and plastron should be examined in addition to the limbs for fractures, ulcerations, pyramiding, abscesses, and external parasites.

The coelom should be palpated for organ enlargement, masses, fluid accumulation, and to identify the presence of eggs. This can be done through the inguinal fossa in chelonians. If it is not possible to restrain the head without sedation, it is still often possible to visualize the eyes, the nares, and even parts of the oral cavity if the patient happens to open its mouth. If this occurs, note the color of the mucous membranes, the quantity and thickness of mucus, and any signs of ulcerations or discharge. Once the head is properly restrained (with sedation if necessary), a full ophthalmic examination can be performed in addition to a more complete examination of the oral cavity.

A deep cloacal temperature can be obtained with specialized thermometers or even indoor/outdoor thermometers equipped with probes.

Basic Diagnostics

As in birds, simple diagnostics, such as a PCV, TP, and white blood cell estimate can be taken with a minimal amount of blood. Blood can be drawn from the jugular vein with varying difficulty in most species. In lizards, the ventral coccygeal vein or the cephalic vein also may be used. In chelonians, the right jugular vein is ideal, as it lowers the likelihood of lymph contamination. Alternative sites include the brachial vein, the subcarapacial sinus, and dorsal tail vein. The anticoagulant used depends on the species of reptile.

Radiographs are a valuable diagnostic tool, as in other species. Boxes or containers can assist the clinician in keeping reptilian patients immobile for radiographs. Ideally, dorsoventral and horizontal beam lateral views are taken. In chelonians an anterior-posterior view also is helpful. Oblique views may be needed to better visualize skull or limb fractures.

Fluid Therapy

Loss of skin elasticity, sunken eyes, stringy mucus, and depression are some common signs of dehydration. PCV and TP are helpful in assessing dehydration, but it is important to remember that many sick patients will be anemic and hypoproteinemic. Ideally, a glucose measurement should also be taken when obtaining a blood sample for a PCV/TP, as a minimal amount of blood is required. This will guide dextrose use in fluid therapy.

Crystalloid fluid preparations, such as Lactated Ringer, Normosol-R, and 0.9% sodium chloride are acceptable for reptiles. Glucose supplementation also can be helpful when indicated.

As in other species, patients with functional gastrointestinal tracts that are less than 5% dehydrated can be given fluids orally. In chelonians, the stomach capacity is approximately 2% of the body weight (100 g turtle, 2 mL stomach capacity). Subcutaneous fluids can be given in any skin fold. In mildly dehydrated reptiles, soaking in fresh water may assist in rehydration. In marine and estuarine turtles, this will also help reduce epibiota, such as barnacles and algae, often found on the carapace and other areas.

In cases of shock or severe dehydration, IV or IO catheters are placed. IV catheters can be placed in the coccygeal or cephalic vein in lizards or in the jugular vein in minimally responsive chelonians. The tibial medullary cavity can be used to place IO catheters in reptiles. In many chelonians, the plastrocarapacial bridge can be catheterized. Remember that medications given parenterally in the caudal half of the body may be filtered through the renal portal system, which may impact choice of catheter site or drugs given. The administration of parenteral fluids and medications intracoelomically is generally no longer recommended in compromised patients.

Maintenance fluid requirements may range from 5 to 15 mL/kg per day in reptiles. Losses should be estimated as in birds and replaced over 12 to 36 hours in an acutely dehydrated reptile, can be as long as 96 hours in a more chronically dehydrated animal.[18]

Drugs Used in Reptiles

Assessing pain in reptiles is often far more difficult than in mammals or birds. It is best to be familiar with the normal behavior of different species to determine if there is a difference in behavior that may indicate pain. Reactions to palpation, moving around an enclosure, appetite, and breathing patterns can all give insight to the degree of pain a reptile patient is feeling. When unsure, it is best to assume that any reptile feels pain in situations that would cause pain in other classes.

Analgesics

Recent studies on analgesic use in reptiles have shown good clinical efficacy of mu-agonists such as morphine and hydromorphone in red-eared sliders.[19] Studies involving buprenorphine have shown less clinical efficacy; however, a pharmacokinetic study using buprenorphine in red-eared sliders shows that the dose reaches levels that would be clinically effective in other species.[20] Nonsteroidal anti-inflammatory drugs (NSAIDs), such as meloxicam and the synthetic opioid tramadol, are also commonly used in reptilian species. A more complete overview of reptile analgesia can be found in the article, "Clinical Analgesia in Reptiles."[21]

Dissociatives

In many species, anesthesia can be induced with inhalant anesthetics. In bright and alert chelonians, injectable anesthetics may be required. Ketamine is often used intramuscularly in combination with dexmedetomidine or medetomidine. Doses for multiple species can be found in the articles "Chelonian Emergency and Critical Care"[22] or "Emergency Care of Reptiles,"[18] in addition to various exotic animal texts or formularies.

Antimicrobials

Antimicrobial selection in reptiles is similar to other animals, but doses and dose frequencies are often different. Reptiles with wounds and chelonians with carapace/plastron fractures should be on antibiotic therapy, as should reptiles with many other conditions in which antibiotic use is indicated.

Supportive Care

Caging choices should be based on the natural history and husbandry needs of the species. Ideally the material is nonporous and easy to disinfect. Examples of appropriate caging include tubs, pools, incubators, aquariums, and pens for grazing.

Appropriate lighting is a requirement, especially for reptiles that will be housed indoors for longer periods of time. Basking lights can help to maintain patients at their PBT and provide a gradient of heating in an enclosure. Caging should have monitoring equipment to be sure the temperature and humidity stay at an appropriate range. Full-spectrum lighting, or time outside in natural sunlight when weather and temperature allows, should be provided to each patient.

Nutritional Support

Patients should be offered food once they are well hydrated and at their PBT. If the animal refuses to eat in captivity after multiple days of offering a variety of foods, placement of a feeding tube may be considered in some species.

Feeding in cachexic reptiles should be initiated at 10% to 20% of calculated requirements for first few days, and then gradually increased to prevent refeeding or overloading an atrophied gastrointestinal tract.[18]

Common Emergency Presentations

Traumatic injuries, especially shell fractures, are very common in chelonians. Because of their location, these fractures are often highly contaminated and can involve significant hemorrhage. Controlling bleeding should be a priority when presented with any patient. Once bleeding is controlled, the patient should be stabilized and treated with fluids, analgesics, and antibiotics as indicated. Initial fracture stabilization often includes bandaging until the patient is stable for surgical repair if indicated. Wounds and fractures should be flushed and debrided as soon as possible. Radiographs always should be taken and may help determine if the fracture penetrates the coelomic cavity or involves the spine. Patients with shell fractures near the spine should be monitored for paresis or paralysis of limbs. Fracture management techniques for various reptilian species have been described.[22,23] Wound management can often be facilitated through the use of negative-pressure wound therapy.

Euthanasia

Euthanasia can be accomplished via IV injection of euthanasia solution. If there is concern over being able to access a vein, the animal can be anesthetized before euthanasia so that an intracardiac injection can be performed. Intracoelomic administration of euthanasia solution also can be effective once the patient is anesthetized. Loss of consciousness and nociception may occur rapidly, but cessation of cardiac function can take longer than it would in birds or mammals.

MAMMALS
Patient Assessment

Wild mammals are often treated similar to domestic small animals; however, even small animals can be dangerous, and proper precautions should be taken when handling. It is important to know which species are common rabies vectors in your area, but remember that any mammal can potentially be a carrier. Gloves, nets, and often sedation may be required to properly examine a wild mammal.

Sedation and Anesthesia

Sedation or anesthesia is often required to assess more aggressive species. Animals may be anesthetized using injectable anesthetics through carrier cages or traps, or they can be transferred to induction chambers where they can receive inhalant anesthetics. As long as the animal is stable, anesthesia can be the safest way to complete a physical examination.

Physical Examination

As in all wildlife patients, it is important to get intake weights on mammals for monitoring and drug dosing.

The animal should be examined for wounds and fractures, masses, skin issues, and other external abnormalities. The head and face should be safely palpated for any signs of skull or jaw fractures and for any dental abnormalities. It is important to determine if the patient is in shock right away and treat accordingly.

Basic Diagnostics

Mammalian blood can be handled similar to any domestic small animal. It is still possible to do basics such as PCV/TP in house and white blood cells can be estimated off a slide, as in other species. Blood can be drawn from any vein normally used in small animal medicine, although this may be difficult in very small mammals.

Radiographs are again one of the most important diagnostic tools. Mammals under general anesthesia can be easily positioned, whereas some conscious mammals may be best radiographed in a box or possibly held in place.

Fluid Therapy

Degree of dehydration can be determined as in other animals. Patients that are less than 5% dehydrated can be given water or rehydration solution orally. Mildly to moderately dehydrated animals will benefit from subcutaneous crystalloid fluids, whereas IV/IO catheter placement should be performed in severely dehydrated patients. PCV, TP, and blood glucose are important values to get initially when creating a fluid therapy plan. Medium-sized to large-sized mammals, such as raccoons, opossums, coyotes, and bobcats, can be treated like domestic dogs and cats as far as doses and types of fluids being used.

IV catheters can be placed in any easily accessible vessel. In small species such as rabbits, squirrels, and neonatal mammals, cephalic catheters often can be placed, but IO catheters in the femur or tibia may be best.

Fluids ideally should be warmed to body temperature before administration. Maintenance fluid requirements for smaller mammals are slightly higher than in dogs and cats at 70 to 90 mL/kg per day or 3 to 4 mL/kg per hour. If boluses are required in severely dehydrated patients, crystalloids can be given at 15 mL/kg and hetastarch at 3 to 5 mL/kg to reach and maintain normal blood pressure. Losses should be estimated as in other species and replaced over 6 to 8 hours in an acutely dehydrated mammal, or up to 24 hours in a more chronically dehydrated animal.[24]

Medications Used in Mammals

Analgesics

Pain can be assessed as it would be in domestic animals, but remember that wild animals, especially prey species, will commonly have much more stoic reactions than companion animals. Reactions to palpation, gait abnormalities, and behavior can give clues to pain. Monitoring heart and respiratory rates also can be helpful.

NSAIDs and opioids are commonly used in mammals at doses extrapolated from dogs and cats. In general, drug dosages for opossums can be extrapolated from cats, squirrels from laboratory rodents, and raccoons from dogs.

Anesthesia in smaller mammals is typically induced by inhalant anesthesia via face mask or induction chamber; however, injectable anesthetics are often more reasonable in larger more dangerous mammals. Ketamine is often used intramuscularly in combination with dexmedetomidine. Tiletamine-zolazepam alone or in combination with other drugs also can be used.

Antibiotics

Antibiotic selection and dosing are similar to other animals, and doses for smaller animals can be extrapolated from smaller exotic animal doses in formularies. Be aware of antibiotics that are not appropriate for oral use in certain species, such as rabbits, that can be prone to dysbiosis and subsequent potentially fatal diarrhea with inappropriate antibiotic choice.

Supportive Care

Caging choices should be based on the natural history and husbandry needs of the species. Ideally the material is nonporous and easy to disinfect. Small, young, or sick animals may require heat support.

Nutritional Support

Patients should be offered food once stable. Many animals will be cautious about eating initially and may require something to make the food more desirable, such as providing a mash, critical care diet, or canned diet that will get them started eating more traditional foods. Most carnivores can be fed whole prey items, whereas omnivorous mammals can do well on dog or cat diets supplemented with fresh meat and produce. Rabbits should be offered plenty of forage, ideally with local plant species. Formulas and manufactured adult diets for specific species can be found through companies like Fox Valley, Lake Zurich, IL and Mazuri, St. Louis, MO.

Common Emergency Presentations

Many mammals come to clinics with histories of having been hit by a car, attacked by a predator, or otherwise wounded. Once bleeding is controlled and the patient is stable enough for sedation, the wounds should be treated as they would be in domestic mammals. It is important to consider how safe or easy it will be for staff to handle this animal for bandage changes or flushing drains. In animals that will be difficult to handle frequently, consider using oral antibiotics or longer-acting injectables that do not need to be given daily. Cefovecin appears to work well in raccoons at the dog dose.

Euthanasia

Euthanasia can be easily accomplished through IV or IO injection of euthanasia solution. In smaller animals in which venous access is difficult, it may be more reasonable to anesthetize the patient with inhalant anesthetic drugs, then euthanize via intracardiac injection.

Legalities Concerning the Medical Treatment of Wildlife

After a physical examination, it may become obvious that the animal has injuries or illness that would negate successful release and survival in the wild. With the exception of animals that are good candidates for a lifetime in captivity for educational purposes, these animals should be euthanized. FWS guidelines instruct that "you must euthanize any bird that has sustained injuries requiring amputation of a leg, a foot, or a wing at the elbow or above, and/or is completely blind. You must not sustain the life of any migratory bird that cannot after medical management feed itself, perch upright, or ambulate without inflicting additional injuries on itself."[25]

Finding educational homes for nonreleasable wildlife can be difficult, and the search for a home should begin right away. Animals may not be kept longer than 6 months in a rehabilitation facility unless there on an educational permit. Animals deemed nonreleasable due to imprinting may not be kept as educational animals by the facility that imprinted them. Federal guidelines can be found online for many endangered species. Many states have specific laws concerning dangerous animals and rabies vector species. In general, it is important to research laws and regulations in your state specifically before you begin treating wildlife.

REFERENCES

1. Desmarchelier M, Toncy E, Firzgerald G, et al. Analgesic effects of meloxicam administration on post-operative orthopedic pain in domestic pigeons (*Columba livia*). Am J Vet Res 2012;73:361–7.

2. Molter CM, Court MH, Cole GA, et al. Pharmacokinetics of meloxicam after intravenous, intramuscular, and oral administration of a single dose to Hispaniolan Amazon parrots (*Amazona ventralis*). Am J Vet Res 2013;74(3):375–80.

3. Paul-Murphy J. Pain management. Clin Avian Med 2006;1:233–9. Available at: http://avianmedicine.net/content/uploads/2013/03/08_pain_management.pdf. Accessed September 19, 2015.

4. Guzman DS, Flammer K, Paul-Murphy JR, et al. Pharmacokinetics of butorphanol after intravenous, intramuscular, and oral administration in Hispaniolan Amazon parrots (*Amazona ventralis*). J Avian Med Surg 2011;25(3):185–91.

5. Guzman DS, Drazenovich TL, KuKanich B, et al. Evaluation of thermal antinociceptive effects and pharmacokinetics after intramuscular administration of butorphanol tartrate to American kestrels (*Falco sparverius*). Am J Vet Res 2014;75(1):11–8.

6. Riggs SM, Hawkins MG, Graigmill AL, et al. Pharmacokinetic of butorphanol tartrate in red-tailed hawks (*Buteo jamaicensis*) and great horned owls (*Bubo virginianus*). Am J Vet Res 2008;69(5):596–603.

7. Ceulemans SM, Guzman DS, Olsen GH, et al. Evaluation of thermal antinociceptive effects after intramuscular administration of buprenorphine hydrochloride to American kestrels (Falco sparverius). Am J Vet Res 2014;75(8):705–10.

8. Tseng F. Pain management in wildlife rehabilitation. In: Tseng F, Mitchell M, editors. Topics in wildlife medicine emergency and critical care, vol. 2. St. Cloud (MN): National Wildlife Rehabilitators Association; 2007. p. 99–111.

9. Guzman DSM, Drazenovich TL, Olsen GH, et al. Evaluation of thermal antinociceptive effects after intramuscular administration of hydromorphone hydrochloride to American kestrels (*Falco sparverius*). Am J Vet Res 2013;74(6):817–22.

10. Pavez JC, Hawkins MG, Pascoe PJ, et al. Effect of fentanyl target-controlled infusions on isoflurane minimum anaesthetic concentration and cardiovascular function in red-tailed hawks (*Buteo jamaicensis*). Vet Anaesth Analg 2011;38:344–51.

11. Souza MJ, Martin-Jimenez T, Jones MP, et al. Pharmacokinetics of oral tramadol in red-tailed hawks (*Buteo jamaicensis*). J Vet Pharmacol Ther 2011;34:86–8.

12. Guzman DSM, Souza M, Braun J, et al. Antinociceptive effects after oral administration of tramadol hydrochloride in Hispaniolan Amazon parrots (*Amazona ventralis*). Am J Vet Res 2012;73(8):1148–52.

13. Paula VV, Otsuki DA, Auler Júnior JO, et al. The effect of premedication with ketamine, alone or with diazepam, on anaesthesia with sevoflurane in parrots (*Amazona aestiva*). BMC Vet Res 2013;9:142.

14. Shaver SL, Robinson NG, Wright BD, et al. A multimodal approach to management of suspected neuropathic pain in a prairie falcon (*Falco mexicanus*). J Avian Med Surg 2009;23(3):209–13.

15. Taylor JW, Zaffarano BA, Gall A, et al. Pharmacokinetic properties of a single administration of oral gabapentin in the great horned owl (*Bubo virginianus*). J Zoo Wildl Med 2015;46(3):547–52.

16. Gaskins LA, Massey JG, Ziccardi MH. Effect of oral diazepam on feeding behavior and activity of Hawai'iiamakihi (*Hemignathus virens*). Appl Anim Behav Sci 2008;112:384–94.

17. Bartlett S. Diagnosing and treating anemia in the wild avian patient. In: Tseng F, Mitchell M, editors. Topics in wildlife medicine emergency and critical care, vol. 2. St. Cloud (MN): National Wildlife Rehabilitators Association; 2007. p. 40–6.

18. Martinez-Jimenes D, Hernandez-Divers S. Emergency care of reptiles. Vet Clin Exot Anim 2007;10:557–85.

19. Mans C, Lesanna LL, Baker BB, et al. Antinociceptive efficacy of buprenorphine and hydromorphone in red-eared slider turtles (*Trachemys scripta elegans*). J Zoo Wildl Med 2012;43(3):662–5.

20. Kummrow MS, Tseng F, Hesse L, et al. Pharmacokinetics of buprenorphine after single-dose subcutaneous administration in red-eared sliders (*Trachemys scripta elegans*). J Zoo Wildl Med 2008;39(4):590–5.

21. Sladky KK, Mans C. Clinical analgesia in reptiles. J Exot Pet Med 2012;21(2):158–67.

22. Norton T. Topics in medicine and surgery: chelonian emergency and critical care. Semin Avian Exot Pet Med 2005;14(2):106–30.

23. Raftery A. Reptile orthopedic medicine and surgery. J Exot Pet Med 2011;20(2):107–16.

24. Lichtenberger M. Critical care of the exotic companion mammal (with a focus on herbivorous species): the first twenty-four hours. J Exot Pet Med 2012;21(4):284–92.

25. What you should know about a federal migratory bird rehabilitation permit. Available at: http://www.fws.gov/forms/3-200-10b.pdf. Accessed September 19, 2015.

Tarantula and Hermit Crab Emergency Care

Cinthia Marnell, BS, BVMS

KEYWORDS

- Tarantulas • Fluid therapy • Biology • Hermit crabs • Diagnostics • Trauma
- Euthanasia • Husbandry

KEY POINTS

- Tarantulas and hermit crabs must have proper substrates, temperatures, humidity, diet, hygiene, and minimal handling to have the best health and longevity.
- Safe handling and physical examination are the first steps in approaching any medical condition in these species.
- Dehydration and blood loss can be treated with fluid therapy, which consists of both oral and injectable fluid treatment, and tissue glue if needed.
- Diagnostics can be done on these species; however, practitioners are limited by lack of diagnostic laboratories, normal values, and standardized tests.
- Euthanasia may be one of the best ways to help these pets, if their condition is advanced or if they are suffering.

 Video content accompanies this article at http://www.vetexotic.theclinics.com

INTRODUCTION

Many emergency practitioners are willing to examine and treat some exotic pet species, such as birds, reptiles, amphibians, rabbits, rodents, hedgehogs, and sugar gliders. However, there are hundreds of other species also in need of emergency care. These species are not necessarily uncommon; they may be considered "classic" children's pets. Tarantulas and hermit crabs are "classic pets" from the 1970s and 1980s. It was not uncommon for one to run across these species in a small neighborhood pet store, and indeed, even today they are still found at such establishments (and also in larger national pet store chains).

Tarantulas and hermit crabs may be "creepy crawly," but they are as deserving of basic veterinary treatment as any other species. This article introduces the practitioner to these families of multilegged critters, so that they can feel confident in evaluating

The author has nothing to disclose.
516 Stockbridge Ct, Salisbury, MD 21804, USA
E-mail address: psittacine@all-animals.net

Vet Clin Exot Anim 19 (2016) 627–646
http://dx.doi.org/10.1016/j.cvex.2016.01.005
1094-9194/16/$ – see front matter © 2016 Elsevier Inc. All rights reserved.

them and providing basic supportive care, if not outright welcoming them into their practice (or indeed homes!) on a more regular basis.

TARANTULAS

Spiders: the very word sends a wave of fear over many people. It is thought that humans possess a cognitive mechanism to detect specific animals that were potentially harmful throughout evolutionary history; for instance, infants have been found to have the ability to detect images of spiders as potentially harmful.[1] It has also been shown that children can learn the fear of spiders from their mothers, further explaining the strength of our fears.[2]

Despite a natural human predisposition to fear spiders, there are plenty of spider enthusiasts. There are arachnology and tarantula societies and organizations, nationally and internationally. "Tarantulas" are the most commonly kept family (*Theraphosidae*) of spiders, although occasionally you may find people who keep widows, wolf spiders, orb weavers, and other species. This portion of the article focuses on tarantulas, although most information is applicable to other families of spiders as well. Some of the benefits of keeping tarantulas are found in the following list.

- Tarantulas can live up to 30 years of age.[3]
- People enjoy caring for spiders (similar to how they enjoy caring for aquarium fish and reptiles/amphibians).
- Owners can firmly bond with their spiders by raising them from spiderling stage (often ≤5 mm in leg span) up to adult size (often ≥13 cm in leg span).
- Tarantulas are probably the easiest pet to care for and are ideal for people who travel frequently.
- If never manually handled, tarantulas can be very safe pets.
- Tarantulas can amaze owners by decorating their enclosures with webbing and/ or digging tunnels.
- Caring for a tarantula creates an increased respect and appreciation for wild spiders.
- Tarantulas take up very little space.

Anatomy

Tarantulas have (in order of length of appendages): 4 pairs of legs, 1 pair of pedipalps, and 1 pair of chelicerae (which contain the paired fangs).[4] They have a prosoma and opisthosoma; the prosoma is where the legs attach and is equivalent to a fused head and thorax.[5] The prosoma contains the esophagus and sucking stomach, which leads to the proximal midgut (that in many species has diverticula that lead into the proximal limbs).[6] There are paired venom glands that exit into the fangs, and a central nervous system (which is divided into 2 ganglions); there is also a large amount of musculature inside the prosoma, for controlling the limbs.[6]

The opisthosoma is the equivalent of an abdomen. It contains more of the midgut and diverticula, the heart dorsally, the book lungs and trachea (respiratory organs) anteriorly, the reproductive organs (ventrally), the spinning glands (posteriorly and ventrally), the Malphigian tubules (excretory organs located mid-to-posteriorly and dorsally), and a stercoral pocket (where excrement from Malphigian tubules and midgut are combined, located posteriorly and dorsally).[6] Externally, at the distal end of the opisthosoma, there are 2 pairs of spinnerets; silk is also produced from the spigots of the tarsi in multiple tarantula species, enabling them to prevent slipping or falling from a smooth vertical surface.[7]

Ecdysis

Ecdysis is the term for molting. Owing to their rigid exoskeleton, spiders cannot grow unless they molt. Molting occurs after a new cuticle is formed beneath the old exoskeleton. The length of time between molts is variable, and in tarantulas the males have a "terminal molt" or ultimate molt; the male emerges from this final molt with enlarged palpal organs and possibly tibial spurs, ready for breeding, and dies within a limited time period.[5] Tarantulas will usually have a period of anorexia before and after molting. They will also often make a bed of silk, or molting mat, before molting. Most tarantulas molt on their back, and the process can take several hours.[5]

Purchasing and Species

Tarantulas are commonly found for sale at pet stores and reptile shows, and there are now several breeders who sell them on the Internet. It is important to encourage potential owners to purchase captive bred spiders, rather than wild caught. Many species of tarantulas are threatened in the wild. The International Union for Conservation of Nature has 19 species of tarantulas listed as near threatened to critically endangered, on its red list.[8] The *Brachypelma* genus and 2 *Aphonopelma* species are on the Convention on International Trade of Endangered Species checklist.[9]

There are more than 800 species of tarantulas (family *Therophosidae*) within 131 genera.[10] When presented with a tarantula patient, it is helpful to first determine which species it is (if possible). Most of the time, owners will be aware of the spider's species (or at least its common name). However, if they are not, you can usually determine whether it is an arboreal versus terrestrial tarantula and often if it is an Old World versus a New World tarantula.

Arboreal tarantulas have longer legs and slimmer bodies. They prefer to be in a vertical position at rest. Terrestrial tarantulas have stockier bodies and usually lie in a horizontal position at rest. There are a few species (*Chromatopelma cyaneopubescens*, for instance) that have no preference between vertical and horizontal resting positions. Old World tarantulas have a smoother appearance than New World tarantulas because they do not possess urticating hairs. On the Internet, there are several pictorial guides to commonly kept tarantula species that can help in the identification a particular specimen. The knowledge of species is helpful to provide the best husbandry advice, and also for research purposes (certain species have been involved in research) and to have better knowledge of a particular species' venom capabilities in case of an accidental bite.

Husbandry

Tarantula husbandry is not difficult; however, if a tarantula's needs are not addressed, it is prone to becoming dehydrated and/or emaciated. Tarantulas (and spiders in general) are not social in nature, and should be housed singly. They are known to cannibalize each other if kept together. Males should be kept separately from females, except during mating, because the female is quick to kill her mate. Only about 20 species of spiders have been known to live together socially in the wild.[6] *Poecilotheria* genus tarantulas are one of these, and have been successfully maintained together in captivity. There is always a risk of cannibalism, however.

Tarantula enclosures are usually made out of glass, clear plastic, or acrylic to permit easily visualization of the pet. Arboreal tarantulas should have an enclosure that is taller vertically than it is horizontally, and both front and top access doors are helpful.[3] Terrestrial tarantulas should have an enclosure that is longer on the horizontal plane than the vertical plane.

Enclosures should be secured against escape, with latched or screwed on lids and doors. Ventilation holes should be smaller than the tarantula's opisthosoma (body); this is especially important for spiderlings, which are easily able to escape through ventilation holes. The size of tarantula enclosures should not be too large; many tarantulas will hide more often when excess space is provided. Spiderlings are often content in tiny pill vials or sauce cups.

Commonly used substrates include vermiculite, potting soil, peat, and coconut coir.[3,5] Moistened paper towels are often used as a substrate in smaller enclosures for transport of tarantulas. The substrate should be fairly deep for terrestrial tarantulas (especially for some species such as Haplopelma lividum, which like to burrow). No matter the type of substrate used, it should be free of chemicals and potential parasites.

Environmental enrichment for tarantulas includes appropriate depth of substrate for burrowing species, and appropriate hiding places for all species.[3] Clay pots turned on their sides, half coconut shells, a variety of logs (solid and hollowed out), and cork flats make excellent hiding spots for tarantulas. Artificial plants offer some privacy and often spiders will cover these in webbing; webbing can be considered a sign of a less stressed spider.[3]

Tarantulas of all species typically do well at room temperature (68°F–75°F). Temperature extremes should be avoided, and supplemental heating may be necessary in the winter.[5] Under-the-tank heating pads seem most appropriate for tarantulas, because they tend to avoid light.[5]

Water should be available at all times, and may be provided in a shallow dish, with or without small stones.[11] Most tarantulas will perch on top of the dish and drink readily from the dish. The use of sponges should be avoided, because sponges will act as a medium for bacterial and fungal growth, and may contain chemicals.[11,12] Arboreal species such as Avicularia spp. may not drink from a dish, because they spend so much time at the top of their webs; it is more common to provide water through a gentle spritz on the web or side of cage for these species.[13]

Tarantulas use their paired fangs to penetrate their prey. Venom aids in killing the prey. To digest, tarantulas' intestinal digestive fluid is injected into their prey.[6] This liquefies the contents and it can be sucked out. At the end of a meal, the tarantula drops the remaining indigestible parts in the form of a bolus, similar to a raptor, which casts its indigestible prey material.

Prey of tarantulas in captivity most often consists of crickets, roaches, wax worms, meal worms, flightless fruit flies, and other commonly cultivated invertebrates used in the reptile trade. The tiniest spiderlings can be fed parts of these if necessary, and may also eat prekilled or freeze dried insect prey.[11] Many tarantula owners have large collections of spiders; having their own cockroach colonies is often more economical than buying crickets. Blaptica dubia (commonly known as Dubia cockroaches) are the most widely accepted of cockroach species, and they breed rapidly. Variety of insect prey types is important to provide sound nutrition.[11]

Frequency of feeding can be variable. In general, tarantula owners should carefully monitor their pets' body conditions and feed accordingly. Overweight tarantulas (recognized by a balloon-shaped, overextended opisthosoma) can safely be fasted (**Fig. 1**).[3] Excessively thin tarantulas should be fed more frequently until they increase in body condition (**Fig. 2**).

Tarantulas will often go through periods of anorexia, most notably before and after a molt. Some species are known to go through phases of anorexia for reasons unknown (ie, Grammostola rosea). It should be noted that mature male tarantulas are nearing the end of their lifespan, and may refuse to eat. Mature males can be identified by having

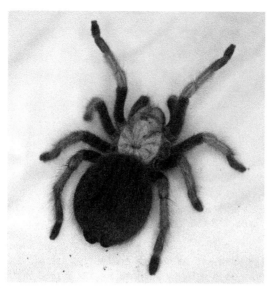

Fig. 1. Overweight tarantula (*Aphonopelma chalcodes*). (*Courtesy of* Heather Bjornebo, DVM, Arizona Exotic Animal Hospital, Mesa, AZ.)

enlarged palpal organs on their distal pedipalps, and potentially (species-dependent) tibial spurs (**Fig. 3**).[5]

Hygiene of equipment and enclosures is very important to prevent bacterial and fungal overgrowth on surfaces (which can lead to secondary infections). It is recommended to remove boluses of digested prey promptly and to clean and sanitize water dishes frequently. The entire enclosure should be cleaned and sanitized at least annually, and sooner if it seems excessively dirty; too much disturbance of the spider can result in stress and hair kicking, potentially leading to disease.[14]

Dangers and Warnings

Tarantulas have 2 defense mechanisms that are potential dangers to their keepers and handlers. The defense that most people immediately think of is biting and venom. Tarantulas are fierce predators. They pounce on their prey at high speeds and use their chelicerae and pedipalps to manipulate it and stab the prey with their fangs (which lie

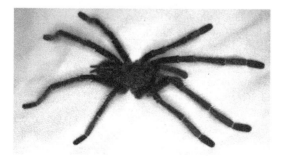

Fig. 2. Underweight tarantula (*Lampropelma violaceopes*). (*Courtesy of* Heather Bjornebo, DVM, Arizona Exotic Animal Hospital, Mesa, AZ.)

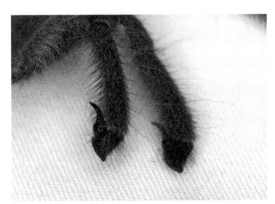

Fig. 3. Palpal organs on distal pedipalps of mature male (*Lampropelma violaceopes*). (*Courtesy of* Heather Bjornebo, DVM, Arizona Exotic Animal Hospital, Mesa, AZ.)

in a groove of the chelicerae).[6] All spiders possess venom glands and envenomate their prey. The venom does not play a significant role in digestion, but aids in killing their prey.

Both Old World and New World species of tarantulas have venom glands and sharp fangs. A recent study found that Old World tarantulas tend to bite quicker than New World tarantulas owing to lack of the second defense (urticating hairs).[15] However, even species that are considered more docile in nature should not be considered safe.

The venom of tarantulas is unique to each species. Several species' venoms have been analyzed, although the toxic effects on humans are not always characterized in these studies.[16–19] The effects of tarantula bites on humans seems to vary by genus of tarantula. On hobbyist websites, there are lists of tarantula bites and corresponding symptoms, but actual medical reports are few. **Table 1** summarizes scientific reports involving the various genera of tarantulas. There are a few reports about domestic

Table 1		
Summary of scientific reports of tarantula bites by genera		
Genus of Tarantula	**Consequences of Bites in Humans**	**Consequences of Bites in Dogs**
Lasiodora	Pain, edema, erythema[20]	—
Poecilotheria	Delayed onset severe muscle cramping lasting several days[21]; localized muscle cramps[22]; muscle spasms[23]; swelling, pain, erythema; numbness of extremities[24]	—
Selenocosmia	Pain, puncture marks, bleeding[25]	Death[25]
Phlogiellus	Pain, puncture marks, bleeding[25]	Death[25]
Phlogius	Pain, swelling, erythema, numbness[26]	—
Lampropelma	Pain, swelling, episodic generalized muscle cramps[22]	—
Pterinochilus	Pain, swelling, episodic generalized muscle cramps[22]	—
Chaetopelma	Pain[27]	Recoverable anaphylaxis[23]
Vitalius	Pain, erythema, edema[28]	—
Chilobrachys	Gangrene of foot[29]; urticaria[29]; death[29]	—
Haplopelma	Pain, erythema, joint stiffness[30]	—

dogs being bitten by tarantulas. Reminding tarantula owners to keep their spiders in a separate room away from other pets is a wise idea.

The second defense that tarantulas have are urticating hairs. Only New World tarantulas have these hairs.[31] The distribution of the urticating hairs varies with the species of tarantula, with the majority of hairs distributed over the opisthosoma, but some are also seen on the palpal organs in *Ephebopus* spp.[32,33] There are 6 types of urticating hairs, also known as true setae, and they are used in 3 types of defense: (1) tarantulas kick them off their abdomens and into the air toward their predator, (2) tarantulas intertwine them with their silk to be used in their webbing or egg sac to defend against parasites, and (3) tarantulas use them to make a defensive sound (stridulation).[33,34]

The urticating hairs of tarantulas can affect 2 areas of their human "predators": their eyes and their skin. The urticarial hairs, when lodged in the human cornea, can cause keratitis, uveitis, and ophthalmia nodosa; some of these disorders may even require surgery to repair.[35–39] It is, therefore, recommended to wear eye protection when handling New World species of tarantula.

When penetrating human skin, urticating hairs cause a mechanical irritation.[31] If the hairs cannot be removed manually, medical care should be sought. Allergy and anaphylaxis are both possibilities after contact with a tarantula, as with any species of animal. Both the urticating hairs and the tarantula's venom can be potential allergens. Therefore, precautions should always be taken when handling these pets: always wear gloves and eye protection.[5]

Safe Handling

Although many species of tarantula are docile in nature (for instance, *G rosea*, *Brachypelma spp.*, and *Avicularia spp.*), it is not in the best interest of the tarantula, owner, technician, or clinician to perform manual handling.[5] The dangers listed as well as the danger to the tarantula if dropped (leading to hemorrhage of hemolymph, or even death) should be taken seriously. Luckily, there are 2 relatively easy methods to handle tarantulas. The first method involves using a glass or plastic container (such as an anesthesia mask or a cup) to place over the spider, and then sliding a piece of cardboard beneath this and under the spider (**Fig. 4**). The spider can then be anesthetized or examined through the container. The second method involves carefully herding the tarantula using a paint brush into a glass or plastic container and then placing a piece of cardboard or other lid over the entrance to the container (**Fig. 5**, Video 1).

Tarantula handling can be more difficult with the faster and/or more aggressive species (examples include *H lividum*, *Pterinochinus murinus*, *Psalmopeus* spp., *Poecilotheria* spp., *Citharischius crawshayi*, *Theraphosa blondi*, *Stromatopelma calceatum*, and *Haplopelma hainanum*). Spiders may be merely defensive, with a threatening body posture (**Fig. 6**), or they may be actively aggressive and chasing toward the offending person or object. It is important to be prepared by performing the handling in a secured room in case of escapes, to never attempt handling these species alone, and to maintain a calm attitude.

Presentation, History, and Physical Examination

Why would a tarantula present on emergency to your office? The most common presentations of tarantulas include weakness, being curled up ("in a death curl"), being nonresponsive, trauma, difficulty molting (dysecdysis), hair loss or skin lesions, hemorrhage, or ataxia.[40] A normally aggressive spider may present in a weak or limp state.

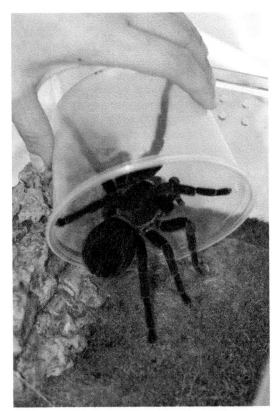

Fig. 4. Putting a spider in a container by placing container over tarantula from above (*Brachypelma vagans*). (*Courtesy of* Heather Bjornebo, DVM, Arizona Exotic Animal Hospital, Mesa, AZ.)

A thorough history should be taken. The use of questionnaires is often helpful to expedite the process and to thoroughly review the husbandry practices of the owner. Proper husbandry is as important in invertebrates as it is in vertebrate species, and most disorders can be directly tied to improper husbandry. Important questions are highlighted in **Table 2**.

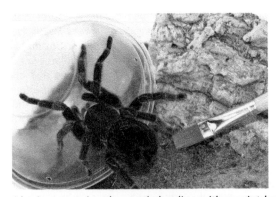

Fig. 5. Putting a spider in a container by gently herding with a paint brush (*Brachypelma vagans*). (*Courtesy of* Heather Bjornebo, DVM, Arizona Exotic Animal Hospital, Mesa, AZ.)

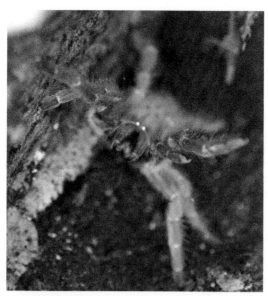

Fig. 6. Defensive spider (*Pterinochilus murinus*). (*Courtesy of* Heather Bjornebo, DVM, Arizona Exotic Animal Hospital, Mesa, AZ.)

The physical examination should be performed cautiously, practicing safe handling techniques as discussed previously. If the tarantula is very dehydrated, it will be too weak to put up much of a response to gentle prodding with a soft tipped object (such as a paint brush or cotton-tipped applicator). If the tarantula is more able to move around, then it is best to anesthetize it for a thorough examination (anesthesia information can be found elsewhere in this paper).

The use of magnification is recommended to examine the various structures of the tarantula. Missing appendages, hemorrhage/open wounds, alopecia, ectoparasites, discoloration of the skin, discharges or parasites near the mouth, and body condition should all be noted (see **Figs. 1** and **2** for body condition evaluation). Examine the gait of the nonanesthetized spider for hypermetria or ataxia. Gently palpate the

Table 2		
Important history questions to include in a questionnaire		
Date	Name of Pet	
Species of pet	Wild caught?	Yes No Unknown
When acquired	Housed alone?	Yes No
Cage material	Dimensions of cage	
Temperature of room pet housed in	Humidity of room pet housed in	
How is water provided?	Is the cage misted and how often?	
Cage substrate	Cleaned how often and how?	
Diet?	Where are insects obtained?	
Last molted when?	Do you handle your pet?	
Is your pet docile or aggressive?	Current problem?	
Other pets treated for fleas or ticks and how?	Exposure to toxins?	

opisthosoma for excessive firmness or masses. Look for signs that the pet may be a "mature male" (therefore potentially dying), namely, palpal organ enlargement and tibial spurs.

Anesthesia and Diagnostics

There are several studies regarding anesthesia in tarantulas. Inhalant gases have been used, including isoflurane, carbon dioxide, and sevoflurane, in Chilean rose tarantulas (G rosea).[41–43] Isoflurane (5% in 1 L/min oxygen) has been studied in wild-caught T blondi.[42] All 3 gases cause anesthesia in the species studied; however, the use of carbon dioxide had adverse effects (stress response, seizures, defecation) compared with both isoflurane and sevoflurane.[41–43] For inhalant gas anesthesia, an induction chamber or a mammalian anesthesia mask (used as an induction chamber, with the whole spider placed inside) may be used, attached to a scavenging system and vaporizer.[4]

More recently, injectable anesthesia agents have been studied in tarantulas.[44] G rosea was the species used during the study. Alphaxalone alone, alphaxalone with ketamine, alphaxalone with xyalazine, and preanesthetic morphine followed by alphaxalone were used in the study, and all were injected into the area of the dorsal heart on the opisthosoma. All protocols were effective and safe; all spiders recovered uneventfully.

For monitoring of anesthetic depth, the righting reflex is the most commonly used test.[42,43] Others have also used muscle tone, response to tactical stimulation, and heartbeat.[44,45] The heart rate can be detected with a special linear output Hall effect transducer and a small magnet, although this is not practical in most private practice situations owing to the cost of the equipment compared with the number of patients that may benefit.[46] Also reported is the use of a Doppler probe placed with a small amount of ultrasound gel on the dorsal opisthosoma to monitor heart rate, which is a much more practical method in private practice.[4,5,45] A normal heart rate is 30 to 70 in large spiders, and up to 200 in smaller spiders (although it may prove difficult to place a Doppler probe on the smaller species).[4]

Hemolymph pressure has been studied in invertebrates, including spiders, using direct methods of measurement; however, the technique is not very practical for private practice.[47,48] Hemolymph pressure also varies widely owing to 2 circulation mechanisms of spiders: "normal" circulation with the heart pumping hemolymph anterior–posterior, and hydraulic circulation where muscles in the prosoma and opisthosoma pump hemolymph into the limbs to aid in locomotion.[49]

Imaging modalities have been studied in spiders. One study on traditional (nondigital) radiography (including gastrointestinal contrast radiographs, plain radiographs, and computed tomography with and without gastrointestinal contrast) was conducted in 2008.[50] Radiography and computed tomography were not very helpful owing to poor detail; however, the use of a mammography radiography machine provided the best images. Tarantulas refused to eat prey that contained contrast agent, so the researchers had to gavage contrast into 1 tarantula (they used Hypaque). Contrast did appear on the radiographs and computed tomography scan; however, individual organs could not be identified. Digital radiography may prove equivalent or better to traditional mammography machine and films; however, further studies are necessary.

MRI has been performed on 3 tarantulas with and without contrast, and revealed good morphology of structures and information about regional perfusion.[51] Pizzi[5] reported that ultrasonography can be useful with a 10-MHz curvilinear probe; however, there will be air trapped between the ultrasound gel and the prosoma cuticle, leading to poor imaging. He noted that ethanol could be used instead of gel, resulting in a better image, but potentially increased anesthetic depth.

Cytology can be useful to examine skin surface, discharges, and feces for evidence of parasites, fungal, and bacterial infections. Skin scrapings, swabs, and touch preparations can be taken similar to these techniques in mammals.[45,52] Bacterial and fungal cultures can also be useful if cytology is supportive of bacterial or fungal infection; culture temperatures may need to be lowered owing to the poikilothermic nature of arachnids.[45]

Histopathology and necropsy have proven to be challenging owing to rapid autolysis of tissues. Ethanol was suggested as the best fixative by Pizzi, and it was recommended to make an incision in the lateral opisthosoma to allow internal fixation as well.[5] A study of fixatives on the tissue of *Loxosceles intermedia* (an arachnid but not a tarantula) found that a mixture of glutaraldehyde and paraformaldehyde was best for that species, although the researchers feel that there may be variation in species' hemolymph osmolality that could require different fixatives.[53] For tissue samples, it is important to use a pathologist who has experience and knowledge of invertebrate histopathology, because it differs markedly from that of vertebrates.

Hemolymph is the arachnid equivalent of blood. Owing to the location of the arachnid heart on the dorsal midline opisthosoma, sampling is not difficult.[52,54,55] It should be performed under anesthesia. However, at this time, there are 4 limitations to its use:

1. There is no specific research of anticoagulants for arachnid hemolymph. There has been minimal research on the effects of various anticoagulants of arthropods with no conclusion as to the most effective anticoagulant.[56,57] The valuable hemolymph sample will most likely clot before it can yield useful information.
2. There is a lack of reference ranges and validated laboratory techniques. There have been studies about biochemistry values, proteins, blood gases, and types of cells in hemolymph, although the results were variable and could not aid in the development of reference ranges.[43,58–60] Variability between species and effects of anesthesia may alter values.[43,58]
3. There are no studies designed specifically to support the amount of hemolymph that is safe to sample; however, there are anecdotal reports that 1% to 10% of body weight is safe.[45,52]
4. There are no commercial laboratories at this time that routinely evaluate hemolymph samples.

Disorders and Treatment

Dehydration is one of the most common disorders of tarantulas. The dehydrated tarantula is unable to extend its legs very well, and has them pulled inward toward its prosoma. The reason for this is that hemolymph pressure is required to move the limbs via hydraulics, because there are not leg extensors in spiders.[45,61] A normally aggressive or fast/fleeing tarantula will be unable to act to defend itself and owners may notice this in addition to the legs being pulled inward.

Treatment for dehydration depends on the tarantula's condition. If the spider still has some ability to move, it will be able to ingest water orally. It can be placed over a shallow dish of water (to prevent water going into its book lungs) or syringe-fed some water.[5,40,45] If dehydration is so severe that the spider is unable to ingest water orally, fluids may be given as an injection into the heart, which is found on midline dorsal opisthosoma.[5,40,45] A 27-G needle and insulin syringe are recommended.[45] Normal saline or lactated Ringer's solution may be used, and 2% to 4% of the spider's body weight should be administered.[45] Fluid may also be injected intracoelomically by injecting from the lateral side of the opisthosoma.[45] At the completion of any injections, a small amount of cyanoacrylate should be applied to the cuticle to seal the hole.[5,40,45]

Dysecdysis is another possible emergency presentation. The owner may bring in a spider that is upside down. It is normal for a tarantula to molt in the upside down position (and the process may take multiple to 24 hours), so this may not require any treatment.[5,40] The tarantula should be examined carefully for any hemolymph leaks (hemorrhage), in which case some cyanoacrylate/tissue glue may be applied to stop the leakage. Minimal interference with the molting process is recommended, because interference often can result in death or deformities of the tarantula.[40]

If excessive time has passed ($\geq$24 hours) and the animal has not molted, attempts can be made to help free the spider from its retained exoskeleton by moistening it with mild detergent solutions or triple antibiotic ointment, avoiding the book lungs.[40] The exoskeleton may also be trimmed with fine iris scissors, but there is a greater risk of hemorrhage with this option.[40]

Some tarantulas may present as an emergency for alopecia. The most common cause of this is a source of stress causing the New World tarantula to kick off its urticating hairs, leaving a bald patch on the opisthosoma.[5,40] It should be determined if the owner is handling the pet too frequently or aggravating it by cleaning its enclosure too often. If so, the owner should be counseled into avoiding creation of these stressors.

Parasites may be a problem with tarantulas. There are a variety of small mites that often live on tarantulas that may not cause problems unless in excess numbers.[5,40] These are often owing to excess humidity in the enclosure and may be treated by manually removing them using a fine-tipped paintbrush or by trapping in ultrasound gel or petroleum jelly.[5,40]

Oral nematodes are an increasing problem in captive spiders, with the most common parasite being *Panagrolaimus spp.* nematodes, although others do occur.[62] The clinical signs of oral nematodes include anorexia, an abnormal posture (standing on the "tips of their toes"), and eventually death.[62] The parasitic infection is localized to the mouth region and may result in secondary bacterial or fungal infection; the mode of infection is unknown.[62] Diagnosis is via thorough examination of the oral region under anesthesia, and via cytology of flushed discharges around the mouth.[5] Treatment has been attempted with various medications, but none have been particularly successful when compared with manual removal or flushing of the parasites from their site in the mouth, which should only be done under anesthesia (particularly because the zoonotic potential of these parasites are unknown).[5]

Trauma is another common emergency presentation. A leg may be torn or lost, or wounds in the exoskeleton may be hemorrhaging. Hemorrhaging can be stopped with gentle pressure and the application of tissue glue or cyanoacrylate, followed by fluid therapy if necessary (all should be performed under anesthesia except in the most critical of patients).[40] Limbs may be amputated with fine iris scissors if necessary, and the resultant wound sealed with cyanoacrylate; the limb will grow back with coming molts.[5] Sutures are not appropriate for spiders because they are ineffective and can damage the cuticle.[5]

Tarantulas may present for an odd gait or ataxia. Tarantula enthusiasts often refer to this collection of clinical signs as "dyskinetic syndrome." There have been no specific etiologies discovered; however, it has been proposed that tarantulas with these symptoms, which are ultimately fatal, may be exposed to a toxin. The environment of the tarantula(s) should be carefully examined for cat or dog flea and tick medications (including spot-ons, collars, shampoos, sprays, and powders), household insecticides, water-borne toxins such as heavy metals, contaminated prey, and other environmental toxins. Supportive care may be administered to these neurologic spiders, but most often, treatment is unsuccessful.[40]

Euthanasia

Euthanasia of spiders has been grouped with euthanasia of terrestrial invertebrates in the American Veterinary Medical Association Guidelines for the Euthanasia of Animals.[63] The recommended method of euthanasia for terrestrial invertebrates is injecting an overdose of pentobarbital or similar agent into the hemolymph (or intracoelomically), using inhalant or injectable anesthesia if necessary. Freezing is not an acceptable method, unless anesthesia is first induced. Potassium chloride injection has been recently studied as an effective method of euthanasia in terrestrial arthropods, and likely falls into the category of "pentobarbital or similar agent."[64]

HERMIT CRABS
Biology

Hermit crabs are entertaining pets. They may be one of the first pets that children are permitted to have, because they are inexpensive, require little care, and are interesting to watch. The majority of hermit crabs sold in the United States as pets are of the genus *Coenobita*, which are a group of terrestrial hermit crabs from tropical regions.[65] Each species has subtle differences in appearance, shell selection preferences, and behaviors. The most commonly imported (wild caught) and sold species include *Coenobita clypeatus* (the "purple pincher" or "purple claw" hermit crab), *Coenobita compressus* (Ecuadorian hermit crab), *Chromatopelma brevimanus*, *Chromatopelma violascens*, *Chromatopelma perlatus*, and *Chromatopelma rugosus*.[40]

Hermit crabs are crustaceans, which are arthropods. They share many of the same features as insects and arachnids, with a cephalothorax and abdomen, a hard exoskeleton, and hemolymph as their version of blood. They are also able to regenerate limbs that are damaged, similar to spiders, and they grow via molting.[66] They are decapod crustaceans, meaning that they possess 5 pairs of appendages and antennae.

Coenobita species hermit crabs begin their lives as planktonic larvae (zoeal stages) that live in the ocean and after several zoeal stages (the number of which is species specific), they become megalopae; megalopae emerge and become entirely terrestrial before they molt into juvenile crabs.[67] They have 3 organs used for respiration: the gills (which are reduced in size and modified for air breathing), the branchiostegal lungs, and the abdominal lung.[67-69] Terrestrial hermit crabs struggle with maintaining hydration owing to the high temperatures and humidity in their natural environment.[70] Because of this, they are mostly nocturnal and seek out a water source to rehydrate every night and usually maintain a certain amount of water (called shell water) within their shells.[70] Shell water can make up 30% to 50% of a hermit crab's weight, and it is used as a reservoir to replace evaporative losses; *Coenobita* species crabs also have 2 distensible sacs in their abdominal wall that they can fill with hemolymph after drinking.[67]

Hermit crabs are scavengers and omnivores, and they find their food mostly through their sense of smell.[71] They have a negative preference for foods that they have recently consumed, instead seeking out foods they have not eaten recently.[71,72] It is thought that this preference is a way to avoid nutritional deficiency or accumulation of toxins that may occur when relying on a single food type.[67] One study found that humidity is critical to the olfactory function in hermit crabs, because their response is mostly to water-soluble odors, although this has been found to be species specific.[73,74]

Coenobita hermit crabs are highly social and do not thrive when isolated.[75] They will change shells when they prepare to grow, and can be highly selective as to shell type; some prefer shells of only certain gastropod species, others prefer a specific shape, weight, or size of shell, and many will reject damaged shells.[76,77] The presence of other hermit crabs enables more shell selection, and when a hermit crab dies, others will seek out its shell via the odor of its dead body.[78] Lifespan of hermit crabs is up to 30 years in the wild and up to 15 years in captivity.[79]

Husbandry

The husbandry recommendations for hermit crabs can be derived from the natural history of the individual species. There are several Internet sites that have guides to identification of commonly kept hermit crab species, and once this is known, more specific advice can be given based on the multiple ecological and biological studies on most of these species. The following guidelines are general and based on the known lifestyles of *Coenobita* hermit crabs.

Hermit crabs should be kept in a glass or plastic terrarium with a solid lid that helps to maintain the humidity at 70% to 80%.[70,79] They are known to climb, so a tight-fitting lid is essential.[67] The size of the terrarium should be large enough for the crabs to move around in, ideally 10 to 20 gallons or larger. They should have a depth of substrate that allows for digging, because they will bury themselves at time of molting. The substrates that are commonly used include sand and coconut coir or a mixture of the 2 materials.[40] The substrate should be slightly damp but not wet; hermit crabs seek out humidity and avoid wet substrates.[67] The temperature of terraria should not be less than 75°F, to simulate their natural habitat. Tank heating pads can be placed on the sides of the terrarium if necessary.

Hermit crabs should be provided with a water dish that is deep enough for soaking, but they should also be able to get out of the water easily. As with tarantulas, sponges are not recommended in water dishes owing to the sponges becoming a medium for bacteria and fungi.[12] Hermit crabs will consume water, and the majority drink dilute fresh water; however, *Chromatopelma scaevola* and *C perlatus* require salt water for drinking.[67] Fresh water must be dechlorinated.

Hermit crabs spend a lot of their daytime hours hiding beneath leaf litter and plant debris found on beaches and inland tropical areas to avoid direct sunlight and preserve hydration; therefore, in captivity it is essential to provide hiding areas other than the substrate alone.[67] Artificial or well-sanitized logs, leaves, and plants will be relished by hermit crab pets. A variety of shells should be available for hermit crabs at all times, and owners should be encouraged to research their particular species of hermit crab to find if there are known shell preferences (gastropod species, size, shape, color, weight) for that species.

There are many commercial diets available for hermit crabs; however, there is little research about hermit crab nutritional requirements and therefore the commercial diets should only make up a small portion of the crabs' overall diet. A variety of fresh fruit and protein sources (such as dried shrimp or dried insects and small pieces of cooked meat with bones) should be offered and replaced on a day-to-day basis.[79]

Diagnostics

Before undergoing diagnostics, one should consider the appropriate handling of hermit crabs. These crabs have large pinchers or claws that are capable of causing pain, and often they will refuse to let go. It is best to keep this in mind and handle them by carefully lifting their shell over a padded table (in case of falls), or to examine them in an enclosed plastic or glass chamber. There are no studies of anesthesia techniques in hermit crabs, but because they breathe air it is suspected they would respond to inhalant gases. This is not recommended until further studies are done.

There are few studies about diagnostics in hermit crabs. Diagnostics such as imaging, cytology, cultures, fecal examination, and hemolymph evaluation can be done, but the use of any information yielded may be limited owing to lack of normal values and standardized tests.

Disorders and Treatment

Most hermit crabs are presented to the veterinarian for lethargy/failure to emerge from their shells, prolonged burial or molting, anorexia, being found without a shell, and limb injuries from fighting. Failure to emerge from their shells may be seen if a crab is kept in isolation, away from other hermit crabs.[75] It may also be an individual response to the presence of perceived danger, because all hermit crabs are wild caught and some may not adapt well to captivity and presence of human "predators"; a normal hermit crab response to threats has been found to be species specific among the Coenobita hermit crabs, with the majority withdrawing into their shells to hide, and 2 species preferring to run and escape, even abandoning their shells.[67]

Dehydration and temperature extremes are another potential cause of lethargy in hermit crabs, so husbandry should be assessed. A lethargic crab may also be preparing to molt. If the crab seems to be wrinkled or shrunken, dehydration is suspected. Fluid therapy can be performed, either orally via placing the crab into a bath of fresh or salt water, or parenterally by injecting with saline solution (using a 27-G needle) at the joint region of a limb.

When Coenobita hermit crabs prepare for molting, they will be lethargic for several days. They bury themselves in the substrate, deeply, and usually molt within their shells.[67] Their new exoskeleton is very soft afterward, and they are vulnerable to injury and dehydration until it hardens. The molting process can take weeks to months (anecdotal reports on the Internet; no scientific studies available). Hermit crabs will eat their exuviae once the molt is complete, aiding in calcium reuptake.

If clients dig up their hermit crabs fearing that something is wrong after months under the substrate, there is potential to harm the crab owing to recent or imminent molt affecting the protective nature of the exoskeleton.[40] Therefore, if the client presents a hermit crab that is in the process or about to molt, it should be immediately and gently placed in a safe habitat with appropriate damp substrate and isolated from other crabs, in hopes this will help it to continue the molting process.

Hermit crabs may be presented without a shell. Occasionally, they will abandon their shell if stressed or frightened.[67] Also, they may undergo the process of molt only to not be able to find a suitable shell in which to rehome. In either scenario, the best treatment is to gently place the crab in very soft, deep, damp substrate with a variety of shells and isolated from stressors such as humans, mammals, and other crabs. The idea is to get the crab to feel comfortable enough to enter a shell, or to find an appropriate shell.

Hermit crabs will "shell fight" or have "shell wars" at times, trying to remove each other from their shells and to antagonize each other to abandon shells.[80] During this process, a crab may have its exoskeleton damaged or a limb torn. If a crab is presented for wounds, the treatment is similar to tarantulas with wounds: pressure is applied to the area of hemorrhage, and a small amount of cyanoacrylate or tissue glue is used to seal the wound.[40] Similar to spiders, crabs will also regenerate limbs with coming molts.

Euthanasia

Hermit crabs fall under the category of captive invertebrates in the American Veterinary Medical Association Guidelines for the Euthanasia of Animals.[64] As such, the acceptable method of euthanasia is injecting an overdose of pentobarbital or similar agent into the hemolymph (or intracoelomically), using inhalant or injectable anesthesia if necessary. Physical means of euthanasia (freezing or concussion) are not acceptable unless the patient is first anesthetized.

SUMMARY

Tarantulas and hermit crabs may seem small and terrifying; however, they are not difficult to help when they are experiencing an emergent condition. Fluid therapy, treatment of hemorrhage and wounds, and assistance with husbandry can help these animals to have an increased quality of life and longevity. If an animal is truly suffering and beyond treatment, euthanasia is something that practitioners can do rather than let the animal suffer a prolonged death at home.

ACKNOWLEDGMENTS

The author thanks Heather Bjornebo, DVM, for providing the figures of tarantulas used in this article.

SUPPLEMENTARY DATA

Supplementary data related to this article can be found online at http://dx.doi.org/10.1016/j.cvex.2016.01.005.

REFERENCES

1. Rakison DH, Derringer J. Do infants possess an evolved spider-detection mechanism? Cognition 2008;107:381–93.
2. Lebowitz ER, Shic F, Campbell D, et al. Avoidance moderates the association between mothers' and children's fears: findings from a novel motion-tracking behavioral assessment. Depress Anxiety 2015;32:91–8.
3. Bennie M, Loaring C, Trim S. Laboratory husbandry of arboreal tarantulas (Theraphosidae) and evaluation of environmental enrichment. Anim Technology Welfare 2011;10:163. Available at: https://www.researchgate.net/profile/Steven_Trim/publication/222089254_Laboratory_husbandry_of_arboreal_tarantulas_%28Theraphosidae%29_and_evaluation_of_environmental_enrichment/links/02faf4f76db29ca325000000.pdf.
4. Lewbart GA, Mosley C. Clinical anesthesia and analgesia in invertebrates. J Exot Pet Med 2012;21:59–70.
5. Pizzi R. Spiders. In: Lewbart GA, editor. Invertebrate medicine. 2nd edition. Hoboken (NJ): Wiley-Blackwell; 2011. p. 187–222.
6. Foelix RF. Functional anatomy. In: Biology of spiders. 2nd edition. New York: Oxford University Press; 1996. p. 12–37.
7. Rind FC, Birkett CL, Duncan BJ, et al. Tarantulas cling to smooth vertical surfaces by secreting silk from their feet. J Exp Biol 2011;214:1874–9.

8. International Union for Conservation of Nature (IUCN) 2015. The IUCN red list of threatened species. Version 2015-4. Available at: www.iucnredlist.org. Accessed November 9, 2015.

9. United Nations Environment Programme World Conservation Monitoring Centre (UNEP-WCMC) (Comps.). The checklist of CITES species website. Geneva (Switzerland): CITES Secretariat; 2015. Compiled by UNEP-WCMC, Cambridge, UK. Available at: http://checklist.cites.org. Accessed November 9, 2015.

10. World Spider Catalog. Natural history museum Bern. World Spider Catalog; 2015. Version 16.5. Available at: http://wsc.nmbe.ch. Accessed November 9, 2015.

11. De Voe RS. Captive invertebrate nutrition. Veterinary Clin North Am Exot Anim Pract 2009;12:349–60.

12. Bechanko R, Hitt N, O'Malley K, et al. Are we aware of microbial hotspots in our household? J Environ Health 2012;75:12.

13. Frye FL. "Tarantulas" and other spiders. In: Captive invertebrates a guide to their biology and husbandry. Malabar (FL): Krieger Publishing Company; 1992. p. 7–17.

14. Schultz SA, Schultz MJ. The pet tarantula. In: The tarantula keeper's guide. China: Barron's Educational Series; 1998. p. 98–172.

15. Blatchford R, Walker S, Marshall S. A phylogeny-based comparison of tarantula spider anti-predator behavior reveals correlation of morphology and behavior. Ethology 2011;117:473–9.

16. Celerier ML, Paris C, Lange C. Venom of an aggressive African Theraphosidae (Scodra griseipes): milking the venom, a study of its toxicity and its characterization. Toxicon 1993;31:577–90.

17. Diego-Garcia E, Peigneur S, Waelkens E, et al. Venom components from Citharischius crawshayi spider (Family Theraphosidae): exploring transcriptome, venomics, and function. Cell Mol Life Sci 2010;67:2799–813.

18. Herzig V, Hodgson WC. Intersexual variations in the pharmacological properties of Coremiocnemis tropix (Araneae, Theraphosidae) spider venom. Toxicon 2009; 53:196–205.

19. Mourao CBF, Oliveira FN, e Carvalho AC, et al. Venomic and pharmacological activity of Acanthoscurria paulensis (Theraphosidae) spider venom. Toxicon 2013; 61:129–38.

20. Hortaa CCR, Chtazakic M, Oliveira-Mendesa BBR, et al. The venom from lasiodora sp.: a mygalomorph Brazilian spider. In: Gopalakrishnakone P, Gerardo AC, Diego-Garcia E, et al, editors. Spider venoms. Netherlands: Springer; 2015. p. 1–17.

21. Fuchs J, von Dechend M, Mordasini R, et al. A verified spider bite and a review of the literature confirm Indian ornamental tree spiders (Poecilotheria species) as underestimated theraphosids of medical importance. Toxicon 2014;77:73–7.

22. Ahmed N, Pinkham M, Warrell DA. Symptom in search of a toxin: muscle spasms following bites by Old World tarantula spiders (Lampropelma nigerrimum, Pterinochilus murinus, Poecilotheria regalis) with review. QJM 2009;102:851–7.

23. Dinamithra NP, Sivansuthan S, Johnson P, et al. Clinical presentation and outcome of Sri-Lankan ornamental tarantula poecilotheria fasciata spider bite: a case report. Anuradhapura Med J 2013;7:10–2. Available at: http://amj.sljol.info/articles/abstract/10.4038/amj.v7i1.6136/.

24. Kim DY, Han SB, Kim JH, et al. A case report of spider bite by tarantula. J Korean Soc Clin Toxicol 2014;12:85–7. Available at: http://www.komci.org/GSResult.php?RID=0137JKSCT%2F2014.12.2.85&DT=1.

25. Isbister GK, Seymour JE, Gray MR, et al. Bites by spiders of the family Theraphosidae in humans and canines. Toxicon 2003;41:519–24.

26. Raven RJ, Covacevich JA. New information on envenomation by a whistling spider, 'Phlogius Crassipes' (family theraphosidae). Queensl Nat 2012;50:19.

27. Srugo I, Aroch I, Bruchim Y. Anaphylactic reaction to a spider (Chaetopelma aegyptiaca) bite in a dog. Isr J Vet Med 2009;7:84.

28. Rocha-e-Silva TA, Collares-Buzato CB, da Cruz-Höfling MA, et al. Venom apparatus of the Brazilian tarantula Vitalius dubius Mello-Leitão 1923 (Theraphosidae). Cell Tissue Res 2009;335:617–29.

29. Banerjee K, Banerjee R, Mukherjee AK, et al. Tarantula bite leads to death and gangrene. Indian J Dermatol Venereol Leprol 1997;63:125–6.

30. Takaoka M, Nakajima S, Sakae H, et al. Tarantulas bite: two case reports of finger bite from Haplopelma lividum. Chudoku Kenkyu 2001;14:247–50 [in Japanese].

31. Cooke JA, Roth VD, Miller FH. The urticating hairs of theraphosid spiders. Am Mus Novit 1972;2498:1–43.

32. Foelix R, Bast B, Erb B. Palpal urticating hairs in the tarantula Ephebopus: fine structure and mechanism of release. J Arachnology 2009;37:292–8.

33. Marshall SD, Thoms EM, Uetz GW. Setal entanglement: an undescribed method of stridulation by a neotropical tarantula (Araneae: Theraphosidae). J Zoolog 1995;235:587–95.

34. Bertani R, Guadanucci JPL. Morphology, evolution and usage of urticating setae by tarantulas (Araneae: Theraphosidae). Zoologica 2013;30:403–18.

35. Mangat SS, Newman B. Tarantula hair keratitis. N Z Med J 2012;125:107–10.

36. Chang PC, Soong HK, Barnett JM. Corneal penetration by tarantula hairs. Br J Ophthalmol 1991;75:253.

37. Hom-Choudhury A, Koukkoulli A, Norris JH, et al. A hairy affair: tarantula setae-induced panuveitis requiring pars plana vitrectomy. Int Ophthalmol 2012;32:161–3.

38. Hered RW, Spaulding AG, Sanitato JJ, et al. Ophthalmia nodosa caused by tarantula hairs. Ophthalmology 1988;95:166–9.

39. Tillotson J, Giddens G. Sight threatening pets? The tarantula tale. Int J Ophthalmic Pract 2013;4:26–9.

40. Dombrowski D, De Voe R. Emergency care of invertebrates. Veterinary Clin North Am Exot Anim Pract 2007;10:621–45.

41. Dombrowski DS, De Voe RS, Lewbart GA. Comparison of isoflurane and carbon dioxide anesthesia in Chilean rose tarantulas (Grammostola rosea). Zoo Biol 2013;32:101–3.

42. Zachariah TT, Mitchell MA, Guichard CM, et al. Isoflurane anesthesia of wild-caught goliath birdeater spiders (Theraphosa blondi) and Chilean rose spiders (Grammostola rosea). J Zoo Wildl Med 2009;40:347–9.

43. Zachariah TT, Mitchell MA, Watson MK, et al. Effects of sevoflurane anesthesia on righting reflex and hemolymph gas analysis variables for Chilean rose tarantulas (Grammostola rosea). Am J Vet Res 2014;75:521–6.

44. Gjeltema J, Posner LP, Stoskopf M. The use of injectable alphaxalone as a single agent and in combination with ketamine, xylazine, and morphine in the Chilean rose tarantula, Grammostola rosea. J Zoo Wildl Med 2014;45:792–801.

45. Braun ME, Heatley JJ, Chitty J. Clinical techniques of invertebrates. Veterinary Clin North Am Exot Anim Pract 2006;9:205–21.

46. Coelho FC, Amaya CC. Measuring the heart rate of the spider, Aphonopelma hentzi: a non-invasive technique. Physiol Entomol 2000;25:167–71.

47. Blickhan R, Barth FG. Strains in the exoskeleton of spiders. J Comp Physiol A 1985;157:115–47.
48. Ward DV. Leg extension in Limulus. Biol Bull 1969;136:288–300.
49. Kropf C. Hydraulic system of locomotion. In: Nentwig W, editor. Spider ecophysiology. Berlin; Heidelberg (Germany): Springer; 2013. p. 43–56.
50. Davis MR, Gamble KC, Matheson JS. Diagnostic imaging in terrestrial invertebrates: Madagascar hissing cockroach (Gromphadorhina portentosa), desert millipede (Orthoporus sp.), emperor scorpion (Pandinus imperator), Chilean rosehair tarantula (Grammostola spatulata), Mexican fireleg tarantula (Brachypelma boehmei), and Mexican redknee tarantula (Brachypelma smithi). Zoo Biol 2008;27:109–25.
51. Pohlmann A, Moller M, Decker H, et al. MRI of tarantulas: morphological and perfusion imaging. Magn Reson Imaging 2007;25:129–35.
52. Van Wettere A, Lewbart GA. Cytologic diagnosis of diseases of invertebrates. Veterinary Clin North Am Exot Anim Pract 2007;10:235–54.
53. Costa-Ayub CLS, Faraco CD, Freire CA. Evaluation of fixative solutions for ultrastructural analysis of brown spider Loxosceles intermedia (araneae: sicariidae) tissues. Braz J Biol 2006;66:1117–22.
54. Veres S, Ciprian OBER, Liviu OANA, et al. Intracardiac hemolymph sampling technique in the domestic tarantula. Bulletin of University of Agricultural Sciences and Veterinary Medicine Cluj-Napoca. Vet Med 2009;66:386.
55. Dyer SM, Cervasio EL. An overview of restraint and blood collection techniques in exotic pet practice. Veterinary Clin North Am Exot Anim Pract 2008;11:423–43.
56. Gupta A. Cellular elements in the hemolymph. In: Kerkut JA, Gilbert LI, editors. Comprehensive insect physiology biochemistry and pharmacology, volume 3: integument, respiration and circulation. New York: Pergamon Press; 1985. p. 401–52.
57. Greegoire CH. Blood coagulation in arthropods. III. Reactions of insect hemolymph to coagulation inhibitors of vertebrate blood. Biol Bull 1953;104:372–93.
58. Zachariah TT, Mitchell MA, Guichard CM, et al. Hemolymph biochemistry reference ranges for wild-caught goliath birdeater spiders (Theraphosa blondi) and Chilean rose spiders (Grammostola rosea). J Zoo Wildl Med 2007;38:245–51.
59. Soares T, dos Santos Cavalcanti MG, Ferreira FRB, et al. Ultrastructural characterization of the hemocytes of Lasiodora sp. (Koch, 1850) (Araneae: Theraphosidae). Micron 2013;48:11–6.
60. Schartau W, Leidescher T, Schartau W, et al. Composition of the hemolymph of the tarantula Eurypelma californicum. J Comp Physiol B 1983;152:73–7.
61. Ellis CH. The mechanism of extension in the legs of spiders. Biol Bull 1944;86: 41–50.
62. Pizzi R. Parasites of tarantulas (Theraphosidae). J Exot Pet Med 2009;18:283–8.
63. American Veterinary Medical Association (AMVA). The AVMA guidelines for the euthanasia of animals. 2013. Available at: www.avma.org/KB/Policies/Documents/euthanasia.pdf. Accessed November 10, 2015.
64. Bennie NA, Loaring CD, Bennie MM, et al. An effective method for terrestrial arthropod euthanasia. J Exp Biol 2012;215:4237–41.
65. Noga EJ, Hancock AL, Bullis RA. Crustaceans. In: Lewbart GA, editor. Invertebrate medicine. 2nd edition. Hoboken (NJ): Wiley-Blackwell; 2011. p. 179–93.
66. Mariappan P, Balasundaram C, Schmitz B. Decapod crustacean chelipeds: an overview. J Biosci 2000;25:301–13.
67. Greenaway P. Terrestrial adaptations in the anomura (Crustacea: Decapoda). Mem Mus Vic 2003;60:13–26.

68. Greenaway P, Farrelly C. Vasculature of the gas-exchange organs in air-breathing brachyurans. Physiol Zool 1990;63:117–39.
69. Farrelly CA, Greenaway P. The morphology and vasculature of the respiratory organs of terrestrial hermit crabs (Coenobita and Birgus): gills, branchiostegal lungs and abdominal lungs. Arthropod Struct Dev 2005;34:63–87.
70. de Wilde PAWJ. On the ecology of Coenobita clypeatus in Curacao with reference to reproduction, water economy and osmoregulation in terrestrial hermit crabs. Stud Fauna Curaçao other Caribbean Islands 1973;44:1–138. Available at: http://repository.naturalis.nl/record/506107.
71. Thacker RW. Food choices of land hermit crabs (Coenobita compressus H. Milne Edwards) depend on past experience. J Exp Mar Biol Ecol 1996;199:179–91.
72. Thacker RW. Avoidance of recently eaten foods by land hermit crabs, Coenobita compressus. Anim Behav 1998;55:485–96.
73. Krång AS, Knaden M, Steck K, et al. Transition from sea to land: olfactory function and constraints in the terrestrial hermit crab Coenobita clypeatus. Proc Biol Sci 2012;279(1742):3510–9.
74. Vannini M, Ferretti J. Chemoreception in two species of terrestrial hermit crabs (Decapoda: Cocnobitidae). J Crust Biol 1997;17:33–7.
75. Bartmess-LeVasseur JN, Freeberg TM. Isolation increases time to emerge from shells in two Coenobita hermit crab species. Acta Ethol 2014;18:221–5.
76. Osorno JL, Fernández-Casillas L, Rodriáguez-Juárez C. Are hermit crabs looking for light and large shells?: evidence from natural and field induced shell exchanges. J Exp Mar Biol Ecol 1998;222:163–73.
77. Hazlett BA. The behavioral ecology of hermit crabs. Annu Rev Ecol Syst 1981;12: 1–22.
78. Small MP, Thacker RW. Land hermit crabs use odors of dead conspecifics to locate shells. J Exp Mar Biol Ecol 1994;182:169–82.
79. Smith SA, Scimeca JM, Mainous ME. Culture and maintenance of selected invertebrates in the laboratory and classroom. ILAR J 2011;52:153–64.
80. Elwood RW, Briffa M. Information gathering and communication during agonistic encounters: a case study of hermit crabs. Adv Study Behav 2001;30:53–97.

Index

Note: Page numbers of article titles are in **boldface** type.

Vet Clin Exot Anim 19 (2016) 647–668
http://dx.doi.org/10.1016/S1094-9194(16)00025-6
vetexotic.theclinics.com

Moving?

Make sure your subscription moves with you!

To notify us of your new address, find your **Clinics Account Number** (located on your mailing label above your name), and contact customer service at:

Email: journalscustomerservice-usa@elsevier.com

800-654-2452 (subscribers in the U.S. & Canada)
314-447-8871 (subscribers outside of the U.S. & Canada)

Fax number: 314-447-8029

Elsevier Health Sciences Division
Subscription Customer Service
3251 Riverport Lane
Maryland Heights, MO 63043

*To ensure uninterrupted delivery of your subscription, please notify us at least 4 weeks in advance of move.

Printed and bound by CPI Group (UK) Ltd, Croydon, CR0 4YY

03/10/2024

01040398-0013